GREEN GUIDE
FAMILIES

GREEN GUIDE
FAMILIES

The Complete Reference for Eco-friendly Parents

BY
CATHERINE ZANDONELLA,
SCIENCE EDITOR,
GREEN GUIDE MAGAZINE

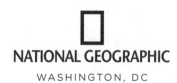

NATIONAL GEOGRAPHIC
WASHINGTON, DC

Founded in 1888, the National Geographic Society is one of the largest nonprofit scientific and educational organizations in the world. It reaches more than 285 million people worldwide each month through its official journal, *National Geographic,* and its four other magazines; the National Geographic Channel; television documentaries; radio programs; films; books; videos and DVDs; maps; and interactive media. National Geographic has funded more than 8,000 scientific research projects and supports an education program combating geographic illiteracy.

For more information, please call 1-800-NGS LINE (647-5463) or write to the following address:

National Geographic Society
1145 17th Street N.W.
Washington, D.C. 20036-4688 U.S.A.

Visit us online at www.nationalgeographic.com

For information about special discounts for bulk purchases, please contact National Geographic Books Special Sales: ngspecsales@ngs.org

For rights or permissions inquiries, please contact National Geographic Books Subsidiary Rights: ngbookrights@ngs.org

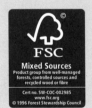

FSC
Mixed Sources
Product group from well-managed forests, controlled sources and recycled wood or fibre
Cert no. SW-COC-002985
www.fsc.org
© 1996 Forest Stewardship Council

Library of Congress Cataloging-in-Publication Data

Zandonella, Catherine, 1968-
  Green guide families : the complete reference for eco-friendly parents /
by Catherine Zandonella.
    p. cm.
  Includes index.
  ISBN 978-1-4262-0542-2 (pbk.)
1. Child rearing--Environmental aspects. 2. Sustainable living. 3.
Environmental health. 4. Environmentalism. I. Title.
  HQ796.Z335 2010
  649'.1--dc22

                         2009046984

Printed in U.S.A.

10/CK/1

Recommendations in this book do not constitute product approvals or endorsements. Our aim is to inform and engage consumers to try those products in the marketplace that have been manufactured to reduce the health and environmental impacts associated with one or more stages in their life cycle, from production through use and disposal. Material in this book is provided for informational purposes only and is not a substitute for professional advice, whether medical or otherwise.

Contents

Introduction

BY WENDY GORDON

There is nothing that compares to the birth of your first child. It's transformative. Up until then, most of us are pretty independent, with few responsibilities outside of work. But at that moment, when you count his tiny fingers or her teensy toes, everything is different. Your life has been changed. You are needed in ways that you've never been before, and for all those things that truly matter—food, shelter, health and well-being.

I remember watching my newborn breathe, his chest quivering as his lungs filled with air. As we brought him home from the hospital, it was hard not to wonder what the street level air, the bus and car fumes and the construction dust, might do to him. At home, as my husband and I struggled with the first diaper change, I pondered the words of a friend who said cloth diapers are really no better than disposables: "So what if all those diapers go to a landfill, the cotton in your cloth diapers is heavily doused with pesticides. Those same pesticides are regularly used on fruits and vegetables, too, the very ones you love to eat and will feed to your kids." Then a few weeks later, a friend told me how she inadvertently boiled away all the water in the pot in which she was sterilizing her baby bottles, and the melted plastic offgassed this strangely sweet smell that lingered in her kitchen for days. Her pediatrician later told her the chemicals she smelled were very toxic.

Though I hold a degree in environmental health and a job at a non-profit advocating for safe drinking water, nothing had prepared me for any of this. It's a basic life truth but at the time (remember I'd just given birth) it seemed profound: Parenting is a responsibility that links us to Earth—to the air we breath, the water we drink, the food we eat, and the homes we create for shelter and security. To best care for my son, to provide a safe, healthy home for him and his brother (who would come three years later), means fundamentally to care for the planet, that place where they would live for decades after me, and their children after them.

There were lots of books on parenting, which I read and read again. One was very helpful when our firstborn was waking too many times in the night and couldn't get back to sleep on his own. Others provided great advice on breast-feeding, naps, introducing bottles, going back to work, day care, and introducing foods. But there were no books that offered parents advice on how to create an environmentally healthy home and how to raise your family in an environmentally responsible way.

This is that book, and though it's 2010 now, *Green Guide Families* reflects the culmination of years of careful research and reporting first started in the late 1980s by a small consumer education organization that I co-founded, called Mothers & Others for a Livable Planet. The original members of Mothers & Others were like me mostly, moms of young children, eager for information about the best ways to keep their families safe from harmful environmental contaminants, such as pesticides that could be found in our food, and toxic chemicals in popular personal care and home products. It was for them that in 1994 Mothers & Others introduced the first *Green Guide*, a short (just four pages) and frequent (we mailed or faxed it bi-weekly) newsletter offering simple solutions to environmental issues that were easy and ready to put into action. Each issue focused on a daily decision—whether to buy organic foods, what sort of containers to store leftovers in, what pest control methods were safest, how to save energy and water, etc.—and offered practical cost-conscious suggestions and advice. We modeled our newsletter after *Consumer Reports*, providing well-researched product recommendations as well as reasonable advice on behavior changes one could make that would protect health, preserve the environment, and save money. By the time National Geographic acquired *Green Guide* in 2007, it had developed into a well-respected resource for eco-minded consumers both online and in print.

Catherine Zandonella, who joined the Green Guide team as the science editor in 2002, is the perfect author for *Green Guide Families*. A mother of two children, with a master's degree in public health from the University of California, Berkeley, she has researched and written dozens of *Green Guide* articles on everything from apples to xeriscaping and everything in between. She goes deep with her research, though she writes as if she were talking to you over a cup of coffee at the kitchen table.

Her expertise and range of knowledge, as well as her perspective as a mom, make her the ideal voice for this book, the ultimate green living reference for the eco-minded parent. There is not a matter she doesn't explore, from your baby's teething ring to the turf at the school's ball fields. If you've read about it, seen it on television, or heard about it from friends, Catherine covers it and offers practical, ready-to-apply solutions to the health and environmental concerns that are a part of the world we live in.

Starting in Chapter 1, Catherine considers with you the fundamentals of setting up a home, beginning with the most basic decisions about where and how to live. How close is home to the school, the park, good places to shop? Can the kids bike? Can you take public transit to work? These are important questions that speak to the healthiness of your community as well as the health of your family and home.

Chapters 2 and 3 deal with food and look at everything from obesity issues to why eating lower on the food chain matters. Start early to establish good eating habits: Stock up on fresh, whole, flavorful foods; make your own snacks and lunches; and take the kids with you to the farmers market to learn together what real food is, where and how it's grown, and why local, seasonal foods are so much better for you and the planet. Find out why eating more homemade meals with less animal protein and more whole grains, nuts and seeds, and fresh fruits and vegetables will put you and your family on the right course. It's not about deprivation, in fact quite the opposite; it's about retaking our food system and our health by reacquainting ourselves with delicious foods that are great to eat and great for health and just also happen to be right for the environment.

In Chapter 4, Catherine looks at ways to keep kids healthy, including how to treat common colds and fevers without overusing antibiotics. She explores most everything on your mind, from mercury in dental amalgams to the epidemics of neurobehavioral disorders, specifically attention deficit/ hyperactivity disorder (ADHD) and autism, that a growing number of scientists and parents think are related to environmental exposures. And she looks at emerging diseases that arise from interactions of humans with the environment. Why are asthma, allergies, and childhood cancer rates on the rise? How strong is the evidence for environmental triggers of these diseases?

Chapter 5 turns the discussion around. Rather than looking at what you can do for the health of your kids, this chapter ponders what your kids can do to make their world a better place for all living things. Wisely, Catherine offers up suggestions for every stage of childhood, from toddlerhood through the teen years. It's a virtual treasure trove of ideas, for fun projects to dinner table talk, so don't skip this chapter.

In Chapter 6, you'll find out what eco-friendly baby care truly means. When it comes to purchasing baby supplies, the choices can seem endless, and sorting out the claims of manufacturers and consumer comparisons becomes a daunting task. It helps simplify matters to think in terms of a back-to-basics approach that emphasizes natural baby care items over synthetic ones, tried-and-true practices over unproven theories, and needs over consumerism. Whatever your questions, from diapers and bedding to sunscreen and toys, this chapter will provide you with a practical guide to healthy baby care that dovetails with best practices for the planet.

Chapters 7 and 8 look at kids at play and kids at school. Catherine investigates what are the right toys for your child's development and what materials in toys can be toxic to health and the environment. She also looks at ways to navigate a culture where kids are expected to stare at screens, and so spends a good amount of time on healthy outdoor activities like gardening, playing on the playground, and caring for a pet. Then she shows ways that you can help your child's school adopt more environmentally conscious and health-protective practices.

Lest you are thinking greening family life isn't going to be fun, I suggest you start at the end of the book, with Chapters 9 and 10. In Chapter 9, you'll learn that it's not just fun but surprisingly easy to integrate eco-friendly practices into your celebrations, from birthdays to holidays. And then there's Chapter 10, which is all about greening your vacation. Whether your idea of a family vacation is packing the kids in the car for a multistate trip to the national parks, or jetting to a Caribbean island to escape the winter blues, you *can* satisfy your travel lust and still tread lightly on the planet. You may have to give extra thought to where to go, how to get there, where to stay, and what to do, but choosing more responsible ways to travel can be immensely rewarding.

There is a lot of wisdom packed into this one book, the practical good sense kind that you can apply to every aspect of family life. It wasn't there for me when I was starting my family, but it's here now as my kids launch into adulthood. The oldest just got his first apartment, had to buy a new bed and some kitchen supplies, and even found some secondhand backyard furniture at a rummage sale. It got us both thinking about wood finishes for the outdoor furniture and the right sort of pots and pans to get. We're a family forever, I guess, making *Green Guide Families* book something all of us should get and keep and refer to over and over again.

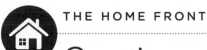

THE HOME FRONT

Creating a Safe and Eco-friendly Home

SOME PARENTS WILL GO TO ANY LENGTHS TO KEEP THEIR CHILDREN safe. They attach harnesses to their children at amusement parks. They give their children cell phones at age six. We can smile at these antics, but we can't really blame the parents. Children are the most precious and vulnerable people in our lives.

Kids need our protection, and protect we do. We do whatever is in our financial power. Marketers know this, which is why so many products are advertised as being necessary for the health and safety of our children.

Yet some of the biggest threats to our children get little attention at all and are featured on few television commercials. In fact, many parents have heard little about them. These are threats such as chemicals in our household products, furnishings, and air, both indoors and out. Sometimes we have been warned of these dangers, but we fail to heed the warnings. We all know that pesticides are deadly, and we would never leave rat poison on the counter where a child could reach it. But we continue to spray weed-killer on our lawns where our kids play.

Study after scientific study demonstrates that exposing our children to even low levels of toxic chemicals can contribute to health risks—from asthma and allergies, developmental delays and learning disorders, to cancer and birth defects.[1]

As parents, many of us only start learning about the connections between chemicals and health *after* a child we know has been affected. We might have a friend who has a child with cancer or know a neighbor whose child has severe asthma. Or it might be our own child who is affected.

Wouldn't it be better if we went through our homes and eliminated these chemicals before they could harm our children? We can, and this chapter and other chapters in this book will show you how.

The steps we take to make our homes healthful and safe for our children are the same steps that clean up and preserve our larger home, Earth. Less toxic cleaning chemicals? Safer for children and better for the environment. Shorter drive times to school or play dates? Healthier for our children because they can walk or bike instead, keeping greenhouse gases out of the atmosphere. Saving energy around the home? When we use less electricity and heat, we keep pollution out of the air that our children breathe.

When making decisions about our children's health—and we parents make hundreds of these decisions each month—we need to ask ourselves two questions: Is this product safe and healthy for my child? And, Is this safe and healthy for the planet? The two questions go hand in hand.

Our home is where we make our most important decisions about our family's health. It is also where we can do the most good for the planet. We spend more than 90 percent of our lives indoors, and a third of it sleeping. And babies sleep the most of any family member.

Keeping our indoor environment as chemical-free as possible is essential to children's health. The simple reason is that babies and children breathe more air than we adults do, on a pound for pound of body weight basis. They also eat more often and bring more toxic chemicals into their bodies during those put-everything-in-the-mouth toddler years.

Babies and children are also more vulnerable to toxic substances than are adults. The infant's and child's brain and body are rapidly growing. The brain undergoes a staggering amount of development from conception through adolescence, with complex growth of neurons and other cell types that need to connect with each other.

This long window of vulnerability explains why exposure to a brain toxicant such as lead early in childhood irreversibly alters mental function, whereas the same exposure in adults may cause no lasting harm. Think of alcohol: A few swigs of whiskey can kill a one-year-old but will only cause a grown man to act a little foolish.

Choosing *where* to live is also important to both our children's health and for the health of the planet. Children who can easily walk or bike to parks and schools tend to be more physically fit than those who rely on automobile transportation. If you live close to where you work or close to public transportation, you can cut your carbon footprint and reduce your commute time so that you can spend more time with your family. Making simple and inexpensive upgrades to your home can conserve energy that will not only reduce your utility bills but also will drive down the amount of pollution your household generates. Cutting your household energy usage keeps climate-warming gases out of the air.

By embracing the three Rs—reduce, reuse, and recycle—we can lessen our impact on the planet's resources and enjoy knowing that we are doing what we can to protect the environment not only for our children but for generations to come.

In this chapter we'll talk about how to maintain a house in a way that keeps our earthly home and our children safe and healthy. We'll chat about common household chemicals and how to clean and green your house. We'll discuss decorating with flair not formaldehyde. We'll ruminate on renovations and *real* green houses. Finally, we'll explore the energy-saving techniques that can shrink your utility bills and your carbon footprint.

Household Chemicals

Homes old and new come with problems that you may not detect until you've lived in them for some time. Most of the environmental problems can be fixed with a little ingenuity and elbow grease.

You've fallen in love with the perfect house or apartment. In your mind's eye you can just picture where you'll put the crib and the toddler bed. You are already envisioning ditching all your college-age furniture and redecorating in style. But wait: Before signing that rental agreement or mortgage, a little investigation is warranted.

Older homes can have problems such as lead paint and asbestos tile or insulation. These homes can slowly release chemicals that could poison your family over the years. Some of these problems are more easily fixed than others, as we'll see in the following sections.

Newer homes come with their own set of potentially harmful chemicals, albeit different ones from older homes. Today, many builders are forgoing the use of expensive lumber in favor of composite materials made from fusing wood chips together with glue. In some ways this is good for the environment because the lumber industry is able to use more of the tree than ever before and discard less as waste. However, some of these composite wood products release form-aldehyde gas, which is not only irritating to many sensitive individuals but has the potential to cause cancer, according to the U.S. Environmental Protection Agency (EPA).

Today's homes are often stocked with chemicals that are either harmful or not adequately tested. These chemicals are not only in bottles on garage shelves or in broom closets but also embedded in our consumer products, from home furnishings to carpets. These chemicals can "offgas" and enter our indoor air, where our children inhale them.

Many of these chemicals have the potential to trigger asthma attacks, irritate sensitive eyes and skin, or cause cancer and harm reproductive organs. Some of these chemicals, such as cancer-causing radon gas that seeps up from the soil beneath homes, are naturally occurring. Other toxic substances, such as formaldehyde, come from the building materials used to construct our homes. And finally there are toxic chemicals in many of the household cleaners, air fresheners, and other consumer products that we use daily.

Humans are not the only ones affected by these chemicals. Many are also harmful to pets, wildlife, and aquatic life, and in some cases contribute to global climate change. Chemicals that run down our drains eventually end up in streams, rivers, and oceans where they can kill aquatic wildlife. Cleaning up toxic chemicals in your indoor air and around your home will benefit not only your family's health but also the environment.

Most health and environmental issues can be tackled without having to uproot the family and move to a new house. Other renovations, such as the removal of lead paint or asbestos, may require the family to relocate while the work is being done. Some solutions are as easy as swapping conventional cleaning products for greener ones—or making your own.

The good news is, many of these environmental problems can be fixed. In this section we'll talk about common hazards found in homes old and new.

WHEN THE CHIPS ARE DOWN Toddlers will put just about anything in their mouths. But paint chips seem like a rather unusual choice of snack. Oddly enough, many children find paint chips—the leaded variety in particular—to be sweet-tasting. Some children even develop a craving for them and will go to great lengths to pry layers of paint off windowsills.

Your child's paint food fetish can be harmful and should be nipped in the bud, whether or not the paint contains lead. But if you live in a home that was built in 1978 or earlier, you should be extremely cautious. If peeling paint contains lead, even a single paint chip could affect the child's developing brain.

Lead causes neurological damage to the developing brain in infants and children, resulting in permanent learning disabilities, behavioral problems, and lower intelligence quotient (IQ). The Centers for Disease Control and Prevention (CDC) have set the definition of an elevated blood lead level at 10 micrograms per deciliter, which many public health officials say is too high to protect children. A 2008 study in the journal *Environmental Health Perspectives* found that six-year-old children with blood lead levels that ranged from 5 to 10 micrograms/deciliter had IQs that were nearly five points lower than children in a comparison study with lower blood lead levels.[2] Five points may not seem like much to some people, but most of us want to avoid anything that reduces our child's potential. Indeed, many studies indicate that there is no safe level of lead exposure in children.[3]

But you may be saying, I live in a suburban home, and lead is an inner city problem. In fact, suburban homes built before 1978 were often painted with lead paint. And even if your child doesn't regularly hit the paint chip buffet, he or she could be getting regular doses of this toxic metal from the air in the house, dust on the floor, toys, and other surfaces.

If you own or rent a pre-1978 home, and you plan to do sanding, painting, and replacing windows, stop right away and test for lead. The moment you put the sander to the paint, you'll create airborne leaded dust that can sicken not only you but your children and pets.

Lead paint can be detected in a couple of ways, but the most reliable method is x-ray fluorescence (XRF). For a few hundred dollars, a certified lead inspector will come to your home with a portable device that can take x-ray images of walls, windowsills, doorframes, and other features. The device can "see" lead even through subsequently applied layers of paint. The EPA maintains a list of licensed lead paint testing companies at *cfpub.epa.gov/flpp*, or you can contact your state or local government.

It is possible to buy cheap lead test kits at paint and hardware stores for just a few dollars. But these tests can be unreliable. The U.S. Consumer Product Safety Commission (CPSC) recommends against relying on these tests, which can miss the presence of lead, especially lead under several layers of paint.

If you live in an older home, consider testing your children's blood lead levels. The CDC recommends that children at high risk for lead poisoning be tested at 12 months and again at 24 months. Some cities and states are more aggressive, requiring tests every six months up to age two, and then yearly after that. Health insurance companies usually cover the test if mandated by law. If not, check with your health department to see if it sponsors clinics where you can take your child for a free test. Your child's pediatrician can also prescribe the test. If all else fails, pay for the test yourself if your house or your child's day care is older than 1978, or the tests you conducted on your house or apartment find anything.

GET YOUR FIBER: ASBESTOS Asbestos was used in many homes up until the 1970s. This tiny mineral fiber can lodge in the lungs and lead to a deadly form of lung cancer called mesothelioma. This disease takes decades to develop, according to the U.S. National Cancer Institute *(www.cancer.gov)*.

Asbestos can be found in insulation for pipes, boilers, and furnace ducts. It was also used in roofing, shingles, sidings, and in the paste used to hang drywall (also called drywall joint compound). It was mixed into vinyl and made into floor tiles and the felt lining under the floor tiles.

Before purchasing or leasing a home, have it inspected for asbestos. This fiber can be very expensive to remove, requiring experts in hazmat suits to come in and your family to move out for a while, so you want to know about it before you sign a mortgage or lease. If the asbestos is embedded in a product like vinyl flooring, it is likely to stay there and removing it could be more dangerous than letting it lie. However, asbestos found in insulation disintegrates over time, releasing the fibers into the air where they can be inhaled. Don't try to remove it yourself because you risk exposing yourself to the fibers.

GET RID OF RADON Radon is an odorless and invisible gas that seeps up from soil beneath homes, the result of naturally occurring radioactive rocks in the ground. Radon is the second leading cause of lung cancer after smoking, accounting for about 21,000 deaths each year, according to the EPA.

Radon can be detected using an inexpensive kit (about $15) that can be purchased at any home improvement store. The EPA recommends radon testing in all homes or apartments below the third floor. If radon is detected, a radon reduction system can usually bring the level below the EPA's action limit of 4 picocuries per liter (pCi/L) of air. The EPA recommends that occupants reduce the radon level to 2 pCi/L or lower if at all feasible. This usually involves installing a fan and pipe system to vent radon to the outdoors.

FRIENDLY FIRE A wood-burning fireplace adds a rustic, return-to-nature sort of feeling, but fireplaces can be potentially unhealthy for occupants and the environment. Wood smoke is a lung irritant that contains carcinogens such as soot and benzene. Wood-burning fires contribute to smog and are banned in some regions of the country. Burning wood generates nitrogen dioxide, an irritant and contributor to acid rain.

Fireplaces if not properly vented can present a health hazard. In poorly insulated houses, warm air can escape through the roof. The escaping air creates a vacuum-like effect that sucks air upward from the lower part of the house.

This exit system competes with the chimney for elimination of smoke. So, while some smoke goes up the chimney, some of it is also drawn into the house where it causes a smoky smell and can trigger asthma attacks and expose children to harmful particles.

Wood-burning heating devices include common fireplaces, masonry heaters, pellet stoves, outdoor wood boilers, and outdoor furnaces. If you must have a wood-burning residential heater, look for the cleanest-burning model available.

Outdoor wood furnaces burn wood or wood-chip bricks and pipe the heat into the living space. These furnaces are big polluters, however. Unlike your car, which has a catalytic converter to completely combust fuel, the furnace emits particles of soot and ash as well as other combustion products that increase the risk of lung cancer and contribute to poor air quality. If the chimney of the furnace is not higher than your house's roofline, the dirty smoke can seep back into your house.

If your memories of childhood include nights reading by the fire, and you want to pass that legacy on to your children, consider installing a clean-burning gas fireplace. The most efficient ones can return 80 percent of the heat to the room and safely vent the smoke to the outdoors. The EPA recommends against ventless models that allow combustion products, including carbon monoxide, to seep into the room.

While you are avoiding wood smoke, also avoid burning candles and incense, which release small particles that can be inhaled. You'll cut down on the risk of a home fire while protecting your family's lungs. Candles older than 2001 may contain lead in their wicks and release lead fumes when burning. You can usually tell if the wick contains lead by looking for dark-colored threads in the wick.

Another common source of smoke in the home is from cooking. Try to avoid overheating pans, especially if they are treated with a nonstick coating, which can release a gas that is toxic to birds. (See more about chemicals from nonstick coatings in Chapter 2.) Gas ranges emit nitrogen dioxide, a gas that can trigger asthma attacks, according to a 2008 study published in the journal *Environmental Health Perspectives*.[4] When cooking, always use your range's fan, which draws the nitrogen dioxide out of the house.

While on the subject of combustion, make sure you protect your family against carbon monoxide, an odorless gas that can be fatal within minutes. If your heating system goes awry, carbon monoxide can build up quickly. Install a carbon monoxide detector and run practice drills with your children so that they recognize the sound of the alarm and know to exit the house quickly.

DON'T GET YOUR DANDER UP Contemplate the dust floating in a sunbeam of light, and you'll realize that your home's indoor air is actually a thick soup of tiny particles through which you and your family move everyday. What is more, you are inhaling this soup daily. Most people experience no harm from this, but babies and children, as well as the elderly, are more sensitive than the rest of us. For sensitive individuals, inhaling these tiny particles can trigger asthma attacks and lung irritation.

Much of what is floating in the air is dander, the dead skin cells shed by pets and people. Dander is prime food for a resident freeloader, the dust mite. These microscopic bugs live in the warm, relatively moist innards of mattresses, pillows, sofas, and anywhere we (and our cats and dogs) love to lounge around. The dust mites create as waste tiny proteins that make their way into the air where they are inhaled and can trigger asthma, chronic congestion (allergic rhinitis), and lung problems in sensitive individuals.

Many families with asthma or allergy sufferers must forgo having furry friends in their lives to reduce dander and other allergy triggers around the house. Covering pillows and mattresses in allergen-reducing covers can help starve the dust mites, as can laundering pillows and sheets regularly in warm (greater than 77°F) water. One recommendation is to leave the bed unmade each morning, which allows the sheets to dry out and kills dust mites. It is worth a try, and your teenagers will love you for it.

Other suggestions for cutting down on asthma and allergy triggers around the home:

- ✓ Wash children's stuffed animals.
- ✓ Look for furniture with removable and washable cushions.
- ✓ Install flooring instead of carpets and rugs, especially in bedrooms.
- ✓ Encase mattresses, pillows, and sofa cushions in natural and untreated woven fiber casings.
- ✓ Dust frequently using a damp cloth. Mop and vacuum regularly. Use a vacuum with a high-efficiency particulate air (HEPA) filter.

DON'T DAMPEN YOUR ENTHUSIASM Damp places in your house or apartment send a loud invitation to two unwelcome guests, mold and mildew. These fungi can grow anywhere moisture lingers, such as on damp basement walls, around leaky pipes, or in poorly caulked areas around the shower. Several studies have linked mold to the onset of allergy and asthma attacks, and some scientific evidence suggests that mold can put children at risk of developing asthma.

ECO-TIP:
VANQUISH VINYL

When allergy proofing, avoid products made with vinyl (polyvinyl chloride or PVC). Vinyl releases volatile organic compounds, or VOCs, that can irritate the eyes and throat and cause headaches, especially in sensitive individuals. Off-gassing can go on for months.

Be vigilant when you see mold developing in a basement or other living space. Promptly remove it using soap and water or, if necessary, chlorine bleach. If using chlorine bleach, mix 1 cup of bleach in 1 gallon of water. Wear gloves and eye protection. Open windows and doors for ventilation. Never mix ammonia and chlorine bleach, which together create a highly toxic gas.

For large tracts of mold, call a mold-removal professional. Be sure to fix the source of the water (a leaky pipe, or rainwater slipping down along an outer foundation wall). Otherwise the mold will be back.

To prevent mold and mildew, use the exhaust fans in your bathrooms and kitchen. Make sure they vent to the outdoors and not to the attic. Keep attic and crawl spaces properly vented and indoor humidity at 40 to 60 percent. If you have a dehumidifier, clean the water pan regularly to keep it free of bacteria and other pathogens.

SMOKING SECTION Smoking is an entirely preventable cause of lung cancer, both for smokers and their loved ones. Environmental tobacco smoke, or secondhand smoke, not only contains cancer-causing chemicals, but it also triggers asthma attacks and allergies. Secondhand smoke increases the number of childhood ear infections and can contribute to chronic cough, persistent runny nose, bronchiolitis, pneumonia, and difficulties with learning and behavior.[5]

Secondhand smoke causes an extra 7,500 to 15,000 hospitalizations annually of children younger than 18 months in the United States, according to the EPA. Parents should also restrict their children from coming in contact with "third-hand smoke," defined as smoke that stays in the hair, clothes, furniture, and personal items of smokers, according to a 2009 study in the journal *Pediatrics*.[6]

Despite a massive public health campaign to notify families of the dangers of secondhand smoke, roughly one-fifth of Americans continue to consume tobacco products regularly, reports the CDC. If you have a smoker in the family, don't give up on urging the person to quit. In the meantime, don't allow the smoker to smoke inside the house or family car.

A ROACH BY ANY OTHER NAME A midnight encounter with a cockroach in your kitchen is enough to make even the staunchest environmentalist wish for a can of bug killer. To protect your family's and your planet's health, reach for a shoe instead. Pesticides are designed to kill bugs, but they can have subtle yet harmful effects on humans, especially children. A number of good alternatives to pesticides exist, but first let's look at why we should avoid purchasing these products.

Pesticides cause two kinds of trouble: short-term toxicity and long-term health impacts. The short-term effects happen when a child grabs a bottle from under the kitchen sink or puts weed-killing pellets into his mouth while playing on the lawn. Large doses of pesticides can cause symptoms ranging from nausea and headaches to rashes, allergic reactions, seizures, coma, and death. Avoid the risk by not purchasing these items in the first place, or storing them in a locked area high above the reach of most kids.

Long-term health issues are harder to pin down and much of what we know comes from animal studies and studies in highly exposed groups like children of farm workers. Long-term potential health risks include birth defects, asthma, neurodevelopmental or behavioral effects, and cancer.[7] Our children are regularly exposed to pesticides. A nationally representative survey published by CDC researchers in 2005 found that 96 percent of children ages 6 to 11 have been recently exposed to organophosphate pesticides.[8]

Instead of using pesticides, try an integrated pest management (IPM) approach that focuses on prevention, safe methods of elimination, and pesticides only as a last resort. IPM methods can be more effective against roaches than conventional pesticides, a 2009 study in the *Journal of Medical Entomology* found.[9]

To keep pests out of the house:

- ✓ Seal cracks in exterior walls and around windows and doors.
- ✓ Fix moisture problems.
- ✓ Clean up crumbs promptly and store food in sealed containers.
- ✓ If you absolutely must use pesticides, avoid the sprays and foggers that broadcast the chemicals into carpets, floorboard cracks, and onto tabletops and toys. Sprayed pesticide residues linger on these surfaces and children can ingest the chemicals through hand-to-mouth activity. Use traps, baits, or gels instead of sprays.

EXTREME VOLATILITY If you've ever developed a headache while painting a room, you've smelled volatile organic compounds, or VOCs for short. You may have smelled VOCs when you first opened a box containing a self-assembly bookcase or when you unrolled a new rug for the first time. VOCs are found in paints, some household cleaning agents, building materials, furniture, carpets, office equipment such as copiers and printers, glues, adhesives, permanent markers, and a great many other products.

Products containing VOCs are hard to avoid, yet we should try to do so whenever we can. The chemicals can irritate sensitive areas of the nose, throat,

ECO-TIP:
FOOTWARE-FREE ZONE

Keep toxic chemicals from being tracked into the house by making your house a shoe-free zone. Have family members and visitors remove their shoes at the door. If you haven't done so already, install doormats outside each entrance.

VOLATILE ORGANIC COMPOUND (VOC)

A chemical that tends to evaporate into the air rather than stay as a solid or liquid. (The use of the term "organic" refers to the chemical structure and is different from the use of "organic" to describe agricultural practices.)

lungs, and eyes, and trigger asthma attacks and allergies. Some VOCs, such as benzene used in shoe manufacture, are known to cause cancer in people who work with these chemicals on a daily basis, according to the EPA.

As with any chemical, the amount and duration of exposure can influence the risk of toxicity. Children are potentially at greater risk than adults because babies and kids inhale a greater volume of air per pound of body weight than adults do.

To avoid VOCs, choose low- or no-VOC paints and other products. If possible choose furniture made of solid wood (see suggestions later in the chapter on where to find it inexpensively). Most of us, however, will not be able to avoid bringing these chemicals into our lives. The best we can do is to let the products offgas the VOCs as much as possible before we bring them into our homes. If you've brought home an item with a strong chemical smell, put it outside for a couple of days to let the fumes escape.

THE RUBBER DUCK CHEMICAL Phthalates (pronounced THAL-ates) are chemicals added to plastics to make them flexible. Household items that contain phthalates include vinyl shower curtains, vinyl flooring, and, until recently, plastic toys such as rubber ducks. Plastic materials may contain up to 40 percent phthalates by weight.

Studies in laboratory animals indicate that long-term exposure to phthalates may disrupt hormonal activity, harm reproduction, and cause birth defects, according to the CDC. Several phthalates have been linked to cancer, and some researchers suspect they play a role in asthma. A 2004 study in the journal *Environmental Health Perspectives* found an association between asthma and allergies in children and phthalate concentrations in dust collected from the children's bedrooms.[10]

Phthalates are called semi-VOCs (sVOCs), because they can either migrate into the air or settle down on dust particles and surfaces. This behavior makes them likely to be inhaled or be transferred into the body via hand-to-mouth activity. They are far more persistent than VOCs, so they can expose and re-expose a child for months.

A study by CDC scientists released in 2004 found phthalate metabolites (breakdown products of phthalates) in 75 percent of the urine samples tested.[11] This reflects recent exposure, since phthalates don't stick around in the body but are rapidly broken down and eliminated. The CDC study revealed that children ages 6 to 11 were more likely to have higher levels of phthalates than were older children. (Children younger than six years of age were not tested.)

In 2009, the United States enacted a ban on three phthalates, di(2-ethylhexyl) phthalate (DEHP), dibutyl phthalate (DBP), and butyl benzyl phthalate

(BBP), in children's toys and child-care articles. Three other phthalates, diisononyl phthalate (DINP), diisodecyl phthalate (DIDP), and di-n-octyl phthalate (DnOP), were also provisionally banned.

To avoid phthalates, limit your purchase of items containing soft plastics. If you purchased baby toys before the phthalate ban, consider replacing them with newer plastics, or choose all-natural solid wood teethers and toys. (See Chapter 7 for more suggestions on eco-friendly toys.)

OUT OF THE FRYING PAN AND INTO THE FIRE Flame-retardant chemicals are meant to save lives, but some of them can take their toll on your children's health. Polybrominated diphenyl ethers (PBDEs) are flame-retardant chemicals that are suspected of causing cancer, liver toxicity, and neurodevelopmental problems, according to the EPA. These chemicals are used in electronics, plastics, and foam cushions manufactured prior to 2005.

Like phthalates, these chemicals fall into the semi-VOC category. The chemicals migrate from household products, attach to dust particles, and float through a room until they settle on surfaces. When children and adults touch objects in their home and then touch their mouths, they transfer and ingest the chemicals.

A CDC survey published in 2008 found that many American adults have phthalate metabolites in their blood and breast milk.[12] American women have some of the highest levels of PBDEs in human breast milk anywhere in the world, according to a report by the Environmental Working Group.[13] A study published in a 2008 issue of *Environmental Science & Technology* found that infants had higher levels of PBDEs in their blood than adults.[14] Infants and young children are at greatest risk because they may be nursing, and they engage in hand-to-mouth activity.

Sofa and mattress manufacturers have voluntarily phased out two PBDEs (penta- and octa-PBDE), but some U.S. electronics manufacturers are still using deca-PBDE, a possible human carcinogen that Europe banned in 2008. New flame retardants are now being used, but many health experts are concerned that the replacements also have worrisome health properties.

To avoid flame-retardant chemicals in electronics, you can find a list of safer products at the Environmental Working Group's website *www.ewg.org/pbdefree*. When shopping for furnishings, look for items made of metal, leather, and natural fibers such as jute, hemp, and wool. When choosing children's sleepwear, look for close-fitting all-cotton pajamas rather than synthetic fabrics, which are more likely to be treated with flame retardants. (See Chapter 6 for more sleepwear suggestions.)

KITCHEN TABLE TALK

A Word About Chemicals

By now you may be asking, if a certain chemical is so dangerous, posing risks to a child's developing brain, nervous system, and reproductive system, then why hasn't the EPA stepped up to ban it? This question will come up over and over as you read this book. Here is the answer.

We live in a society that allows chemicals into consumer products without fully understanding their toxicity. When chemicals *are* found to be toxic, the U.S. government agencies often take decades before they enact a ban. For example, lead was known to be toxic when it was introduced into gasoline to fix engine knock in the 1920s, yet the U.S. government allowed it to be sold until 1986.

Common sense dictates that manufacturers and chemical companies should discover and document any harmful effects of chemicals *before* they go on the market. The United States does require testing of chemicals used in food, pharmaceuticals, and agriculture. However, most other industrial chemicals enjoy an "innocent until proven guilty" status. The EPA has rigorously tested only about 200 of the roughly 80,000 industrial chemicals listed under the U.S. Toxic Substances Control Act (TSCA), according to the Government Accountability Office (GAO).

With so many untested chemicals around, we consumers need to take responsibility to learn about health hazards and make informed decisions about what products to purchase. When the science is inadequate or unavailable, many consumers choose to err on the side of caution, adopting what is known as "the precautionary principle." This means that when concerns exist about a particular chemical, and less toxic choices are available, the consumer should use the less toxic option.

In many cases, consumer outcry effectively forces companies to reformulate their products, simply because companies do not want to lose customers. That is why it is important to make your desire for a cleaner and healthier environment known through your purchases. Let your preferences be heard through phone calls and e-mails to companies as well.

But, you counter, don't most companies have an economic interest in providing safer ingredients? Well, yes, and no. If a toxic reaction is immediate (a skin rash, a common report of allergic reactions), those complaints get addressed in short order. But health problems like reproductive difficulties and cancer crop up years down the road, making it hard to attribute the health problem to a specific product or chemical.

CLEARING THE AIR Commercials for room air purifiers lure us with the promise of sleep-filled nights and relief from congestion due to allergies. But do they really work? Many people report that room air filters help them breathe better. But before you spend $100 or more on an air purifier, you should first reduce the source of irritants. As mentioned above, frequent vacuuming, mopping, and dusting with a damp cloth can reduce pet dander and other allergens. Regularly washing sheets in warm water and putting allergen barriers on pillows and mattresses can diminish dust mites. Remove carpets and cushions where dust mites burrow. Avoid burning candles, smoking indoors, and lighting improperly ventilated wood stoves. In addition to removing the source of irritants, ventilate your home regularly. Open windows and run fans that can circulate fresh outdoor air with stale indoor air.

If you've taken all these steps and you are still miserable, you may want to try a room air purifier. There are three basic kinds.

OZONE PURIFIERS Steer clear of purifiers that advertise that they generate ozone. Although ozone plays a much needed role high up in the atmosphere in protecting the planet from ultraviolet radiation, at ground level this chemical is a lung irritant. It can trigger asthma attacks and weaken your ability to fight off respiratory infections.

IONIC FILTERS AND ELECTROSTATIC PRECIPITATORS Electrostatic precipitators work by charging (ionizing) particles as they pass through the nearby air and then collecting them on an oppositely charged metal grid or plate. Ionic purifiers also charge the particles but generally have no collector plate or grid and instead rely on the principle that the charged particles will cling to walls and other surfaces, possibly causing stains. A *Consumer Reports* evaluation found that some ionic and electrostatic purifiers generate small amounts of ozone.

GREEN DICTIONARY

THE PRECAUTIONARY PRINCIPLE

Taking action to reduce threats to human health or the environment even if some cause-and-effect relationships have not been fully established scientifically.

HEPA FILTERS Instead of opting for ozonation or ionization, choose a good quality purifier containing a high-efficiency particulate air (HEPA) filter. These filters are usually made of pleated fiberglass sheets and are good at capturing larger airborne particles, such as dust, pollen, dust mites, cockroach allergens, dander, and some molds. These accordion-pleated filters can remove about 99.97 percent of airborne particles down to 0.3 microns in diameter, less than 1/1000 the diameter of a period on this page. Some air purifiers use even finer filters called ultra-HEPA (ULPA) filters. These filters can trap 99.999 percent of all airborne particles 0.12 microns and larger. You'll need to replace the filter annually or according to the manufacturer's directions.

You'll want to choose a filter that removes very small particles because they lodge deep in the lungs and can lead to chronic lung problems. Particulate matter (PM) can be produced by cigarette smoke, candles, and wood fires. It can also consist of viruses, bacteria, and some molds.

When buying an air filter, look for one certified by the Association of Home Appliance Manufacturers (AHAM). Each certified purifier has a maximum clean air delivery rate (CADR), a measure of cleaning speed. Learn more about CADRs at *www.cadr.org*. Choose a purifier that is rated for a bigger area than the room you plan to use it in.

If your house is equipped with a ventilation system, keep it well maintained and change the filters regularly according to the manufacturer's recommendations. These ventilation systems can be added to homes that have forced-air heating and cooling systems. Installation usually must be done professionally because it involves adding to existing ductwork and connecting the ventilation system to your home's electrical system. Duct-cleaning, advertised in the fliers that get left on your doorstep, can stir up more dust than it eliminates, according to the EPA, and should be used only if substantial duct contaminants are entering the home.

Home Renovations

Whether updating a 1950s bathroom or just applying a coat of paint, renovating a home is a labor of love that can add value and personality to your home. For the good of the planet and your family, opt for safer and more environmentally friendly paints and furnishings.

A new addition to the family often prompts a new addition to a home, whether it is adding on a room or just giving a nursery-like look to the corner of a bedroom shared with siblings. When considering home renovations with a baby on the way or young children in the home, pay special attention to the furnishings and chemicals you'll be introducing to your new space. It is impossible to avoid chemicals in today's world, and indeed, many are perfectly safe when applied in ventilated areas with proper skin and eye protection. But you'll want to avoid products that contain chemicals that continue to offgas long after the renovations are done.

The best time to renovate is before conception of a child. Most parents don't plan that far in advance, however. If you want to do major renovations with children around, you might consider relocating to an extended-stay hotel or taking a long vacation. Depending on the scale of the project, you might consider postponing renovations until the children are older and can be sent for a week to camp or grandmother's house.

WALL FLOWERS Paints and wallpapers can transform a room from a space into a sanctuary. Kids can help pick colors and get involved in designing the look of their room. But keep in mind that some paints and home improvement products are safer than others.

If your home is older than 1978, don't do any sanding or painting until you've tested for lead paint. (See the section earlier in this chapter on lead paint.) If you are pregnant, have someone else do the painting. Most paints contain volatile organic compounds, which give the paints that distinct "new paint" smell. Even the low-VOC varieties can give you a headache after several hours, so always paint in well-ventilated areas. Pregnant women should avoid painting with even low-VOC paints. A number of no-VOC brands are now available.

If you do paint the nursery, wait several days before moving your new baby in. Keep windows open, run fans, and circulate as much fresh air into the space as possible. VOCs are irritating and can serve as allergy triggers. It is possible that sensitizing infants and young children causes allergies and asthma later in life, although studies are not conclusive.

Wallpaper can add flair and unique style to a room, but wallpaper glue can contain formaldehyde, a VOC that is irritating to the eyes and lungs and is considered a probable carcinogen by the EPA. Low-VOC glues are available.

DECORATING WITH FLAIR, NOT FORMALDEHYDE Whether you are prepping the nursery for a new baby or redecorating a child's room into a teen's retreat, you'll want to take time over each decision about the materials you plan to use. A trip to a home improvement store will yield numerous options

POSTCONSUMER WASTE (PCW)

PCW is waste paper from your home or office that you've tossed into the recycling bin. Not all recycled paper products are made from PCW, however, but instead contain preconsumer wastes such as manufacturing scraps and by-products. The more we can use PCW, the more we can return used paper to the supply chain and keep it out of landfills.

for building products, but many products emit potentially harmful chemicals (discussed in the sections above) that offgas for months or even years.

When redecorating, try to avoid buying new furniture made with particleboard. Particleboard consists of wood fibers glued tightly together, usually with formaldehyde-emitting glue. If you must go with particleboard, choose U.S.-made particleboard, which according to the Composite Panel Association meets new limits on formaldehyde emissions set by the state of California in 2009. You can also seal particleboard with products designed to prevent offgassing. Give new furniture time to offgas by putting the items in a garage or on a porch until they no longer smell prior to installation.

Another option is to look for gently used solid wood furniture. You can find furnishings made of solid wood at garage sales, thrift stores, antique stores, and online at sites such as *www.freecycle.org* and *www.craigslist.org.* (Buyer beware that some used furnishings may harbor bedbugs, which can be very hard to eliminate once they've taken up residence in your house. Inspect items carefully prior to purchase.) When buying new wood furniture, check for the country of origin. Many areas of the world, such as Southeast Asia, are being rapidly deforested of old-growth rain forest trees. Look for products bearing the Forest Stewardship Council (FSC; *www.fsc.org*) label, which certifies wood as being harvested from well-managed forests.

Bamboo is an attractive material that is becoming popular for flooring and furniture. This hardy grass grows rapidly, so it potentially is more sustainable than wood. However, the bamboo in many stores is imported from China or Vietnam, raising concerns about the sustainability of growing practices, equitable labor conditions, and the greenhouse gases generated when products are shipped around the world. Look for bamboo products certified by the FSC. You may be able to find domestically grown bamboo. Bamboo flooring must be treated with finishing agents to give it durability, so look for low-VOC formulations.

KITCHEN ENCOUNTER Kitchens are places to gather, and a bigger family needs more gathering space. If you are renovating your kitchen with young children in the house, choose natural products whenever possible. Consider installing flooring made from tile, hardwood, cork, low-VOC bamboo, or natural composite flooring.

For kitchen counters, consider all-wood butcher block, stone, or granite. Some stores offer eco-friendly options like recycled paper composites. If opting for granite, make sure the piece you are installing has been tested for radioactivity. Some granite is naturally radioactive and emits enough radiation to substantially increase your risk of lung cancer.

Kitchen cabinets are often made of particleboard coated with a wood veneer. The veneer reduces formaldehyde emissions on the surface that faces the kitchen. The interior cabinet surfaces may be unfaced and capable of releasing VOCs. It is possible to paint them with a sealant marketed for the purpose of sealing in toxic chemicals. The state of California has enacted new limits on formaldehyde emissions from composite wood products. Given the state's large population of consumers, California's ruling is likely to force manufacturers to reformulate their products for the entire nation. A bill has already been introduced in the Senate that would enact the equivalent standard nationwide.

GREEN ROOM ADDITIONS When you are ready for a major home renovation, such as adding a room, many resources are available to help you design and build an ecologically friendly room addition. The U.S. Green Building Council *(www .usgbc.org)* has a green building rating system known as Leadership in Energy and Environmental Design (LEED), which considers the impact of the building site on local ecology, the building's energy consumption, use of renewable energy sources, water usage, use of healthier building materials, and recycling. If you are a do-it-yourselfer, check out the Building for Environmental and Economic Sustainability (BEES) software, which helps builders select cost-effective, environmentally sound building products, at *www.bfrl.nist.gov/oae/software/bees.*

High-quality wood can sometimes be salvaged when older homes are torn down. Depending on the home's age, the wood may be high quality locally grown hardwoods that are better than what builders have available today. The price can be high, however, and the recycled wood may not build an entire room addition. The Rainforest Alliance's SmartWood *(www.smartwood.org)* program certifies wood from teardowns through its "Rediscovered Wood" label.

After renovating, donate extras to a charity or facility that finds new uses for discarded housing and renovation materials. You can search for facilities near you that accept recycled construction materials at *http://earth911.com.*

Clean and Green

Keeping house involves endless cleaning, especially with kids around. But cleaning with harsh chemicals is rarely if ever necessary and can be harmful to your family's health and the environment. Choose natural cleaners, or make your own.

BETTER LIVING THROUGH CHEMISTRY Chemicals have made our lives better in numerous ways, but toxic ones in cleaning products are best avoided. Several common ingredients in household cleaners have been linked to poisonings and long-term health problems. Some of the most toxic substances in the home are dishwasher detergents, drain cleaners, and toilet bowl cleaners.

Cleaning products are the second most common cause of household poisonings, resulting in 7.5 percent of poisonings of children under five, according to the American Association of Poison Control Centers. (Cosmetics and personal care products are the most common, causing 10.7 percent of poisonings.) When we finish using these chemicals, we wash them down the drain, and from there they flow into lakes, rivers, and the ocean, where they can kill or harm aquatic life.

Some of the chemicals in cleaners have the potential to cause long-term reproductive harm such as decreased fertility, changes in the onset of puberty, miscarriage, premature birth, and cancers of reproductive organs. As mentioned above, these chemicals also harm the environment.

By switching to safer cleaning products you can make your home healthier and reduce the risk of accidental poisonings, long-term health effects, and harming wildlife in the environment. You can either buy brands specifically marketed as being green and less toxic, or you can make your own cleaners out of inexpensive materials. See below for tips on how to make cleaners at home.

When ridding your home of toxic chemicals, check with your local government to see if they accept chemicals. Your town may sponsor a "household hazardous waste day" to collect toxic trash.

LABELS—SOME READING REQUIRED To avoid bringing toxic chemicals into your home, some label reading is required. Some products advertised as green are anything but. Avoid the following:

× **ALKYLPHENOL ETHOXYLATES (ALL-PURPOSE CLEANERS, DETERGENTS)** Hormone disrupting chemicals that can alter sexual development in aquatic organisms. Examples include nonylphenol and octylphenol.

× **AMMONIA (FLOOR, BATHROOM, AND TILE CLEANERS, AND SOLD ON ITS OWN)** Irritating to the skin, eyes, and lungs. Can be fatal if swallowed. Never mix with chlorine bleach, as toxic fumes can result.

× **ANTIBACTERIALS—TRICLOSAN AND TRICLOCARBAN (DISINFECTANTS, DETERGENTS)** May contribute to antibiotic resistance; may break down into more toxic by-products that are linked to cancer.

ECO-TIP:
TRULY GREEN PRODUCTS

Manufacturers are not required to list ingredients in cleaning products. Call the company or look for cleaners certified by Green Seal or EcoLogo, recommends the Environmental Working Group.

For example, in water treatment plants, triclosan can form chloroform; in sunlight it may form dioxin.

× **CHLORINE BLEACH (DISINFECTANTS, LAUNDRY DETERGENT, SOLD ON ITS OWN)** Causes skin, eye, and respiratory irritation and can be fatal if swallowed. Chlorine bleach is toxic to fish and wildlife. Avoid if possible. Sometimes, however, it is needed against mold.

× **DIETHANOLAMINE (DEA) AND TRIETHANOLAMINE (TEA) (DETER-GENTS, CLEANSERS)** Can combine with preservatives or contaminants to produce nitrosamines, cancer-causing chemicals that can penetrate the skin. DEA is linked to brain toxicity in animal studies.

× **ETHYLENE-BASED GLYCOL ETHERS (GLASS CLEANER)** 2-butoxyethanol (butyl cellosolve) is a suspected hormone disrupter linked to reproductive problems. High levels of exposure cause headaches, vomiting, and skin, eye, and lung irritation.

× **PHOSPHATES (DISHWASHING DETERGENTS)** Used to soften water, but encourage algae overgrowth in water, contributing to aquatic dead zones.

× **PHTHALATES (CLEANERS, DETERGENTS)** Used to prolong the release of fragrance but have hormone-disrupting effects at very small doses. Have been linked to liver, kidney, thyroid, and reproductive problems in animals.

× **SODIUM HYDROXIDE OR LYE (DRAIN AND OVEN CLEANERS)** Extremely irritating to eyes, nose, and throat. Can burn on contact.

GREEN ON A SHOESTRING

Environmentally friendly cleaning products are great time-savers because you can squirt and wipe without having to worry that you are spritzing toxic chemicals. However, they can be expensive.

Here are some tips to cut your cleaning costs:

✓ Look for coupons online.

✓ Shop the sales and stock up.

✓ Stop buying paper towels. Use washable cloth rags for your cleaning jobs.

Or try making your own cleaners from the following safer products:

✓ Baking soda acts as a gentle scouring powder; it fizzes when it comes in contact with vinegar or lemon to help loosen dirt. It also works as a deodorizer.

✓ Borax deodorizes, disinfects, and bleaches.

✓ Distilled white vinegar cuts grease, breaks up dirt, and has disinfecting power. (Do not combine vinegar with chlorine bleach.)

✓ Hydrogen peroxide bleaches and disinfects. It also can remove stains.

✓ Lemon juice cuts grease and adds a lemony smell.

✓ Olive oil collects dirt and leaves wood looking polished.

✓ Vegetable-based (liquid castile) soap is a gentle all-purpose cleaner.

✓ Washing soda (found in the laundry aisle) removes stains and dirt, but it is caustic, so wear gloves when using.

With a few of these working in combination, you can tackle almost any household chore.

✓ **TOILET BOWLS** 1/4 cup of baking soda plus 1/4 cup of vinegar. Let sit for 30 minutes, scrub, and flush. Use borax on stubborn stains.

✓ **DRAIN CLEANER** Pour 1/4 cup of baking soda followed by 1/2 cup of vinegar. Let sit for 20 minutes, then follow with 1/2 gallon of boiling water.

✓ **MOLD AND MILDEW** Spray hydrogen peroxide and vinegar one right after the other. Use chlorine bleach only after less toxic methods are tried. (See the mold and mildew section earlier in this chapter for precautions when using chlorine bleach.)

✓ **WOOD FLOORS** 1/2 cup of white vinegar in 2 gallons of warm water.

✓ **LINOLEUM FLOORS** 1 cup of white vinegar in 2 gallons of warm water.

✓ **FURNITURE POLISH** 1/2 cup of white vinegar plus 1 teaspoon of olive oil.

✓ **HOUSEHOLD ALL-PURPOSE CLEANER** 1/2 cup of borax plus 1/4 cup of castile soap in 1 gallon of hot water.

BREATHING LESSONS Air fresheners usually contain chemicals that can cause lung irritation and skin sensitivity. A better strategy is to eliminate the sources of smells in your home. Is a water leak causing mold? Does the pet's bed need washing more regularly? Eliminate the source, and you won't need the air freshener. Open windows when feasible. In midwinter, you can open the windows for a few minutes, and the temperature difference between outside and inside will draw fresh cold air into the house.

Saving Energy

Running a household takes energy—not the kind busy parents seem never to have enough of, but the kind that comes from power plants. The energy that keeps the house warm and the baby monitor running often comes from pollution-generating resources such as oil, natural gas, or coal. Cutting down on your household energy use is a good way to save money and conserve natural resources.

The biggest energy consumer in the home is its heating system. The typical household furnace accounts for 31 percent of the average family's energy usage. The next biggest user is the water heater, which soaks up 12 percent of energy expenditures. Air conditioners use about the same amount of energy as water heaters. Next come lighting (11 percent), computers (9 percent), appliances (9 percent), and refrigeration (8 percent), according to the U.S. Department of Energy's Office of Energy Efficiency and Renewable Energy (EERE).

Weaning your home completely off energy dependence is nearly impossible, but there are ways to substantially reduce your home's energy needs. Heating takes the largest chunk of energy, so it makes sense to start by ensuring that your home is adequately insulated and sealed. Once you've fixed the biggest problems, you can work your way down the list, replacing lightbulbs and appliances as needed with energy-saving models. And don't forget to adopt energy-saving habits such as taking shorter showers, setting your thermostat two degrees cooler, and turning off lights and computers when they are not in use.

HEATING AND COOLING SYSTEMS There is nothing like a warm cozy house in winter, but when your furnace is turning on every few minutes just to keep the house at a livable temperature, you know you have a problem. Homes built before 1980 are especially likely to be poorly insulated, either because the insulation has degraded over time or because very little was installed in the first place. During the 1980s homebuilders began making homes airtight, but it is still possible to find newer homes that were not built to keep in the heat.

Your home's need for insulation will depend on the climate you live in, of course. A heavy-duty heating system is not needed for nights in balmy Florida. But many of the same principles that apply to keeping warm air indoors also apply to keeping cooled air indoors. The money you spend on insulating your home most likely will be repaid several times over by your savings from reduced energy utility bills. Before embarking on expensive renovations, however, you can identify the best way to save energy in your home using online tools such as the Lawrence Berkeley National Laboratory's Home Energy Saver (hes.lbl.gov) or the EPA's ENERGY STAR Home Energy Audit (www.energystar.gov).

The first step in fixing a drafty house and reducing those heating bills is to find out how the warm air is escaping. Although poorly sealed doorframes and rattling single-pane windows are sources of leaks, in fact they are nearly always a symptom of a bigger problem. The majority of homes leak heat through the roof, foundation, and walls.

Why the roof? Warm air tends to rise, and as it does, it finds ways to exit the poorly insulated house through holes between rafters and roofing shingles. As the warm air rises, it creates a vacancy of air in the lower part of the house. This vacuum effect draws cold air from the outside into the house through those rattling windows mentioned earlier. Homeowners who are considering replacing their windows should first make sure that their house is not vacuuming air out of their homes and dollars out of their wallets.

The addition of insulation and airtight boundaries can shut down the vacuum effect. Some of the areas requiring insulation are the attic, exterior walls, basement walls and ceiling, floors, spaces between stories, and crawl spaces. A number of new insulating materials are available as an alternative to the classic fiberglass materials, which can shred over the years and release glass fibers into the air. New insulating materials include ones made from leftover scraps from manufacturing blue jeans or hemp fibers, or even recycled newspapers.

THE FACTS

The heating and cooling of homes in the U.S. generates roughly 150 million tons of the climate-altering greenhouse gas carbon dioxide each year, according to the EERE.

Another option is spray polyurethane foam, which is not a natural product but does come in low-VOC formulations. If installed by a trained professional, the foam polyurethane provides excellent insulation.

Once you've fixed the major holes and restored the insulation, your work is still not done. Another major area of heat loss is the duct system that carries warm or cooled air to and from the living spaces. These ducts should be sealed not only in basements but also within walls and crawl spaces. Finally, seal the cracks around windows and doors, as well as light and plumbing fixtures, electrical outlets, and light switches.

To determine where the holes in your walls, attic, and roof are, you may want to have an energy professional conduct a blower door test. Some municipalities offer free energy audits that include this test. Once you know where the problems are, you can fix problems yourself if you are handy or hire an insulation expert. Look for a contractor who advertises that he or she is environmentally responsible. Ask about the health and safety of the insulating materials and caulks. Sealing should be done with low-VOC caulk or sealant.

Use a programmable thermostat to turn down your heater at night and during the day, when the children are at school and the adults are at work. Contrary to what you may have heard, it takes more energy to maintain a warm house all day than it does to let the house cool and then heat it up just before you return. The colder the climate, the truer that statement becomes. The advantage of programmable thermostats is that they can be set to come on before you wake up or return home, so the house is comfortable when you need it to be.

Use ceiling fans and portable fans to circulate air. Compared to running the air conditioner, electric fans use little electricity and allow you to set the thermostat at a higher temperature that still feels comfortable. In the winter, keep drapes closed at night to keep drafts out, and open them during the day to allow the sun's warmth into the house. During the summer, close the drapes to keep cool air in and the warm sun out.

When it is time to buy a new heating or cooling unit, don't buy too big. Select a furnace with an annual fuel utilization efficiency (AFUE) rating that is 90 percent or better. Choose air conditioners with the best seasonal energy efficiency ratio (SEER) of 14.5 or more.

GREEN DICTIONARY

BLOWER DOOR TEST

A test conducted to determine how airtight a home is. A fan installed in a doorway pulls air out of the house, creating a vacuum that sucks new outdoor air into the house through cracks around windows and doors. The tester uses a smoke pencil to "see" the air coming in through the cracks.

WINDOW WISDOM   About 31 percent of the warm air that leaks out of homes does so through cracks and holes in floors, walls, and ceilings, whereas only about 10 percent leaks out around the windows, according to the EERE. Once you've sealed the floors, walls, and ceilings, it is time to address the windows. Seal around windows with low-VOC caulk and weather stripping.

When buying new windows, consult the climate region map on the ENERGY STAR label or website to make sure the window is right for your climate. Look for the NFRC (National Fenestration Rating Council) label that provides the U-factor. The lower the U-factor, the better the insulation.

Replacing single-pane windows with double-pane windows can save up to 15 percent of your energy bill. You can get even more savings by buying windows with inert gases between the two panes. Low-emissivity (low-e) coatings can reduce energy loss even further. Since replacing windows is relatively expensive and not done often, it pays to purchase the most energy-saving, climate-appropriate windows that you can afford, according to the experts at the U.S. Department of Energy's Lawrence Berkeley National Laboratory.

A TANKLESS JOB The hot water heater is another home energy hog. A lot of the energy expended by water heaters is used to keep the water hot and ready for use. Wrapping the tank in an insulation blanket can reduce this heat loss. Tanks less than five years old are built with better insulation and don't require blanketing. Water heaters powered by electricity can be fitted with a timer to turn off the heater at night and when you are not home.

When it is time to replace your existing unit, choose a water heater with an efficiency factor (EF) of 0.63 for gas-fired heaters and 0.93 for electric heaters, as recommended by the American Council for an Energy-Efficient Economy (ACEEE). Consult the yellow and black EnergyGuide label for an estimation of energy usage per year. ENERGY STAR–rated water heaters have been available since January 2009. On-demand water heaters, or tankless systems, are an excellent environment-friendly option. These units heat water only when it is needed, so they don't waste energy keeping water hot all day long. They are available in both gas and electric models.

To save money on utility bills and reduce your hot water usage, take shorter showers and fewer baths. Wash clothes in cold water as much as possible and use warm water only when needed. Set your hot water heater thermostat to 120°F, which on most water heaters is the midpoint between the low and medium setting.

GREEN ON A SHOESTRING

Inexpensive ways to cut your utility bills by 25 percent:

✓ Add insulation and plug any holes in the attic.

✓ Weather-strip all windows and doors, and caulk around areas where utility wires and pipes enter the house, even in the basement.

✓ If you have single-pane windows, add storm windows (about $100 each) or apply special plastic shrink-wrap (about $2 per window) available at home improvement stores. Replacing windows with ENERGY STAR–qualified windows is pricey, but will save energy and should improve the resale value of your home.

✓ If your water heater is older than five years, it may need a blanket. Special insulated jackets can be wrapped around the tank to keep heat in. Put pipe insulation around the hot water pipe everywhere it is exposed.

✓ Feel for hot air around the heating ducts in the basement, if you have a forced air system. Apply an inexpensive, nontoxic sealant wherever you feel leaks.

✓ Replace your lightbulbs with compact fluorescent lightbulbs (CFLs).

For more tips, see the American Council for an Energy-Efficient Economy (ACEEE) *Consumer Guide to Home Energy Savings***, available at** *www.aceee.org/consumer.*

A LIGHT TOUCH Lighting accounts for 11 percent of a home's energy usage. Switching your incandescent bulbs to compact fluorescent lightbulbs (CFLs) can cut your energy usage substantially. CFLs are four times more efficient than incandescent bulbs, because they don't waste as much energy as heat.

CFLs can last for years, but they do not work as efficiently in locations where you are always switching the lights on and off. Also, they can take several minutes to achieve their maximum brightness and energy efficiency, so you should install them in places where you know you will have the lights on for long periods of time.

The bulbs now come in a variety of shapes and work with most existing lighting fixtures. However most do not work with motion detectors. Some but not all of them work with dimmer switches and timers, so check the package before purchase. For outdoor lighting, consider light-emitting diode (LED) lights. They work better than CFLs in cold temperatures.

CFLs are great energy savers but, because they contain a small amount of mercury, bulbs must be handled and disposed of properly. (See The Science Behind It on page 49 for more information.)

ECO-TIP: **SAFE USE OF CFLS.**

Here are some tips for using CFLs in ways that minimize risks to the environment and you:

✓ **Buy CFLs with the lowest mercury content. The Environmental Working Group maintains a list of low-mercury bulbs at *www.ewg .org/reports/compact-fluorescent-light-bulbs*.**

✓ **Place CFLs in locations where they are unlikely to break, such as ceiling fixtures instead of floor lamps in high traffic areas.**

✓ **Screw CFLs in by the base, not by grasping the glass.**

✓ **Don't use CFLs in rooms frequented by pregnant women or children (bedrooms, playrooms).**

✓ **Dispose of broken and burned-out CFLs through your municipal collection program or check the EPA's website at *www.epa.gov/ bulbrecycling* for nearby disposal sites. Never throw them in the trash.**

IF A CFL BULB BREAKS, TAKE THE FOLLOWING STEPS:

✓ **Open windows to allow volatile mercury vapors to escape.**

✓ **Keep people and pets away for 15 minutes.**

✓ **Don gloves, a dust mask or other facial covering, and old clothes.**

✓ **Scoop up bulb fragments, then pat the area with sticky tape to collect tiny splinters and dust. Wipe with dampened paper towels.**

✓ **Place towels in a glass jar with the bulb and seal.**

✓ **Properly dispose of the jar and its contents, and also dispose of any materials (bedding, etc.) that came in contact with the bulb or its dust. Towels, bedding, and clothing that come in contact with the broken bulb should be discarded—not laundered. Mercury particles** could contaminate the washing machine or the water flowing into the sewage system.

If a bulb breaks on a carpet, the EPA recommends vacuuming it and then cleaning the vacuum. However, the Maine Department of Environmental Protection (DEP) conducted several tests and concluded that vacuuming stirs up room air and can result in elevated mercury levels in the air. Using the vacuum elsewhere in the house could spread the mercury to other rooms. The Maine DEP suggests removing the carpet altogether, especially if pregnant women or children spend time in that area. If the carpet is not removed, be sure to ventilate the area frequently since mercury vapors can release from the carpet over long periods of time.

HOUSEHOLD HELP Appliances (including refrigerators) account for about 17 percent of household energy usage. The biggest user is the refrigerator, followed by the washing machine and clothes dryer, according to the EERE. Most appliances are electricity driven, but some run on natural gas. The average U.S. household uses about 11,000 kilowatt-hours (kWh) per year. (One kWh is the amount of electricity it takes to cook a pot of rice in an electric cooker for one hour.) At an average residential rate of 9.4 cents per kWh, the annual cost of running your appliances is about $1,034.

ECO-TIP: CUT YOUR UTILITY BILL *AND* YOUR CARBON EMISSIONS, WITH TIPS FROM WWW.ENERGYSTAR.GOV

REFRIGERATORS

✓ Set your refrigerator temperature at 37° to 40°F and keep the freezer at 0° to 5°F.

✓ Defrost manual-defrost refrigerators and freezers on a regular basis. Ice buildup decreases the energy efficiency.

✓ Check your refrigerator door seals by closing them over a piece of paper that is half in and half out of the unit. If you can pull the paper out easily, the seal may need replacing.

- Refrigerators with the freezer on top are usually more efficient than side-by-side models. On-door ice dispensers usually make the refrigerator less efficient.

- When buying a new unit, choose an ENERGY STAR model. These use at least 15 percent less energy than required by federal standards.

LAUNDRY TIPS

- Wash most clothes in cold water instead of warm. If you feel that certain clothes require hot water, try using warm water instead.

- Wash full loads whenever possible to save energy and water.

- When ready to replace your unit, choose an ENERGY STAR model. These appliances will save you an average of $50 a year on your utility bills compared to non-qualified models. ENERGY STAR washers also use 18 gallons less water per load. This is about the amount of water used in a daily shower.

DRYER TIPS

- Dry heavy towels and cottons separately from lighter weight fabrics.

- Don't leave your clothes drying for too long. Use your machine's moisture sensor, or use a timer.

- Use a lower heat setting if your dryer has one.

- Clean the lint filter before every use. Regularly inspect your dryer's vent to make sure it isn't blocked.

- Air-dry your clothes on clotheslines or drying racks whenever possible.

- Ironing clothes when they are slightly damp can make ironing easier.

- When replacing your dryer, choose one with a moisture sensor that shuts the machine off when clothes are dry. (ENERGY STAR does not rate dryers.)

DISHWASHER TIPS

- Run full loads.

- Scrape food off plates rather than rinsing or prewashing dishes with water before putting them in the dishwasher.

- **Use an eco-friendly dishwashing detergent without phosphates.**

- **Turn off the drying cycle. Open the door after the wash cycle is complete to aid air-drying.**

- **When buying a new unit, look for ENERGY STAR models. These use at least 41 percent less energy than required by federal standards, and they use a lot less water than non-qualified models.**

GREENHOUSES A typical house emits more than twice the amount of carbon dioxide as the typical car, according to the Environmental Protection Agency. When considering purchasing your next home, you might look for an ENERGY STAR–qualified new home. These homes meet strict EPA guidelines for energy efficiency. They are typically at least 15 percent more energy efficient than standard homes and feature energy-saving appliances that make them 20 to 30 percent more efficient than standard homes. These homes may cost about 3 to 5 percent more to purchase, but advocates say the savings on utility bills more than offset the price after a few years. Plus, an ENERGY STAR home can keep 4,500 pounds of greenhouse gases out of the air each year, according to the EPA.

ENERGY STAR–qualified homes have more effective insulation, high-performance windows, tight construction, nonleaky ducts, efficient furnaces and air conditioners, and ENERGY STAR–qualified lighting fixtures, ventilation fans, and appliances such as refrigerators, dishwashers, and washing machines. The homes are independently certified.

Two other green building standards are the nonprofit U.S. Green Building Council's Leadership in Energy and Environmental Design (LEED, *www .usgbc.org*) program, and the National Green Building Standard (*www.nahb green.org*), created by the National Association of Home Builders, a membership-based trade group. Construction and renovations are aimed at situating homes to maximize natural heating and lighting, improving energy efficiency, and using renewable energy sources. Other factors include water efficiency, environmentally sound building materials, waste reduction, reduction of toxic chemicals, protection of indoor air quality, and smart growth and sustainable development. Proponents of green building say that simply putting more windows on the south side of a home and fewer on the north side can save 10 to 40 percent on winter heating bills. Now that is smart.

There is green, and then there is green. If you are truly concerned about the sustainability of modern building practices, you might want to consider

KITCHEN TABLE TALK

Line Dry Your Clothes

As a child I was mortified by my mother's clothesline. I was sure she was the only person in the civilized (suburban) world who still hung clothes out to dry. Before friends would come over I would rip all the clothes down and stash them in the garage.

Today I am a firm convert to the practice. Sunlight is gentler than dryer heat on fabric, and I don't have to worry about static cling. But most important, my utility bill has shrunk. Hanging clothes outdoors saves about $85 a year, or $1,530 over the 18-year life span of a typical dryer, according to the California Energy Commission. So I save money and help the environment. What is more, I enjoy the five meditative minutes in the warm sunshine that it takes to hang clothes.

Sometimes I pity my children, who will surely be as embarrassed as I was, once they are old enough to notice. Or maybe they won't. A new feature is popping up in the backyards of many of their friends in the neighborhood: clotheslines.

building a home of entirely renewable materials. For example, some families are choosing to build homes with walls made of straw bales, which have excellent insulating properties. Particleboard for interior walls can be made from straw, agrifibers, and bagasse, a by-product of sugarcane.

Conventional homes built today usually have asphalt shingle roofs. Greener alternatives include natural clay, slate, and even living roofs. A living roof supports the growth of plants such as wildflowers or a vegetable garden. Check the structural soundness of your roof before starting to plant—not all roofs can take the extra weight. You'll have to install a mechanism for draining the plot, too.

SUN WORSHIP Take advantage of the sun's power when you are ready to renovate. If you are adding a room or making substantial renovations, you can choose a design that captures the sun's warmth. For example, place large windows facing south where the sun is the strongest year-round.

GREEN ON A SHOESTRING

A number of federal and state tax incentives for solar power have been enacted in recent years. You can view a list of all the state and federal incentives for solar and other forms of renewable energy at the Database of State Incentives for Renewables & Efficiency (DSIRE) at *www.dsireusa.org.*

Installing a solar power system can reduce your dependence on fossil fuels, which provide roughly 85 percent of all energy consumed in the United States.

When considering solar, it is a good idea first to make sure you've done all you can to make your house energy efficient. As mentioned above, improving your home's insulation, installing compact fluorescent bulbs, taking shorter showers, and washing clothes in cold water are all ways to reduce fossil fuel use and save money on utility bills.

Most solar systems use one of two ways to harness the sun's energy:

PHOTOVOLTAIC (PV) CELLS These devices convert sunlight to electricity. They are made of silicon semiconductor materials that are not unlike the chips in your computer. These PV cells convert incoming particles of light (photons) into electrical current. You can store the electricity in a battery and use it later to power lights and appliances. Advances in technology are improving photovoltaic cell efficiency and bringing down the cost. Although installing photovoltaic systems is costly up front, you will realize savings over time and several states offer tax incentives. Additionally, you can offset your bill by contributing the excess electricity you generate back to the electrical grid.

THERMAL SOLAR PANELS Compared to photovoltaics, thermal solar panels are a relatively low-tech approach. These solar panels contain collectors that soak up the sun's warmth and use it to heat water or an indoor space. One of the simplest types uses rooftop flat-panel collectors that contain tubes of a heat-absorbing liquid such as glycol, the same chemical as in antifreeze. The sun warms the glycol and a pump circulates it into the house to a heat exchanger that transfers heat from the glycol to water in a tank. The hot water can then be used for washing clothes, cooking, and bathing.

GREEN DICTIONARY

PHOTOVOLTAIC CELL
A semiconductor device that converts incoming sunlight into electric current.

Installing thermal solar panels is relatively inexpensive compared to photovoltaics. Many companies are in the business of installing these systems. Some systems are simple enough to be done by a capable do-it-yourselfer.

ECO-TIP: TEACHING YOUR CHILDREN TO BE GREEN

Get your children in the habit of saving energy, saving the environment, and saving you money. Here are some tips:

✓ **Make it fun. Turn your kids into "energy detectives" who seek out and take care of energy wasters like a TV left on when no one is watching.**

✓ **Help your kids learn about energy conservation using websites such as the U.S. Energy Information Administration's Energy Kids' website at *www.eia.doe.gov/kids*.**

✓ **Older kids can generate their own electricity using human powered generators available from *www.windstreampower.com*.**

✓ **Have your kids go around the house and see how much electricity each appliance uses with the Kill A Watt electricity usage monitor (available at major stores and online).**

✓ **For older kids, show them online tools like the Embodied Energy Database (EED) created by WattzOn *(www.wattzon.com/stuff)*. The WattzOn EED allows you to see how much power is consumed during manufacturing, shipping, using, and disposing of products and toys like a flat panel LCD television or skateboard.**

✓ **Solar battery rechargers, solar calculators, and solar-powered toys can reduce your need to buy batteries while teaching your kids about energy conservation.**

✓ **Make energy-saving devices with your kids, like a homemade outdoor shower stall.**

✓ **Get your children in the routine of turning off lights when they leave the room.**

✓ **Don't let your kids stand in front of the open refrigerator while they decide what they want to eat.**

✓ **Make sure your children close doors and windows when heating and cooling systems are running.**

✓ **Get your kids used to wearing warm pajamas, robes, and slippers during the winter.**

✓ **Have your children help you with energy-saving chores like hanging laundry.**

Places to Live

Most parents put their children's needs first when choosing where to live. We are looking for safety, good schools, and fresh air. Yet sometimes these locations come with hidden costs to the environment. One of the most significant ways you can help "green the planet" is by choosing to live in a place that reduces the need to drive a car. In this section we'll contemplate a variety of living situations and evaluate their impact on the planet and our children's health.

An old jingle goes, "You are what you eat," but another apt one could be, "You are where you live." Your location shapes numerous other aspects of your lifestyle. Your area's climate determines what outdoor activities your family is involved in and at what times of year you do them. Your home's proximity to school determines whether your children will walk, take the bus, or be driven in your car. The distance to your workplace affects the amount of greenhouse gases and air pollution you generate and how many hours you spend commuting when you could be exercising, resting, or tossing a ball with the kids.

Not everyone has control over where they live, of course, but many of us at some point in life must decide where to settle our families. When that time comes, it is a good idea to consider not just the immediate environment (crime stats, school quality, aesthetics of the neighborhood), but also the way your new home will shape your family's health and the health of the environment.

Several studies indicate that the layout of a community or town directly influences the activity level of children. Children who live in walkable communities with playgrounds nearby tend to get more exercise than children who live in isolated housing tracts where they require parental transportation to reach playgrounds.

The busy schedules of today's kids, combined with the distances between homes in the suburbs and even in cities, means that playdates, as they are now called, need to be orchestrated by parents, who usually must drive children to the other houses and to the park. In many households, both parents work full-time, so they are unable to supervise children after school. As a result, the after-school street play many of us remember from childhood has been replaced by indoor TV time.

Some areas are known as "obesogenic" because they foster a lifestyle that precludes physical activity and healthful eating. These areas can be rural,

THE FACTS

The average American pays 54 cents per mile to operate his or her automobile. For every 15,000 miles traveled, that works out to about $8,100, according to the U.S. Department of Transportation.

exurban, suburban, or urban. For example, the 2,000-person town of Kettleman City in California's Central Valley, a major agricultural area, has no supermarkets but is home to several fast-food outlets.[15] In both urban and rural areas, gang-related and drug-related crime can make it unsafe for children to walk to school or play outdoors.

When choosing a new home, think about the impact of your new lifestyle on the health of your family and the planet, which, after all, go hand in hand. Some questions to ask are:

- Will my children be able to walk or bike to schools and parks?
- Can my children walk or bike to other children's houses for playdates?
- Is the street safe for riding bikes? Are there sidewalks?
- Can my children and I do errands without getting into a car?
- Will I be concerned about crime when my children are outside playing?

EXITING FOR THE EXURBS The exurbs are communities built far from cities, usually on former farm fields. Parents tend to choose the exurbs because of the perception that they provide a higher quality of life for children.

However, exurban living takes a toll on the environment. The reliance on the car for every task, from getting to work to (for some families) getting the newspaper, means that exurban driving produces air pollution and greenhouse gases.

Perhaps the greatest impact, however, is the loss of farmland. As more farmland outside big cities gets converted to housing, more produce needs to be trucked in from other states and countries. Those "food miles" traveled take their toll on the environment in terms of fossil fuels consumed and emissions that contribute to climate change.

If you choose the exurbs, here are ways to reduce your ecological footprint:

- ✓ Plant an organic vegetable garden. You'll save money on your grocery bill and reap high-quality produce for your family.
- ✓ Convert some of your lawn into groundcover using native plants. You'll cut down on the money and time you devote to lawn care.
- ✓ Switch to organic lawn care methods instead of "weed and feed" products.
- ✓ Grow a wildflower meadow on part of your property. You'll attract butterflies and help trap and return rainwater to the soil.

EXURBAN SMALL-TOWN LIFE The advantages of moving far outside the cities can be had without destroying farmland, getting stuck in your car, and losing all sense of community. New densely clustered housing

THE FACTS
Today's typical single family home is 45 percent bigger than homes built in the 1970s, according to the National Association of Home Builders.

developments are springing up that feature handsome row houses situated within easy walking distance of shopping, dining, schools, and public transportation.

These communities combine the quiet country environment with benefits such as the opportunity to exercise by building walking into one's daily routine. There are numerous environmental benefits as well. People drive less and generate fewer carbon emissions. The smaller homes consume less energy and require less energy, water, and chemicals for the maintenance of large lawns.

SETTLING IN THE SUBURBS The suburbs are the environment of choice for a large percentage of Americans. These areas were often built in the post–World War II era of increasing prosperity.

Like the exurbs, these communities were built to suit the needs of the car at the expense of the needs of the human. City planners anticipated that families would use the car for every need, forgetting that even the archetypal stay-at-home mom of the 1950s needed a sidewalk on which to push the baby carriage.

Suburban life has many of the same drawbacks of exurban life, but the houses and properties are smaller and the distances to schools and shops are shorter. Schools are usually a little easier to walk to because many are situated in neighborhoods.

If you choose such a neighborhood, here are some suburban survival tips:

- Advocate to make your town more pedestrian friendly. Petition the town to install sidewalks, crosswalks, and bike lanes.
- Organize a "walking school bus" to help your children and their friends walk safely to school. (See more about walking school buses in Chapter 8.)

THE FACTS

Of all the land developed in the first 225 years of our nation's history, 25 percent was developed in the last two decades of the 20th century, according to a 2001 study by the USDA.[16]

OPTING FOR URBAN LIFE Cities have always provided many kid-friendly diversions such as museums, zoos, and parks. But pollution, crime, and congestion drove many people out of the American cities in an exodus that started as far back as the mid-1800s.

In the last few decades, however, many families have realized there are many advantages to cities, including walkability for kids and shorter commute times for parents. When families move back to cities, crime tends to decline because parents demand better police presence. Schools tend to improve as more parents move into the area and get involved.

Of course, cities have many environmental impacts and create massive air pollution problems as well as water and land pollution. Some cities have made more of a commitment than others to creating opportunities for public transportation, walking and biking, and recreation. To learn about cities that are making strides toward greater environmental stewardship, check out Smarter Cities *(www.smartercities.nrdc.org)*, a project of the Natural Resources Defense Council.

Things to consider when going urban:

- Look for houses sited away from major roads, where air pollution and pedestrian-automobile accidents are of concern.
- If you are buying in a new development built on a former industrial site, try to find out what chemicals were used in the past and find out what cleanup measures were used.
- Find out what opportunities exist for public transportation, walking, and biking.

Whether you go urban, suburban, exurban, or rural, it is a good idea to explore any history of environmental contamination. Before you purchase a house or sign a lease, check with your state's department of environmental quality or *www.scorecard.org* for nearby sources of pollution, such as power plants, Superfund sites, and other sources of air, water, or soil pollution.

Take Action

▸ Choose to live in a neighborhood within walking distance of schools, shops, and public transportation.

▸ Test your home for lead paint, radon, and asbestos, especially if you live in an older home.

▸ Don't paint your home when you are pregnant or have infants around. Choose low- or no-VOC brands of paint.

▸ Avoid buying furniture made from particleboard, or choose items made with safer glues, not formaldehyde.

▸ Look for electronics that do not use deca-PBDEs or other toxic flame-retardants.

▸ Regularly vacuum, mop, and dust with a damp cloth to cut down on allergens such as dander and pollen, as well as toxic phthalates and other chemicals.

▸ Make your own cleaners from natural ingredients like vinegar and baking soda.

▸ Rid your home of toxic cleaners. Avoid antibacterial soaps.

▸ Air-dry your laundry.

▸ When renovating or building a home, choose a builder trained in one of the green building standards established by the nonprofit U.S. Green Building Council or the National Association of Home Builders.

▸ Save energy by insulating your home and sealing drafts around windows and doors.

▸ When you need to replace appliances, choose ENERGY STAR appliances.

▸ Replace incandescent bulbs with low-mercury compact fluorescent lightbulbs (CFLs).

▸ Clean up broken mercury-containing CFLs promptly.

▸ Teach your children energy-saving habits such as turning off lights and taking shorter showers.

▸ Choose a place to live where you and your children have opportunities to build walking and biking into your daily routine.

THE SCIENCE BEHIND IT

CFLs

Finding an alternative to mercury-containing CFLs is a major research focus for lighting companies. Until they come through, we are stuck using mercury simply because it is the best material for the job. Let's take a look at how a CFL works, and we'll see why mercury is so important.

A CFL consists of a plastic-encased base unit, or ballast, and two or more long glass tubes coated inside with a white powder. Inside the ballast is an electronic circuit and an electrical transformer that boost and regulate the incoming electricity. When you switch on the light, the circuit passes the electricity to a set of metal plates called electrodes that in turn release free electrons, which shoot into the glass tubes. The glass tubes contain mercury gas. The electrons collide with mercury atoms, and this collision causes mercury atoms to give off photons (light particles) of invisible ultraviolet light.

If this were the end of the story, we wouldn't see any light at all, so we need another component, the white coating inside the tubes. This white coating is made up of chemicals called phosphors. When the invisible ultraviolet photons strike the phosphor atoms, they give off energy in the form of visible fluorescent light.

While CFLs are energy efficient, mercury is not environmentally friendly. It is a brain toxicant proven to cause problems with learning and memory as well as lower IQ scores in children, according to the EPA. It is also toxic to fish and wildlife, so discarding CFLs in landfills is not a good idea.

The good news is that CFLs contain little mercury and pose little risk of neurological damage from breakage of a single bulb, according to the EPA. The amount of mercury vapor that a small child might inhale from a broken bulb would depend on the location of the breakage (a child's bedroom versus a utility room) and whether the room is carpeted (because it is difficult to completely remove mercury from a carpet). See Eco-Tip: Safe Use of CFLs in this chapter.

Reducing the need for electricity, which is often generated by coal-fired power plants, removes far more mercury from the environment than bulbs introduce into it. The U.S. releases 50 tons of mercury into the air each year from coal-fired power plants. By contrast, CFLs sold in 2004 contained a total of 1,479 pounds of mercury, according to the EPA.

CFLs contain about five milligrams of mercury, which is far less than other household items. Oral glass thermometers have 100 to 200 times more mercury in them, which is a good reason to dispose of them and switch to digital ones right away. Silver-colored dental fillings have 60 to 200 times more mercury, which is a good reason to choose less toxic white (composite) fillings (more on these in Chapter 4). Old-fashioned thermostats also contain mercury. Contact your municipality to find out how to dispose of these items.

GREEN AND LEAN

How to Raise a Healthy Eater in a Toxic World

SEA OTTERS SHOW THEIR YOUNG HOW TO CRACK OPEN SCALLOP shells. Snow leopards teach their cubs how to stalk prey. We humans also need to teach our children eating patterns that will ensure them a long and healthy life.

Yet feeding our children seems more complex than ever. The cereal aisle alone is filled with enough choices to keep a slightly sleep-deprived mom in an agony of indecision, at least until the wails of the child in the supermarket cart remind her to move on. And if choosing a cereal isn't complex enough, there are numerous other questions: How do I convince my child to eat fresh fruits and vegetables in a world of fast food? Should I avoid artificial sweeteners and dyes? How long will it take this plastic packaging to degrade in a landfill?

With so much complexity built into the simple decisions we make daily when feeding our kids, it is tempting to just throw in the proverbial dish towel and reach for a box of macaroni and cheese (nonorganic, with artificial dyes and flavors). Who could keep mental tallies of the health and environmental impacts of each and every food choice we busy parents make?

No one can possibly track the impacts of every item we serve to our children. Luckily we don't have to. Using a simple rule of thumb, parents can choose healthy and delicious foods that are grown using sustainable methods that don't strip more from the land than we put back into it.

What is this rule of thumb? *If it is good for the planet, then it is probably good for my child.* Foods that are grown or raised without harmful chemicals, processed as little as possible, and served fresh are good for children and the environment.

Healthy eating is essential to living an environmentally conscious life. "Going green" means not only embracing the three Rs (reduce, reuse, recycle), but also greening your diet—literally. Green-colored foods are some of the healthiest foods available. Garden-fresh sugar snap peas, lightly steamed broccoli florets, and crisp celery sticks (topped with peanut butter) are three green, kid-friendly favorites.

Whole foods such as these give kids energy without loading their bodies with sugar, salt, and fat. In contrast, prepackaged conventional snacks such as chips and cookies are best saved for special occasions rather than everyday use. The packaging waste contributes to an already massive waste-disposal problem, while the energy consumption that goes into processing foods takes its toll on our planet's natural resources.

It is the exceptional parent who can raise a child to maturity without buying some junk food. We all need to take shortcuts now and then. But it *is* possible to raise kids that like the taste of *real* food, rather than oversugared, oversalted, high-fat foods. Do this and you'll not only cut down on the family food fights, but you'll set your child up for a lifetime of health in a culture where one in three children will go on to develop adult-onset diabetes.

In this chapter we'll talk about how to teach kids to be lifelong healthy eaters in a world of unhealthy choices. We'll discuss practical tips such as how to feed kids a healthful meal in the car, how to package fresh fruits in reusable snack containers, and how to choose whole foods that kids *love*. (We'll explore the environmental impacts of food production in Chapter 3.) We'll round out the chapter by covering food additives, eco-conscious food preparation and storage, and how to raise a child who is green *and* lean.

Health Comes First

Children love sweet fruits and vegetables such as crunchy snap peas, baby carrots, brightly colored raspberries, and sweet melon slices. Serve fresh fruits and vegetables instead of packaged sugary and salty snacks and you'll set your children up for a lifetime of healthy habits. At the same time you are teaching them to appreciate the bounty of the earth and the role of nature in sustaining all living things.

TOO MUCH ON OUR PLATES Unlike most animals, we humans have an amazing choice of foods. As omnivores we will eat practically anything as long as it doesn't make us sick. Our brains get a pleasurable jolt from sugary snacks. We get a sated feeling from fat. High-caloric foods activate our innate pleasure sensors, a trait that helped our ancestors store energy during times of plenty in preparation for times of famine.

The energy-storage mechanism that served our ancestors so well has proven to be a disaster in today's industrialized nations, where we have enjoyed a long and continuous time of plenty. The United States produces a truly staggering amount of food. Add up all the corn, potatoes, and other crops that are grown, and toss in the chickens, cows, pigs, and other animals that are raised and slaughtered each year, then you'll find that our great country produces 4,000 kilocalories (or just simply calories) per person per day, according to figures published by the U.S. Department of Agriculture in 2008. The average active adult requires 2,000 to 2,500 calories per day. Kids typically need 1,000 to 2,000 calories, depending on age and activity level.

Although much of this surplus gets exported or discarded, many of these excess 1,500 to 3,000 calories per day get eaten, which explains why the American waistline is expanding. We are tempted to overeat because the corn, sugar, wheat, soy, dairy fat, and meat are packaged into scrumptious offerings like stuffed crust pizza, quarter-pound cheeseburgers with fries, and chocolate-chip cookie dough ice cream. Blame our brains for wanting to store up energy, blame food-marketers for broadcasting commercials during children's TV shows, or blame the person who invented the double-crust cheese-stuffed pizza. Whomever you blame, America has an eating problem.

Not only do we Americans eat too much, but we also eat too many of the wrong foods. The typical American diet is fundamentally unhealthy. It is high in the types of fat that increase the risk of heart disease. It is high in sugar, predisposing people to type 2 diabetes. It is deficient in vitamins and other nutrients found in vegetables and fruits. The prevalence of obesity has tripled in school-age children over the past three decades.

Today, nearly a third of all children in the United States ages 6 to 19 are overweight or obese, and today's generation of children has the potential to have a shorter life span than their parents. Many children lack access to healthy foods because they live in neighborhoods that have few or no supermarkets or other places to buy fresh produce.

The body mass index (BMI) is a reliable measure of a person's fatness that is calculated as weight in kilograms divided by height in meters squared. To find your child's BMI, visit *www.cdc.gov/healthyweight/assessing/bmi* and enter your child's age, sex, height, and weight. The calculator of the Centers for Disease Control and Prevention (CDC) will tell you your child's BMI and compare it to national averages for your child's age and sex. Overweight children are those who have a BMI in the 85th to 94th percentile range. Obese children have a BMI at or above the 95th percentile.

EATING HABITS FOR HUMANITY Many parents are concerned that their children have a genetic propensity toward weight gain. Genetics do play a part in body shape and size. However, genes do not change dramatically over a period as short as three decades.

Dietary habits, however, have changed. Many parents today think a fruit roll-up is as nutritious as eating fresh fruit or that a 100-calorie package of chocolate sandwich cookies is a good daily snack. Among two-year-olds, the most commonly ingested vegetable is the French fry. Nearly half of all two-year-olds regularly drink sweetened beverages such as soda or fruit punch, according to an article in a 2006 issue of the journal *Pediatrics*.[1]

Some health experts blame our nation's fatness on the uptick in carbohydrate consumption over the last 30 years, which in part was driven by official dietary advice to forgo fats in favor of carbs, according to nutritionists who study the issue. However, carbs cannot take all the blame. Any diet that reduces calories will result in weight loss regardless of whether the diet emphasizes protein, fat, or carbohydrates, a study published in a 2009 issue of the *New England Journal of Medicine* found.[2] The blame for weight gain lies squarely on increased intake of calories and reduced energy expenditures.

Unhealthy eating patterns begin to seem normal when everyone else is doing the same. It can be challenging to raise a child with healthy eating habits in today's world unless you join a commune of like-minded parents or send your children to a private school such as the Waldorf School, where healthful eating is an integral part of the educational philosophy. But it is not impossible. You and your family can choose health-conscious, environmentally friendly foods that satisfy toddler and preteen taste buds alike. And along the way you and your children can serve as role models and gentle educators and, eventually, perhaps change the eating behaviors of others around you.

EATING 101 Teaching your kids to eat right does not mean introducing them to the food pyramid before they are out of diapers. You and your family can eat right without ever reading a label. As journalist and food expert Michael Pollan points out in his book *In Defense of Food* (Penguin, 2008), the focus on individual nutrients has diverted our attention from the age-old cultural practice of

GREEN DICTIONARY

FOOD DESERT

An urban area that lacks supermarkets and stores where people can buy fresh and healthy foods. Instead, area residents buy food from convenience stores and fast-food restaurants.

consuming delicious and satisfying whole foods, most of which have everything we need to keep our bodies healthy.

The more time and effort you spend on teaching your child good eating habits from age zero to six, the less time you'll have to spend in the preteen years on enforcing diets, depriving your kids of treats, and despairing when your child blows an entire week of dieting by purchasing cookies from the school vending machine. If you teach your kids that a normal human diet is one rich in fresh, whole foods prepared at home, and not a continuous stream of fried and sugared foods, then they will be able to enjoy the occasional ice cream cone, slice of birthday cake, or Halloween candy binge without a care.

Children are not small adults, and their dietary needs are different from ours. It is a little known fact that, at just six months old, the majority of babies in the United States already receive 10 to 20 percent more calories than they need. The average child between the ages of one and four years old is taking in 20 to 35 percent more calories than they need, according to the American Academy of Pediatrics (AAP).

To grow up healthy, children need to eat lots of fruits and vegetables, whole grains, and fat-free or low-fat dairy foods, including lean meats, poultry, fish, beans, eggs, and nuts. They should not eat too many saturated fats, trans fats, cholesterol, salt (sodium), or added sugars. (For complete advice, see the 2005 Dietary Guidelines for Americans at *www.healthierus.gov/dietaryguidelines*.)

The U.S. government's food pyramid has changed over the years. Today's pyramid recognizes that calorie requirements vary depending on age and activity. The "percent daily values" on food packages are based on a 2,000-calorie diet, but a six-year-old sedentary child will need only 1,200 calories. The website *Mypyramid.gov* can tell you exactly how many servings from each food group your child should be eating. (See the section "Calories vs. Activity Level" in this chapter to find out how many calories your child should be getting.)

TIPS ON GETTING KIDS TO EAT RIGHT

✓ Introduce whole grains at a young age. Reserve foods made from refined flour for special treats and desserts.

✓ Offer children a variety of foods—especially fruits and vegetables—from an early age.

✓ When introducing a new food, offer it to children ten times or more. Studies show a child is more likely to try a new food when it is offered several times.

✓ Don't forbid sweets; simply don't have them around.

✓ Parental attitudes matter. If you dislike vegetables or prefer cookies to fruit, for your own sake, try to change your behavior. At the very least, conceal your attitude from your children.

✓ Limit mindless snacking in front of the TV. You may want to have a no-eating rule during TV time.

✓ Avoid stocking your car with packaged convenience foods. The wrappers pile up in landfills and the foods are often loaded with sugar, salt, and fat. See the "Eco-Tip: Snacks on the Go" for more ideas.

✓ Go easy on the juice. While 100 percent juice contains vitamins, it is high in sugar and the American Academy of Pediatrics recommends children five and younger drink no more than 6 ounces of juice per day.

✓ Choose healthier breakfast cereals containing whole grains, high fiber, and low sugar. A children's cereal with 12 grams of sugar per serving has the equivalent of 3 teaspoons of sugar (4 grams of sugar equals 1 teaspoon). Beware of high sugar in adult cereals, too. One of the cereals highest in sugar is raisin bran.

BURNING IT OFF The CDC recommends that children get 60 minutes of exercise per day. Many kids get far less, however. The newest version of the U.S. government's food pyramid takes kids' activity level into account when stating how many calories kids need each day. Nutrition labels are based on a daily 2,000-calorie diet, but most children need far fewer calories. Here are the recommendations.

DAILY CALORIE INTAKE		Sedentary	Moderately Active	Active
Male or Female	Ages 2-3	1,000	1,000-1,400	1,000-1,400
Female	Ages 4-8	1,200	1,400-1,600	1,400-1,800
	Ages 9-13	1,600	1,600-2,000	1,800-2,200
	Ages 14-18	1,800	2,000	2,400
Male	Ages 4-8	1,400	1,400-1,600	1,600-2,000
	Ages 9-13	1,800	1,800-2,200	2,000-2,600
	Ages 14-18	2,200	2,400-2,800	2,800-3,200

Source: Dietary Guidelines for Americans 2005, U.S. Department of Health and Human Services, U.S. Department of Agriculture, www.healthierus.gov/dietaryguidelines

A sedentary child is one who does little exercise other than what it takes to get out of bed, get dressed, sit on a school bus and at a desk for six hours, then spend the afternoon watching television. A moderately active child engages in activities equivalent to walking 1.5 to 3 miles per day. He or she might walk to school, spend all recess playing tag, and ride a bike after school. An active child pursues activities that are equivalent to walking more than 3 miles per day. He or she might play one or more sports after school in addition to walking to school and running at recess.

ECO-TIP: SNACKS ON THE GO

Cut down on wasteful packaging by placing your own snacks in reusable containers. Pieces of fruit, cut vegetables, and various nuts make great on-the-go snacks. Make it easy on yourself by taking a few minutes on a Sunday night to pack snacks for the whole week. Fill reusable snack containers with measured amounts of unsalted roasted nuts, blueberries, cherry tomatoes, or baby carrots. All those foods come in small individual pieces so there is no chopping involved.

Fresh fruit is a bit tricky to pack in advance because cutting it up makes it more likely to spoil. For example, apples, pears, and peaches turn brown, making them less palatable to children. Sprinkling lemon juice on apples helps preserve them. Avoid bottled lemon juice because it contains preservatives. Dried banana chips, dried apricots, and dried papaya are usually popular with children. Read labels and avoid preservatives and artificial colors whenever possible. Also try frozen fruit pieces (they'll thaw by the time your child is ready to eat them).

Pretzels and crackers are often marketed as a low-fat healthy snack. However, most pretzels and other crackers are made with refined white flour. Look for whole grain varieties.

Other portable kid-friendly healthy snacks include brown rice cakes, sweet bell pepper slices, broccoli pieces, grapes, sugar snap peas, and cheese cubes. Yogurt is also a favorite, but check the label for high sugar content. Try low-fat plain yogurt instead. Stay away from yogurt that contains artificial sweeteners, flavors, and colors.

Juice boxes are convenient and recyclable, but most of them end up in the garbage. Water is a better choice because it rehydrates and refreshes without contributing to tooth decay and weight gain. Help your child become accustomed to drinking water when thirsty rather than craving the sugar jolt of juice.

ECO-TIP: **PASS ON THE PALM OIL**

Peanut butter can be a delicious protein-rich food for children who are not allergic. Choose "natural" or organic peanut butter that contains only peanuts (a little salt is OK, too). The peanut oil collects at the top, so you'll need to stir the peanut butter the first time you open it, and then store it in the refrigerator. Some organic brands now use palm oil, which does not separate from the peanut butter. However, the global demand for palm oil is driving the deforestation of the island of Borneo, so think twice before adding to the consumer demand for palm oil.

HOME ON THE GRAIN A lot of what we hear about healthy eating involves getting kids and their families to eat more whole grains and fewer refined ones. So what is the difference? Whole grains are made from the entire grain seed, which consists of the bran, germ, and endosperm. To make white flour, processors remove the bran and most of the germ. With these go the dietary fiber, vitamins, and minerals. To make up for these losses, the U.S. government requires that refined white flour be enriched with thiamin, riboflavin, niacin, folic acid, and iron.

Wouldn't it be better if we just ate whole wheat flour instead of going to all the trouble of taking out the bran and germ and then putting back in all the lost nutrients? The answer is, yes, it is probably healthier because the nutrients that the government requires to be added back are just the ones we know about. There may be other nutrients that can contribute to our health. Also, the process of stripping out the bran and germ, then adding back nutrients takes a far greater toll on the environment than just using the whole grains as they are.

Although many whole-grain breads are available, you may need to do some careful label-reading to find them. Look for the words "whole wheat flour" rather than simply "wheat flour." The latter term can be confusing because most flour is made from wheat. The term "enriched wheat flour" means white flour. And remember, whole grains don't have to be wheat at all. Other whole grains include brown rice, millet, sorghum, quinoa, popcorn, whole oats, buckwheat, whole rye, and whole barley.

So now that we know what they are, how do we get our children to eat whole grains? If you raise your children eating whole grains from an early age, they'll never question the taste or color of whole wheat bread, pasta, or crackers.

KITCHEN TABLE TALK

Car Trips

We've talked about the ideal way that children should eat, but now let's talk about reality. You are rushing home from work to pick up your child at her after-school program, and you want to get a filling and nutritious meal in her before her scout meeting starts. You don't have time to stop home for dinner, and fast food is on the way, takes only minutes to buy, and can be eaten in the car. If you stop at a fast-food place, your child is happy because she gets a tasty meal, you are happy because she is in a good mood instead of being hungry and cranky, and the scouting leader is happy because she is on time and ready to participate.

You know in the back of your mind that the nuggets are laden with cholesterol, sodium, and fats. You know, the accompanying packet of French fries is practically devoid of nutrients. You've heard that children should be eating fresh leafy salads, steamed broccoli, low-fat meats, and whole-grain bread for dinner, but you don't know how to serve that sort of food in a moving vehicle without having to pick dropped bits from between the seats for the next few months.

Every parent has to take shortcuts. We start out idealistic, and maybe we even raise our first child that way, but eventually we begin to compromise as we find that time-saving tricks give us an extra minute during the day to simply exhale. The image of the supermom who works 50 hours a week, feeds her children home-cooked organic meals at the family dinner table, always smiles, and speaks kindly to her children is *not* reality. No parent could keep that up for more than a few days at a time.

So yes, shortcuts are wonderful. But try to take shortcuts that preserve your child's health. Instead, try to find ways to eat healthy and quick. Bring dinner along in a cooler. Choose healthier brands of convenience foods: whole-grain freezer waffles instead of conventional ones; low-fat frozen chicken nuggets that you bake at home and bring with you; precut carrot sticks; a container of blueberries for desert. With a little practice, you can make dinner in the car a healthy and tasty experience.

Despite the best intentions to plan for in-car meals, most parents will find themselves headed to the drive-through at some point. If you make a practice of feeding your children healthy foods most of the time, these occasional trips will do little to harm your child's health. Many fast-food restaurants have revamped their child-friendly meals and now offer milk as an alternative to soda and fruit slices as an alternative to fries. To help reduce packaging waste, go lightly on the plastic utensils, straws, and condiment packages.

But if you are trying to switch from white to whole wheat, a gradual change may be what is needed. Several brands of bread contain both types of flour, so you may want to use these during the transition. If you like to bake, substitute a portion of the white flour in recipes with whole wheat flour. Serve oatmeal for breakfast and popcorn for a snack.

GREEN ON A SHOESTRING

You'll pay a premium for whole wheat bread, which is more costly than white bread. Consider saving money by making your own bread at home. It is not as hard as you think, especially if you happen to own a bread machine. Yes, you remember. Someone—probably your mother-in-law—gave you one for Christmas years ago when they were the latest must-have. Eventually these appliances fell off the must-have list when busy parents realized that they actually have to buy flour and yeast, toss some ingredients in it, and turn it on. But these machines are easier to use than you might realize, and they do a pretty good job, so pull your breadmaker out of retirement, and try a few recipes.

MILK IN THE RAW Today all industrially produced milk is pasteurized, a process of heat sterilization that kills off disease-causing bacteria including enterotoxigenic *Staphylococcus aureus*, *Campylobacter*, *Escherichia coli*, *Listeria*, *Salmonella*, *Yersinia*, *Brucella*, and *Mycobacterium tuberculosis*.

THE FACTS

Only eight states allow
raw milk to be sold
in stores for human
consumption—Arizona,
California, Connecticut,
Maine, Pennsylvania,
South Carolina, New
Mexico, and Washington.

But some health advocates say pasteurization kills off valuable nutrients in milk. Proponents of raw or unpasteurized milk say that raw milk is healthier and can boost metabolism, strengthen the immune system, and alleviate digestive problems, skin problems, rheumatism, asthma, and other ailments. According to scientists, however, these health claims are not backed up with data.

What is more, consuming raw milk and milk products puts your child at risk of acquiring a severe case of food poisoning with symptoms such as stomach pain, diarrhea, fever, and muscle cramps. Fatalities can result. Consuming raw milk or cheese caused 1,007 cases of food poisoning and two deaths during the years from 1998 to 2005, according to the CDC.

The U.S. Food and Drug Administration (FDA) advises against the consumption of raw milk by everyone, but notes it can be especially dangerous to the young, pregnant, elderly, and immunocompromised.

PICKY EATERS There are a variety of reasons for children to be picky about what they eat. First, it is normal in childhood for growth to occur in spurts and for appetites to fluctuate accordingly. Many children have unrecognized food sensitivities that cause stomach pains or irritation. Your child's pediatrician can help identify these. Other children are overly sensitive to smells, textures, or flavors. Many children will grow out of their picky stage. Continue to offer a variety of foods and encourage but never force your child to eat them. Resist the temptation to serve only the foods he likes, especially if they are unhealthy. Consult with your pediatrician about whether to give your child a multivitamin to make up for any nutrients he or she is not getting in the diet.

PORTION DISTORTION Serving sizes on packages can vary. You may think you are buying a single-serving-size bottle of lemonade only to find that it contains 2.5 servings at a total of 60 grams of sugar, which is equal to 15 teaspoons of sugar or 240 calories. (Keep in mind that these serving sizes are based on a 2,000-calorie diet, which is likely far more than your child needs.) Don't make the mistake of feeding the entire bottle to your child in a single sitting. If you are at a restaurant or food stand, ask for a cup and split the bottle across two or even three children. Or give your child one cup and save the rest for later.

FAMILY (DINNER) FEUDS Fewer children are eating dinner around the family table, so familiar from old sitcoms. The shift to two-income families, single-parent families, and the "overscheduling" of children contributes to this change. Yet research shows that family dinners can promote better grades among high school students. Family dinners help keep family members in touch with each other and can provide a time when children can develop their abilities to present and defend a point of view. They probably promote better table manners, too.

Family dinners are relatively easy to have when your children are young. If both you and your spouse work, or if you parent alone, try to prepare meals in advance so that you can quickly defrost a healthy offering instead of grabbing fast food on the way home. As kids get older, they may spend more nights at basketball practice and school play rehearsals than they do at home, so try to set aside one or two nights where you can eat as a family. If family dinners simply don't work for your household, try family breakfasts.

GREEN ON A SHOESTRING

Save money with reusable bottles and packaging. Today a variety of reusable bottles and food containers are widely available for purchase. These are usually made of stainless steel or aluminum that is coated with a nonleaching polymer resin. Reusable water bottles and food containers are easy to use, cut down on wasteful packaging, and keep warm foods hot and cool drinks cool. However they are pricey, and children occasionally lose them. Here are some tips to get the most for your money:

✓ Put a sticker on the bottom of the container with your phone number or e-mail address on the bottom.

✓ Ask grandma if she has any containers left over from when she raised her kids. These items last for years.

✓ To ensure quality, buy reputable brands.

AND NOW FOR A WORD FROM OUR SPONSOR Children's TV shows are peppered with commercials for high-sugar breakfast cereals, fast-food restaurants, cookies, candy, and sweetened beverages. Few commercials tout the delicious taste of baby carrots or bananas. Research has shown that the amount of time children spend watching television is directly tied to the types of foods they crave—and pester you for—in the supermarket.

When children are young, it is relatively easy to limit the amount of commercials they see. Instead of letting kids channel-surf, parents can put on videos, on-demand shows, and previously recorded shows. As children get older, these methods become more difficult because kids start wanting to watch the shows their friends tell them about.

Parents need to fight these unhealthy advertisements by turning their kids into savvy media consumers. Around the age of five or six, most children can begin to understand that the purpose of commercials is to encourage parents to buy things. Tell your children that while commercials are fun to watch, they seldom deliver the happiness that they promise. Remind your children that the kids they see in the commercials are paid actors and actresses who are pretending to enjoy the product. Tell them that children who eat the advertised foods on a regular basis tend to become unhealthy and unable to play or run as fast as they used to.

For more about TV's effects on child development, see Chapter 7.

SCHOOLS—JUST ONE PART OF THE PROBLEM Schools have taken a lot of flack for peddling unhealthy snacks and meals to our children through vending machines, cafeterias, and fast-food franchises in schools. In response, many states have beefed up school nutrition standards and are eliminating junk food. Unfortunately many schools continue to provide unhealthy choices alongside the salads and fruit.

But schools are only part of the problem. A study in a 2007 issue of the *American Journal of Public Health* found that weight gain in kindergartners and first graders was faster during summer break than when school was in session.[3] While reforming schools is essential, good eating habits start at home.

Once your children start school, provide healthy snacks in their lunches, and avoid sending money that they can use for buying cookies or potato chips. Find out what your child's lunchroom sells, and speak to the principal or school district about eliminating unhealthy options. You may find that you are not the only parent who has such concerns.

For more on school cafeteria offerings, see Chapter 8.

Food Additives

The living world is dependent on chemicals like sodium chloride (table salt) and dihydrogen monoxide (water) that are essential for life, but others—natural and synthetic alike—are nonessential and not very healthy.

FOOD DYE BLUES Take food dyes, for example. Food dyes are pervasive in children's packaged foods due to the widespread belief that children do not like food that comes in its natural color, with its natural taste.

Ironically these dyes are added to make the food look like the fresh, healthy, colorful foods that people crave. You'll find Blue 2 added to make dried blueberries in freezer waffles look blue or Red 40 making a fruit roll-up look raspberry red. To some animals, brightly colored foods signal that the contents are good-tasting. It is the same for children, only in today's packaged foods, the sugar is high-fructose corn syrup (HFCS), and the dye is artificial.

A natural approach to living means steering clear whenever possible of artificial dyes and additives. One of the main reasons to do so is health. Studies have linked some food dyes and additives to cancer in rodents.[4]

A long-running debate has centered on whether food additives and dyes can contribute to behavioral problems. In the 1960s, Dr. Ben F. Feingold developed an additive-free approach that became known as the Feingold Diet. This diet appeared to help children calm their behaviors and increase their ability to pay attention. However, scientific evidence for the diet was lacking, so the medical establishment never really got behind the diet. Many psychologists jumped from diagnosis to drugs without counseling parents to try dietary changes.

With the publication of new studies of the additive-free approach, however, attitudes are slowly changing. In 2004, researchers at Columbia University concluded that food dyes could worsen attention deficit/hyperactivity disorder (ADHD) symptoms in some children. According to the study published in the *Journal of Developmental and Behavioral Pediatrics*, behavior improved when artificial colorings were removed from the children's diets, and worsened when the chemicals were added back to their diets.[5] The dyes, which are FDA approved, were Citrus Red 2, Yellow 5, Yellow 6, Red 3, Red 40, Blue 1, Blue 2, Green 3, and Orange B. Similarly, a study funded by the British government also found that dyes and the preservative sodium benzoate adversely affected kids' behavior.[6] (See more about sodium benzoate later in this chapter.)

The use of food dyes has risen dramatically over the last several decades. According to the FDA, in 1955 the amount of food dye certified for use was 12 milligrams per person per day. By 2007 the amount of dye per person had risen to 58 milligrams per day, or nearly five times as much, according to the Center for Science in the Public Interest (CSPI). The dyes are found especially in the foods marketed to kids, such as sugary cereals, candies, sodas, and snack foods. Many of these products prominently display the word "fruit" as if in an attempt to get parents to think they'll be satisfying their child's daily requirement of fruits and vegetables.

In response to these and other studies, many of these dyes are being phased out in Europe. In fact, according to the CSPI, certain brands of lunch and snack foods contain artificial dyes in the versions sold in the United States, but they contain natural colorings in the ones sold in the United Kingdom. For example, the CSPI states that the red color of the strawberry sauce on sundaes at a major fast-food chain is from strawberries in England but from Red 40 in the United States.

Pediatricians and public health officials here in the United States are beginning to recognize the potential impact of artificial colorings and preservatives on behavior. Many pediatricians are finding that a trial of a preservative-free, food coloring–free diet is a reasonable intervention for hyperactive children.[7]

CHILDREN OF THE CORN SYRUP Only 50 years ago, most sugary foods contained exactly that: sugar from cane or beets. Then came the discovery that the same sugary taste could be produced from corn, and high-fructose corn syrup (HFCS) was born.

The discovery meant that a crop that the United States has an abundance of—corn—could be put to use in a variety of new ways. HFCS started showing up in sodas and other products in the early 1980s, and it is now found in nearly every product where sugar was once used, including some you wouldn't think of, such as ketchup and chicken broth.

For a number of years, some scientists have worried that HFCS was driving the obesity epidemic. They suspected that because fructose, one of the sugars in HFCS, is broken down differently in the body than good old refined sugar (sucrose), HFCS somehow drove people to put on weight. In reality the two types of sweeteners are not all that different. High-fructose corn syrup is made up of 55 percent fructose and 42 percent glucose, whereas refined sugar, or sucrose, is made of 50 percent fructose and 50 percent glucose.

In fact, the real culprit in the rising rates of obesity is consumption of too many calories, combined with lack of exercise, whether from HFCS or any other source. Children and adults in the United States are eating more calories than ever before, and many of these calories are from HFCS and table sugar in nutrient-deficient foods like sodas.

Some studies indicate that HFCS may worsen obesity in already overweight people. For most of us, however, HFCS may be no worse than table sugar when it comes to packing on the pounds, but that isn't saying all that much, because sugar itself is no health food. Any product that lists HFCS or sugar listed as a first or second ingredient should be considered to be a dessert, according to many nutritionists.

GREEN ON A SHOESTRING

When traveling, skip fast-food stops by packing lunch ahead of time or stopping at a supermarket to load up on preservative-free lunchmeats, fresh fruit, whole-grain bread, and pasta salad.

SWEET DECEPTION Most of us like to have our cake and eat it, too, but without the calories. We've discovered that artificial sweeteners can make that possible. Yet, food scientists and health advocates battle over whether artificial sweeteners are good or bad for you. Rather than try to follow the scientific tennis match, forgo the debate and the artificial sweeteners altogether. If you simply provide whole foods, yummy fresh fruits in season and frozen ones the rest of the year, blended into delicious smoothies or just served in their own sweet juice, you can avoid having to follow the confusing science.

Read on to find out what we know about these artificial sweeteners:

× **ACESULFAME-K (SUNETT, SWEET ONE)** Found in baked goods and diet sodas. Some studies conducted in the 1970s linked the additive to cancer in rodents, according to the CSPI. Critics charge that this sweetener has been inadequately tested for safety.[8]

× **ASPARTAME (EQUAL, NUTRASWEET)** Used in sodas and diet foods, including yogurt and low-calorie frozen deserts. This sweetener is made of a combination of two amino acids (phenylalanine and aspartic acid) and methanol. It is highly toxic to people with phenylketonuria (PKU), a genetic inability to metabolize the amino acid phenylalanine. Many people complain that aspartame causes headaches or dizziness. As to whether it causes cancer, the topic has caused disagreements over the years. An Italian scientist at the Ramazzini Foundation in Bologna, Italy, found that rats exposed to aspartame in utero at eight weeks of age developed white blood cell cancers (lymphomas and leukemias).[9] However, the European Food Safety Authority found no statistically significant increase in the tumors. The Italian researchers also found that rats exposed to aspartame in utero developed mammary (breast) cancer late in life. However, in a study of adult volunteers monitored for five years by researchers at the U.S. National Cancer Institute, there was no evidence that aspartame caused cancer. However, these people were in their 50s and 60s and were not exposed to the chemical as children.[10]

× **NEOTAME** Used in diet soft drinks and other diet foods. This chemical is similar in structure to aspartame, but it is far sweeter and less of it can be used to achieve the same level of sweetness.

× **SACCHARIN (SWEET'N LOW)** Found in diet products, soft drinks, and sweetener packets. Several studies have found that saccharin caused bladder cancer in laboratory rats by mechanisms that do not occur in humans. Some health advocates still recommend avoiding it, however, since it may cause cancer by other mechanisms.

× **SUCRALOSE (SPLENDA)** Used in baked goods, frozen desserts, ice cream, and soft drinks, and as a tabletop sweetener. Sucralose is made by adding chlorine atoms to sugar molecules. It does not cause cancer in laboratory animals. However, a 2008 study found that Splenda (comprised of 1.1 percent sucralose plus maltodextrin and glucose) killed off the good kinds of bacteria that live in the gut and interfered with gut enzymes involved in absorption of oral medications, as reported in the *Journal of Toxicology and Environmental Health, Part A: Current Issues*.[11]

For more information on food additives to watch see *www.cspinet.org/reports/chemcuisine*

PROCESSED SWEETENERS The following sweeteners are naturally occurring, but they go through industrial processing that can take its toll on the environment.

× **INVERT SUGAR** Found in candy, soft drinks, and many other foods. Invert sugar is an equal mixture of two sugars, dextrose and fructose. It can occur naturally but is also produced industrially. Like other sugars, it contributes to tooth decay and obesity.

× **RAW SUGAR** This brown-colored sugar is a less processed form of sugar (sucrose) that retains some of the minerals that are usually stripped during processing. It still contributes to weight gain and tooth decay.

× **STEVIA (REBIANA OR REB A)** A natural sweetener found in a plant called *yerba dulce*, or sweet herb. The FDA in late 2008 declared rebiana, a sweetener derived from stevia, to be "generally recognized as safe," or GRAS, for use as a general-purpose sweetener in foods. However, the CSPI called for further testing of the sweeteners because stevia compounds caused reduced sperm production in male rats and small offspring in female rats. Stevia does not cause weight gain or tooth decay.

× **SUGAR (SUCROSE)** In sweetened foods. Sucrose occurs naturally in sugarcane, sugar beets, and fruit. Although not toxic in the sense of causing cancer or acute disease, sucrose promotes tooth decay and obesity.

× **TAGATOSE** Although tagatose occurs naturally at low levels in milk, it is produced commercially from other types of sugar so it is not considered a natural sweetener. It is approved for use in the United States and elsewhere, but it is not yet widely used. It is not well absorbed in the intestines, so it tastes sweet but isn't as fattening. However, it can cause diarrhea, nausea, and flatulence. Like xylitol, it does not promote tooth decay.

× **XYLITOL** Sugar-free chewing gum, low-calorie foods. Xylitol is a naturally occurring sugarlike molecule made from hardwood or corn. It is safe for humans but can be toxic if ingested by dogs. It has about 80 percent of the calories of sugar and does not produce tooth decay, but it can have a mild laxative effect. Other similar compounds include lactitol, maltitol, mannitol, and sorbitol.

So which types of sweeteners are best for children? Whenever possible choose naturally occurring sugars that are minimally processed. These can be found in molasses, honey, evaporated cane juice, rice syrup, barley malt, and fruit juice. These sweeteners are relatively unprocessed, so their production presumably makes a smaller impact on the planet's resources. It is important to note, however, that they still promote tooth decay and weight gain.

HOLD THE PRESERVATIVES, PLEASE While we are on the subject of chemicals in food, we cannot ignore the ever ubiquitous preservatives found in today's foods. Again, wherever possible, the health-conscious head of the family will forgo foods that contain preservatives in favor of foods eaten at the peak of freshness.

Let's look at preservatives and other food additives and find out why the CSPI recommends avoiding them.

× **BUTYLATED HYDROXYANISOLE (BHA)** Antioxidant: Found in cereals, chewing gum, potato chips, vegetable oil. Study results vary as to whether this chemical causes cancer in laboratory animals. Some researchers question whether the cancer findings apply to humans since the cancer developed in the rodent forestomach, an organ humans do not have.

× **BUTYLATED HYDROXYTOLUENE (BHT)** Antioxidant: Found in cereals, potato chips, oils, chewing gum. Studies in rats were mixed: Some found it reduced cancer risk and others found it increased cancer risk. BHT residues have been found in human fat.

× **CARMINE, COCHINEAL EXTRACT** Artificial coloring: While not toxic, these chemicals, which occur naturally and are extracted from the cochineal insect in equatorial locations, can trigger severe allergic reactions.

× **DIACETYL** Butter flavoring: In microwave popcorn. Diacetyl occurs naturally in butter. When airborne as in a factory setting, diacetyl can lodge in the lungs and cause potentially fatal disease. Its use is more highly regulated now, but microwave popcorn bags may contain other hazardous chemicals, and it is easy and cheaper to make popcorn on the stovetop or in a reusable microwave container.

× **MONOSODIUM GLUTAMATE (MSG)** Flavor enhancer: Restaurant foods, soups, frozen and packaged entrees. Like salt, MSG enhances the flavor of foods. However, studies in animals indicate that MSG damages the developing brain.

× **OLESTRA (OLEAN)** Fat substitute: In potato chips. This synthetic fat is not absorbed in the digestive system, so it has the flavor and texture of fat without the calories. Olestra can cause diarrhea, abdominal cramps, flatulence, and other adverse effects. Olestra reduces the body's ability to absorb fat-soluble micronutrients such as alpha- and beta-carotene from fruits and vegetables.

× **POTASSIUM BROMATE** Flour improver: In white flour, bread. Bromate causes cancer in laboratory animals and has been banned in many other countries. Although it is still legal in the U.S., many bakers no longer use it.

× **SODIUM BENZOATE, BENZOIC ACID** Preservative: In fruit juice, carbonated drinks. These two preservatives are naturally occurring in plants, and for many people are harmless. Sensitive individuals may have allergic reactions, however, and some studies have linked sodium benzoate to ADHD-like behaviors. (See section on food dyes.) Also, sodium benzoate in combination with ascorbic acid (vitamin C) can react to form small amounts of benzene, a chemical linked to leukemia and other cancers. Most soda companies have reformulated their products, but it is worth checking the label to be sure.

× **SODIUM NITRITE, SODIUM NITRATE** Preservative, coloring, flavoring: In hot dogs, lunch meats, bacon. These chemicals are linked to the formation of cancer-causing chemicals called nitrosamines. Several studies indicate a link between nitrites in meats and cancer in pregnant women, children, and adults. These chemicals are also harmful to babies. Nitrate- and nitrite-free lunch meats, hot dogs, and sausages are available in many stores.

× **SULFITES (SULFUR DIOXIDE, SODIUM BISULFITE)** Preservative, bleach: In dried apricots and other fruits, shrimp, processed potatoes. Sulfites can cause reactions in allergic and asthmatic individuals.

× **VANILLIN, ETHYL VANILLIN** Substitute for vanilla: In ice cream, baked goods, beverages, chocolate, candy, gelatin desserts. Avoid purchasing vanilla in Mexico and other Latin American countries. According to the FDA, it can contain a toxic blood-thinning compound called coumarin.

SAFER FOOD ADDITIVES Not all additives are bad for you. The following ingredients give little cause for concern, according to the CSPI.

✓ **ALPHA-TOCOPHEROL** (Vitamin E) Antioxidant, nutrient: In vegetable oils, breakfast cereals, beverages. This antioxidant may help reduce the risk of heart disease and cancer.

✓ **ASCORBIC ACID** (Vitamin C) Antioxidant, nutrient, color stabilizer: In cereals, fruit drinks, cured meats. This important vitamin helps prevent loss of color and flavor in lunchmeats. Some people find that vitamin C reduces the severity of colds.

✓ **BETA-CAROTENE** Coloring, nutrient: In margarine, shortening, beverages, breakfast cereals. This additive is both a food dye and a nutrient supplement. The body converts it to vitamin A, an important vitamin for light-detection in the eye. Beta-carotene is also an antioxidant and may protect against cancer and heart disease.

✓ **CARRAGEENAN** Thickening, gelling, and stabilizing agent: In ice cream, jelly, chocolate milk, infant formula, cottage cheese. Made from seaweed. Some studies have found large amounts are toxic to the digestive system in laboratory animals, but the tiny amounts in food are safe.

✓ **CITRIC ACID, SODIUM CITRATE** Acid, flavoring, chelating agent: In ice cream, sherbet, fruit drink, candy, carbonated beverages, instant potatoes.

Citric acid is an important antioxidant and occurs naturally in citrus fruits and berries.

✓ **GUMS (ARABIC, GUAR, LOCUST BEAN, XANTHAN)** Thickening agents, stabilizers: In beverages, ice cream, frozen pudding, salad dressing. These gums are obtained from natural plant or seaweed sources. They may be used to replace fat in low-fat foods. Some gums may have a laxative effect.

✓ **LECITHIN** Emulsifier, antioxidant: In baked goods, margarine, chocolate, ice cream. This naturally occurring chemical is found in egg yolks and soybeans and is a source of the nutrient choline.

✓ **THIAMINE MONONITRATE** Vitamin B_1: Safe, but adds minuscule amounts of nitrate to food.

ECO-TIP: WHAT YOU CAN DO TO AVOID DYES AND ADDITIVES

✓ Make your own packaged snacks.

✓ Make cakes and frostings from scratch instead of buying mixes.

✓ Dye frostings and other foods with fruit juices.

✓ Make your own gelatin desserts from fruit juice and gelatin, available in every grocery store, instead of buying the brand name versions.

✓ Freeze your own ice pops made from 100 percent juice rather than buying ones containing HFCS.

Food Preparation and Storage

Nonstick coatings work great the first few times you use them, but over time the surface starts to scratch a little, or even peel, despite your best efforts. Given this lack of durability and the fact that nonstick coatings are made with potentially toxic chemicals, it might be time to think about alternatives.

NONSTICK CHEMICALS Nonstick pans contain a coating that keeps food from sticking. Unfortunately one of the ingredients that goes into making the nonstick coating is a harmful chemical called perfluorooctanoic acid (PFOA), or C8. A 2005 study tested 299 newborn babies and found that all of them had the chemical in their blood.[12] The babies were born at Johns Hopkins University Medical Center, located in Baltimore, Maryland, not far from a PFOA plant. In fact, this chemical, which does not occur naturally, is found in nearly all Americans and in wildlife, drinking water, and the air, according to the EPA.

The reason the chemical is so pervasive is that it *never breaks down* in the environment, according to the Environmental Working Group (EWG). It is also toxic. Laboratory animals exposed in the womb to PFOA experienced delays in sexual maturation and reduced organ weights. PFOA in test animals was also linked to increased risk of testicular, breast, liver, and prostate cancer. In animals, PFOA was linked to hypothyroidism. The chemical and a related compound, perfluorooctane sulfonate (PFOS), have been linked to infertility in humans, according to a 2009 article in the journal *Human Reproduction*.[13]

Cooking with nonstick pans can release PFOA and related perfluorinated compounds, or PFCs for short. Manufacturers say these products are safe when used as directed. But if you are like most cooks, especially ones juggling cooking duties with child care, you may occasionally overheat your pans. The EWG found that heating to 680°F causes nonstick coating to give off six toxic gases, including two that have been shown to cause cancer in animals. Fumes from nonstick cookware are particularly toxic to birds and can kill pet birds at temperatures as low as 325°F. The flakes of nonstick coating that come off into your food when you accidentally use that metal spatula are supposed to be inert, but few studies have thoroughly explored the issue.

Since perfluorinated compounds are so long-lasting and toxic, it makes sense to avoid them by switching to safer cookware (see below). However, PFCs are also used in some burger wrappings, pizza boxes, and microwave popcorn bags. PFCs are found in furniture, cosmetics, household cleaners, and clothing. The major manufacturers of PFOA have promised to reduce by 95 percent the level of the chemical in products and facility emissions by 2010 and phase it out entirely by 2015, according to the EPA.

GREEN DICTIONARY

ACRYLAMIDE

Acrylamide is a toxic chemical that is produced naturally in carbohydrate-rich foods during frying, baking, and grilling. It is known to cause cancer in humans exposed to the chemical on the job, so public health officials were concerned when it was first found in foods in 2002. Foods with high levels of acrylamide are French fries, potato chips, and toasted crackers.

ECO-TIP: COOKING HEALTHY AND FAST

Once you've grown, hunted, gathered, purchased, or otherwise procured your food, you have to do something with it. But cooking

whole foods takes longer than ripping open a package of frozen chicken nuggets. Here are some tips on cutting down the time you spend in the kitchen.

✓ Do all your chopping of vegetables at once. Get your kids involved. They can use dull tableware knives to cut the ends off green beans, or they can snap the ends off with their fingers. Make chopping vegetables a weekly event during the growing season. Bring everything to a large table and work your way through it in an hour. Package everything in resealable bags for use during the week. Then on busy nights after school and work, you can pop precut broccoli into the microwave just as you would have done for a store-bought bag of frozen ones.

✓ Meal plan. Work out a schedule of what you will serve and when you will serve it. This will help you avoid last-minute runs to the store, which chew up time and money.

✓ Make two or even three meals in a single night. On nights when you are less busy making sure homework gets done and kids get bathed, cook several meals at once: Have pasta boiling, sauce simmering, chicken roasting in the oven, a pot roast in the slow cooker. If you are a good multitasker, which most parents are, you can get a lot of cooking done at once.

✓ Have your kids cook one or two nights a week when they are old enough. This not only gives parents a break, but it also ensures that your kids will survive on more than just ramen noodles when they go off to college.

✓ Cooking doesn't have to take away from family time and other activities. Modern homes often have large kitchens where children can do homework while Mom or Dad cooks. If you can't all fit in the kitchen, find other ways to incorporate family time into cooking instead of putting the kids in front of video games or the TV while you cook. Show your children that work needs to be done to keep a household running, and involve them in the process whenever possible.

STICK TO SAFER ALTERNATIVES Instead of nonstick, cook with tried-and-true materials such as cast iron, enameled iron, glass, or stainless steel.

Cast iron is an excellent surface for frying, sautéing, and many other types of cooking. These pans distribute heat very well, cook evenly, and are naturally nonstick if properly cared for. Proper care of a cast-iron pan is easy. Just clean the pan with a stiff bristle brush and hot water without soap. Dry the pan immediately to prevent rusting, and apply a thin coat of cooking oil before putting it away.

Enameled iron cookware is cast iron that is coated in enamel. It distributes heat slowly and evenly and can be used for frying, braising, sautéing, roasting, and lots of other types of cooking. Choose a pan with a cooking surface that is either white- or cream-colored enamel because deep red or orange enamel may contain cadmium, a toxic metal.

Glass-ceramic cookware is a good choice as well. It is nonporous so it doesn't absorb food odors or flavors, and it can withstand high temperatures. It can be used on the range top, in the oven, in the microwave, or in a broiler, and be placed in the refrigerator or freezer. Cooks like its see-through quality because they can check on boiling water without lifting the lid, which saves energy since heat does not escape.

Stainless-steel pots and saucepans are great for rapidly heating water to boil pasta or potatoes, and they work well for heating sauces and other foods.

Of the four types of cookware, stainless steel is the least expensive, followed by glass-ceramic cookware, cast iron, and high-end enameled cast iron. Always buy high-quality cookware when possible (it doesn't have to be the best, just as good as you can afford). This can actually save you money in the long run, since these materials last for decades.

GREEN DICTIONARY

MELAMINE

Melamine is an industrial chemical that poisoned pets and has been detected in infant formula. Melamine is also used to make the durable plastic in children's plates and bowls. Some studies have found that melamine and formaldehyde can migrate from the plates into food.[14]

ECO-TIP: POPCORN FROM A KETTLE

Remember popcorn before microwaves? It used to pop in a large stovetop pot. Yes, sometimes it burned, but it was just as tasty and crisp as microwave popcorn, once you got the hang of it. Microwave popcorn is convenient, but some brands use grease-resistant bags containing perfluorinated coatings that can end up on the popcorn, according to a study conducted by the FDA published in a 2005 issue of *Food Additives and Contaminants A*.[15] Once ingested these chemicals may be metabolized to form toxic PFOA. Because PFOA

remains in the body for years, even small levels from eating popcorn can build up over time.

Lots of families are switching from microwave popcorn back to popping it in a stovetop kettle. Avoid popping popcorn in a paper bag in the microwave, because it can cause a fire.

PLASTICS ARE FOREVER The chemical bonds that hold plastic together are very hard to break and the most that will happen is that over time—hundreds of years, in fact—the plastic will break down into dust.

Plastics clog up landfills and roadsides and end up in the ocean, where they may be eaten by marine animals that mistake them for food. A 3.5-million-ton island twice the size of Texas is floating around in the Pacific Ocean between Hawaii and the U.S. mainland. Toxic chemicals like PCBs can stick to plastics, making them more hazardous when eaten by birds or marine animals.

The only way to get rid of giant floating islands of garbage is to reduce the amount of packaging and plastic waste you generate. One way to do this is by placing your child's sandwich in a reusable container rather than a single-use plastic bag. Purchase reusable sandwich boxes or improvise with a plastic container that had been headed for the recycling bin.

Another sandwich-wrapping option is the reusable plastic sandwich wrappers that shops sell for about $6 each. These come in beautiful designs and bright colors, and when unfolded can be used as a placemat. Some of these, however, are made of polyvinyl chloride (PVC), so check before you buy them. (See Eco-Tip: Types of Plastics on page 76.)

If you must go disposable, wax paper and butcher paper are great alternatives to plastic sandwich bags. The wax originates from petroleum products but does not leave residue on food. If you can afford it, chose parchment paper, which is not coated with petroleum products. Although these papers are disposed of after a single use, they are more biodegradable than plastic. Wax or parchment papers work great for those days when your child has a field trip and the school requests that only disposable lunch bags be sent.

SAFER STORAGE Our nation has been enslaved to plastic for the last few decades, and indeed it is an amazing material with many important uses. But food storage, reheating, and serving are not among them. To reduce the risk that plastic chemicals will leach into food during heating, avoid cooking in plastic containers, even if the label says "microwave safe," or "oven safe."

GREEN ON A SHOESTRING

Why buy storage containers when you can reuse yogurt and butter plastic tubs with resealable lids? They are great for storing kids' craft items, game pieces, and small toys. Or cover them with scrap cloth to make a vase.

THE FACTS

The floating island of plastic waste known as the Great Pacific Garbage Patch has been expanding tenfold every decade since the 1950s.

If you are stuck and you absolutely *must* microwave in plastic, follow the manufacturer's directions carefully. For example, some brands of plastic wrap advise to avoid letting the plastic wrap touch the food during microwaving.

Pyrex glass containers with lids are good alternatives to plastic food storage containers. They are widely available in stores and are ideal for food storage because they can move from freezer or refrigerator to microwave and table with ease.

When it comes to plastic food containers, some are safer than others. You can tell what kind of plastic you have by looking at the "resin identification number" located in a triangle on the product. Note that the triangle by itself *does not* mean that the plastic is recyclable. You need to look at the number in the triangle and check with your local recycling company to see what types of plastic they accept.

ECO-TIP: TYPES OF PLASTICS

Some plastics are safer than others.

SAFER PLASTICS

✓ **#1 Polyethylene terephthalate (PET or PETE) (water, juice, and soda bottles, peanut butter jars): PET is usually accepted by municipal recyclers. PET bottles can be reused if cleaned with hot soapy water and dried thoroughly between uses. However, environmental groups advise against washing the bottles repeatedly due to concerns that toxic chemicals can migrate from the plastic into the water. Recycle them when they become cloudy or cracked.**

✓ **#2 High-density polyethylene (HDPE) (miscellaneous food containers, milk jugs, water jugs, cereal box liners): Containers made with HDPE do not leach chemicals into food and are sometimes accepted by municipal recyclers.**

✓ **#4 Low-density polyethylene (LDPE) (sealable sandwich bags, plastic cling wrap, squeezable condiment bottles): These plastics do not leach toxic chemicals into food, but some municipal recyclers do not accept them.**

✓ **#5 Polypropylene (PP) (yogurt containers, reusable plastic snack containers): These containers do not leach toxic chemicals into food.**

Many municipalities do not accept them for recycling, but you can find a list of recycling spots at *www.preserveproducts.com/gimme5.*

✓ **#7 Bio-plastics (picnic plates, cups, utensils):** #7 is an "other" category that sometimes is used on bio-based plastics such as polylactic acid (PLA). Bio-plastics are made from renewable resources such as corn, potatoes, sugarcane, and other materials with a high starch content. Although they are compostable, few facilities exist that can compost large amounts of them.

PLASTICS TO AVOID

✗ **#3 Polyvinyl chloride (PVC) (miscellaneous containers, cling wrap for deli meat and cheese):** PVC is manufactured using processes that release dioxins, which the EPA classifies as likely human carcinogens. PVC also contains plastic softeners called phthalates that harm hormonal systems in animal studies. Cut away the part of the meat or cheese that came in contact with the cling wrap and store in a safe type of plastic.

✗ **#6 Polystyrene (PS) (cups, take-out containers, egg cartons, picnic utensils):** The iconic white foam cup is made of polystyrene, as are many clear or solid plastic picnic utensils and cups. (It is not made of Styrofoam, which is actually a registered trade name for polysterene foam used in construction.) Polystyrene manufacture involves the formation of toxic chemicals, and these products should be avoided in favor of reusable picnic items or safer plastics. Many alternatives now exist, including compostable, plant-based plastics.

✗ **#7 Polycarbonate (PC) (baby bottles, hard plastic cups, 5-gallon water cooler bottles):** #7 is an "other" category but it often refers to polycarbonate, a plastic that is made with bisphenol A (BPA), a suspected hormone-disrupting chemical. Polycarbonate may also be labeled "PC." Some BPA-free PC plastics are available.

SHOULD YOU WASH PLASTICS IN THE DISHWASHER?

Many plastic containers now contain a symbol that indicates they are safe to be washed in the dishwasher. However, you'll get more use out of your plastics and be assured that the hot water and abrasive detergents aren't degrading the plastics and releasing chemicals if you wash them by hand. To make it easy, keep a large tub near the sink. When the kids come home from school or when you return from an outing, set the plastic items to soak in warm soapy water for 20 minutes, then wash briefly with a sponge, rinse, and set in a drying rack.

Take Action

▸ Choose whole foods instead of prepackaged and processed snacks.

▸ Provide a variety of fruits and crunchy vegetables as snacks instead of high-fat, high-salt crackers and cookies.

▸ Teach your kids that cookies, candy, and sodas are treats, not everyday foods.

▸ Make your own prepackaged snacks using reusable containers and foods that come in naturally bite-size pieces (like nuts, cherry tomatoes, and blueberries).

▸ Plan ahead to bring along a healthy meal if you know you'll be eating in the car.

▸ When on long car trips, stop at the supermarket for fresh fruits and sandwich materials rather than the drive-through.

▸ Have family meals together whenever possible.

▸ Opt for less processed sweeteners such as honey and molasses instead of refined sugar.

▸ Avoid artificial sweeteners and dyes.

▸ Make your own ice pops, gelatin desserts, and other kid-friendly favorites that do not contain artificial colors and flavors.

▸ Plan meals in advance, and do prep work (like chopping vegetables) in advance so that you can prepare meals quickly.

▸ Get your kids involved in helping you prepare dinner.

▸ Replace nonstick pans with cookware made of stainless steel, glass-ceramic, or cast iron.

▸ Store food in glass or ceramic containers, which can be used in both the refrigerator and the microwave oven. Avoid microwaving in plastic containers.

THE SCIENCE BEHIND IT

Fats

Despite all the negative press, fats do us a lot of good. Fats provide the body with energy and fatty acids are essential for building cell membranes. Fats are the building blocks of hormones that regulate numerous body functions. And, fats carry the fat-soluble vitamins A, D, E, and K.

Not all types of fat are healthy, however. Trans fats and saturated fats contribute to elevated low-density lipoprotein (LDL) cholesterol, the so-called bad cholesterol implicated in artery blockage and heart attacks, while lowering the "good" high-density lipoprotein (HDL) cholesterol. Only 10 percent of the fats you consume should be trans or saturated fats. Trans fats are primarily found in processed foods or animal fat.

Saturated fats are animal fats and tend to be solid fats such as butter, lard, or the white fat at the edge of a cut of meat.

The healthiest fats are the polyunsaturated and monounsaturated fats found in fish, nuts, and vegetable oils. Monounsaturated fats are usually liquid at room temperature and include canola oil, olive oil, sunflower oil, and high oleic safflower oil. Nuts are also rich in monounsaturated fatty acids.

Two health-promoting types of fats are omega-6 and omega-3 fatty acids. We get lots of omega-6 fatty acids from vegetable oil sources, but many Americans do not get enough omega-3s. Omega-3s are crucial for normal growth and development, and may help alleviate the symptoms of attention deficit/hyperactivity disorder (ADHD). Numerous studies suggest that omega-3s reduce the risk of developing chronic diseases such as heart disease, cancer, and arthritis.

The three most important omega-3s are alpha-linolenic acid (ALA), eicosapentaenoic acid (EPA), and docosahexaenoic acid (DHA). They cannot be manufactured in the body, so we must ingest them in food. ALA converts to EPA and DHA once in the body. Good sources of ALA are vegetable oils, nuts, and flaxseed. Food sources of EPA and DHA are fatty fish such as salmon, trout, and herring. Whenever possible try to introduce your children to fatty fish such as wild-caught salmon, which is naturally low in contaminants such as mercury. See the section on seafood in Chapter 3 for guidance.

GREEN FOODS

Eating Right for the Planet

IN THE CHILDREN'S CLASSIC *CHARLOTTE'S WEB*, WILBUR THE PIG spends his days lolling around in his muddy pen and chatting with geese, spiders, and other barnyard friends. Today's farm animals have moved to the animal equivalent of high-rise apartments. Cattle that once roamed pastures now live in feedlots. Chickens that once pecked at seeds thrown by aproned farmer's wives now live in tiny cages or are packed shoulder to shoulder in chicken houses. And pigs, well, Wilbur would not have recognized the modern swine's digs with their rows upon rows of stainless steel pens.

Food production has changed over the past 50 years. Some of these changes have led to greater availability of food and lower supermarket prices, but these benefits come with a cost. Animal welfare has suffered, crops are grown with chemical pesticides that can harm the environment and our health, and seafood stocks are dwindling due to overfishing.

To continue to be able to feed the six billion plus people on the planet, we will have to pay greater attention to the sustainability of our modern food supply. If we harvest all the cod or sea bass from the oceans, few such fish will be left for our children to enjoy, and perhaps none for our grandchildren. If we pollute our waterways with pesticides or animal wastes, we will jeopardize our drinking water and harm the habitat for animals that depend on that water for survival. If we smother the land in weed-killing herbicides, we will lose fish, frogs, and other wildlife, and we risk losing the biodiversity of the very ecosystem that provides us with food.

A "green" approach to eating involves choosing produce that was grown using methods that maintain soil health instead of stripping it of nutrients and beneficial insects. It involves eating products from animals that were raised on natural diets without added growth hormones or antibiotics. And it involves choosing seafoods from well-managed fisheries and fish farms. Through our purchases we can communicate our demands for safer, more sustainable crops and animal products.

In this chapter, we'll tour the factory farm and find out why a single pig farm in Utah makes more sewage each year than the entire population of Manhattan. We will discuss why you should buy organic food and how you are going to pay for it. We'll talk about supermarket strategies for selecting seafood that is neither overfished nor contains toxic substances such as mercury and polychlorinated biphenyls. We'll talk about why you should avoid milk from cows given hormones, and why a lot of parents are finding locally sourced foods for their family dinners.

Meat in the Making

Children love hamburgers and hot dogs, but today's methods of raising food animals rely on artificial diets, hormones, antibiotics, and confinement in small chambers. However it is easier than you think to provide healthy meats from animals that were raised humanely, and in the process teach your children to appreciate where their food comes from.

Today's farm animals are kept in high-density housing and fed engineered diets formulated to make the animals grow quickly to maturity. Life in these confined animal feeding operations (CAFOs) is a far cry from life on the traditional family farm. Confinement practices include keeping pigs in crates too small to turn around in and keeping egg-laying hens in cages isolated from each other and the outdoors.

The crowded conditions of CAFOs are not just an issue for animal rights activists, however. Our modern ways of raising food animals create several environmental and health problems as well. Hormones and antibiotics in our food have potential health effects for both animals and the humans who eat them. CAFOs create massive piles of animal waste that pollute water, air, and land.

FROM CAFO TO CAFETERIA You don't have to go back far in time to find animals raised in traditional ways: cattle grazing in pastures, chickens clucking in outdoor yards, and pigs wallowing in mud. Many of these farms raised crops to feed animals and used the waste to fertilize crops.

The farms of Charlotte's era began to be replaced in the 1950s by operations that raised only one type of animal, typically housed in the least amount of space and raised on the cheapest food available. Farm labor was replaced with technology. Diversity was replaced with specialization.

These changes led to tremendous increases in food production. American farmers now produce three times as much meat, twice as much milk, and four times as many eggs as they did in 1960. Animals are fed special diets containing growth-promoting hormones and antibiotics. On these diets the animals grow faster to maturity and can be slaughtered and replaced more quickly. For example, in 1950 it took 84 days for a chick to grow into a 5-pound chicken. Today it takes 45 days.

Modern industrial meat production has also brought down the price of food. American consumers spent on average 4.2 percent of their income buying 194 pounds of red meat and poultry in 1970 versus 2.1 percent to buy 221 pounds in 2005, according to a 2008 report by the Pew Commission on Industrial Farm Animal Production.[1]

Some of the decrease in prices is indeed due to increased animal industrialization. However, another important factor is the artificially low price of corn and soybeans, according to a 2007 study by researchers at Tufts University's Global Development and Environment Institute.[2] Prices of these commodities have stayed very low, sometimes lower than the cost of production, due to farm subsidies, according to the report.

The low price of corn and soybeans created incentives to try new types of feeds in farm animals. Cattle that evolved over centuries to graze on grasses are now feeding from troughs filled with a sophisticated blend of corn flakes, protein and fat supplements, hormones, antibiotics, and vitamin supplements. Picture a cow trying to pull the husk off an ear of corn and you can see how absurd this diet is.

But the absurdity factor is not the main problem with this diet. The bovine digestive system is equipped to digest grasses, not corn. Corn turns the first stage of the bovine stomach (the rumen) highly acidic. The acid can eat away at the rumen lining and allow bacteria to pass into the bloodstream. As a result, the cattle are more likely to develop infections, so they are given preventative antibiotics.

Nor is corn the only unusual ingredient in cattle feed. The diet includes liquefied fats from animals. Cattle are herbivores and normally would not eat animal parts. In fact, feeding animal parts to cattle is what caused the outbreak of mad cow disease, more properly known as bovine spongiform encephalopathy

(BSE), in England in the 1990s. The cattle feed contained infected brain and spinal cord parts, transmitting disease-carrying particles called prions. Some people who ate meat from cattle with BSE developed a human version of the disease, variant Creutzfeldt-Jakob disease (vCJD). The outbreak resulted in the slaughter of 4.4 million cattle in an effort to control the disease.

The United States banned the feeding of cattle parts (except for blood and fat) to other cattle in 1997. In the U.S., only two prion-infected cattle have been discovered, but the U.S. Department of Agriculture (USDA) tests less than one percent of the cattle slaughtered. The USDA has blocked individual meat producers from conducting their own tests. One meat producer has sued the USDA for the right to test its meat, and the matter is being decided in the courts.

Instead of testing cattle for BSE, the United States has set up regulations that restrict the likelihood that BSE-infected cattle could enter the food supply. One of these regulations, instituted in 2004, banned the slaughter of sick cattle, or "downer cattle." The regulation was suspended in 2007, however, allowing some crippled cattle to be slaughtered. The largest beef recall ever in the U.S. involved a meat-packing house that in 2008 was slaughtering and processing cattle that were so sick they could not walk. Unfortunately, by the time the practice was publicized by an undercover Humane Society worker, the meat from the downer animal and others before it had already been folded into the meat supply and distributed to school lunch programs and supermarkets. The ban on slaughtering downer cattle has now been restored.

GROWTH SPURT Hormones are given to 90 percent of feedlot beef cattle in the United States, according to the USDA. Six different hormones are permitted as growth-promoting additives to beef cattle. Three are synthetic, and the other three (estradiol, progesterone, and testosterone) exist naturally in humans and cattle. At normal levels these hormones perform important functions in the body, but excess levels have been linked to cancer. Estradiol is a form of estrogen, a hormone implicated in breast cancer in women. Progesterone increases the growth of breast, ovarian, and uterine tumors. Testosterone is linked to prostate cancer. The European Union forbids the addition of hormones to animal feed, citing the potential health risks to consumers.

While no specific studies have been done to address whether added hormones in beef are dangerous to kids, some experts worry that they may be contributing to the declining age of puberty in the United States. However, the U.S. Food and Drug Administration (FDA) states that the amount of added natural hormones (estradiol, progesterone, and testosterone) is negligible compared to the amount naturally produced by the human body.

GREEN DICTIONARY

PRION

An infectious agent that transmits mad cow disease, properly known as bovine spongiform encephalopathy (BSE). Prion diseases have been identified in humans, cattle, sheep, deer, elk, and other animals. These diseases are always fatal, according to the Centers for Disease Control and Prevention (CDC).

Federal regulations prohibit giving hormones to poultry or pigs because the hormones are detectable at significant levels in the meat. Chicken producers that advertise their product as having "no added hormones" are not providing anything special.

DARE TO KEEP YOUR CATTLE OFF DRUGS A glance at a pharmacist's shelf gives the impression that there are hundreds of different kinds of antibiotics. But in fact a limited number of classes of antibiotics are available to treat human diseases. Many of the antibiotics used in animal feed are the same types that we use in humans.

Whenever antibiotics are used, bacteria have an opportunity to mutate and develop ways to evade the drugs' lethal properties. These bacteria become antibiotic-resistant. When the bacteria strike humans, the drugs no longer work against them. Of the 1,400 or so microbes known to cause disease in humans, about 64 percent are able to infect both people and animals, according to the Pew Campaign on Human Health and Industrial Farming. Antibiotic-resistant bacteria have been found on industrialized pig farms, according to the Pew Campaign.

Antibiotics are used not only to treat diseases that spread easily in industrialized farming operations, but also to promote growth. Why do antibiotics cause animals to grow faster? In the case of chickens, it is because the animals harbor bacteria in their guts that consume some of the food that would normally be digested by the chicken. In other words, bacteria are siphoning off a small percentage of the food that the chickens eat. Antibiotics kill off bacteria, so the chicken digests more food and can grow faster.

The FDA and USDA have the unfortunate task of regulating food producers while also supporting them. The agencies do not always follow the best practices recommended by other government scientists. For example, the Institute of Medicine, a government organization of renowned scientists who comb all available data and make recommendations on medical and health practices, recommended in 1999 that farmers minimize the use of antibiotics in food-animal production.[3] The American Medical Association, American Public Health Association, and many other national organizations support the move to phase out nontherapeutic uses of medically important antibiotics in farm animals. The European Union has banned the use of growth-promoting antibiotics since 2006.

Yet the FDA has been slow to move on these recommendations. In mid-2008 the FDA banned the use of the cephalosporin family of antibiotics from animal feed for cows, swine, and chickens. Later in the year, however, the FDA

rescinded the ban, citing the need to review comments made by animal producers regarding the need to keep using these drugs on the farm.

MOUNTAINS OF MANURE In Charlotte's day, manure was collected from
animal pens, dried and aged, and applied as fertilizer in the fields. In today's
industrial animal feeding operations, the amount of waste is so great that it
has become an environmental crisis. A single pig farm in Utah generates as
much waste per year as does the island of Manhattan, according to a report by
the Pew Charitable Trusts. Yet Manhattan has several sewage treatment plants,
whereas farms often are not required to treat waste.

Food corporations in some cases have washed their hands of all this waste
by outsourcing the raising of animals to small-scale growers or individual farmers. This is common in the poultry industry. The poultry corporations supply
baby chicks and chicken feed, and the farmers do the rest. The farmers grow the
chickens to maturity in colossal chicken houses, each the size of a football field.
A single supersize chicken coop can hold 20,000 chickens at once.

In these cases, the farmer is usually responsible for disposing of the waste.
Waste disposal laws are set by a combination of federal and state regulations
and can vary from state to state. Some farmers dump the waste into a shallow
lagoon to let the water evaporate. But evaporation leaves behind concentrated
nitrogen that can seep into groundwater, spread within the underground aquifer,
and contaminate wells used by nearby farmers or neighbors. The cleanup costs
are often borne by the local taxpayers, not the grower or the poultry corporation.

When so many animals are raised in close quarters, it becomes difficult to
dispose of the huge amounts of waste. One option is to spray the animal waste
on fields, but this risks creating airborne contaminants such as ammonia that can
irritate and sicken farmers and their neighbors. Animal waste can contain disease-causing bacteria such as *Escherichia coli* O157:H7 or *Salmonella enterica*.
The waste is very high in nitrogen, which is the main ingredient in fertilizer. In
the amounts generated on a single industrial farm, however, nitrogen levels are
so high that they can damage the plants.

As manure decomposes, it produces at least 160 gases, including lethal
hydrogen sulfide, ammonia, carbon monoxide, nitrous oxide, methane, and
carbon dioxide. The first three are toxic, and the last three are greenhouse
gases. Hydrogen sulfide has killed animals when the gas built up under the
surface of waste slurry and was accidentally released when the slurry was disturbed. According to the U.S. Environmental Protection Agency (EPA), animal
agriculture operations are responsible for nearly three-quarters of the ammonia
air pollution in the United States.

PASS THE (GREENHOUSE) GAS Let's face it: Cattle are flatulent. They also belch. These pungent productions naturally contain methane, a smelly gas that contributes to global warming. Cattle belches are actually a more significant source of methane gas than the stuff that comes out the other end. The digestive system of ruminants such as cattle, sheep, and goats involves a fermentation process in the rumen, or first section of the stomach. As a result the cattle burp a lot of methane and nitrous oxide, two climate-warming gases. Compared to carbon dioxide, methane is about 20 times more potent and nitrous oxide is about 300 times more potent at causing global climate change, according to the U.N.'s Intergovernmental Panel on Climate Change (IPCC).

Greenhouse gas emissions from livestock operations make up 18 percent of all man-made emissions globally, surpassing emissions from cars, trucks, and all transportation methods combined. In the United States, agriculture accounts for about 7 percent of the release of greenhouse gases, according to the EPA.

Raising beef cattle generates far more greenhouse gases than does producing other kinds of foods. An estimated 14.8 pounds of greenhouse gases is generated per pound of beef, which is more than 36 times the climate-changing gases emitted by producing asparagus. Producing a pound of pork generates the equivalent of 3.8 pounds of greenhouse gases; a pound of chicken generates 1.1 pounds, according to a February 2009 article in *Scientific American*.

GREEN DICTIONARY

CO_2 EQUIVALENTS

Methane, nitrous oxide, and carbon dioxide (CO_2) are three gases that contribute to global warming, yet they vary in their potential to raise global temperatures. Climate scientists use the term carbon dioxide equivalents to compare climate emissions from cattle (methane and nitrous oxide) to emissions from automobiles emissions, which are primarily carbon dioxide.

ECO-TIP: BETTER BEEF

Protect your family's health and reduce your ecological footprint when you eat beef:

✓ **Eat beef less often. Try to substitute a protein-rich nonmeat meal such as vegetarian chili.**

✓ **Choose grass-fed beef if and when you can afford it.**

✓ **Look for beef from cattle raised without antibiotics or added hormones (see food label section later in this chapter).**

STOMACH BUGS Reports of deadly foodborne illnesses are becoming more commonplace. Disease-causing bacteria from beef or chicken can persist all the way through processing to turn up in consumer products or fast-food hamburgers and nuggets. Some of the causes include the bacteria *E. coli* O157:H7,

Salmonella, and Campylobacter, as well as calicivirus, also known as Norwalk and Norwalk-like viruses.

E. coli are common bacteria in cattle gut, and cause the animals no harm. But if feces mingle with meat at the processing plant, the meat can become contaminated. Human digestive systems don't take kindly to E. coli O157:H7 and we react with diarrhea, stomach cramps, nausea, and vomiting. In severe cases, the bacteria can cause kidney failure and death. Although E. coli O157:H7 is not limited to industrial farms, the crowded nature of these facilities makes it more likely that more animals will be exposed.

Crowded conditions can foster disease among poultry, as well. Chickens infected with Salmonella have no symptoms, so growers have no way of identifying infected birds. Laying hens can be vaccinated against Salmonella to prevent eggs from becoming contaminated. Even so, in 2000 the Centers for Disease Control and Prevention (CDC) estimated that eggs contaminated with Salmonella caused approximately 180,000 illnesses in the U.S.

Although laying hens are often vaccinated, chickens raised for meat are not always vaccinated. Cooking chicken thoroughly will kill Salmonella as well as Campylobacter, which according to the CDC is the most common cause of diarrheal illness in the world.

The crowded industrial animal feeding operations may be a factor in the development of new diseases that can cross from animals to humans. Pigs can carry a type of antibiotic-resistant bacteria called methicillin-resistant Staphylococcus aureus (MRSA) that has been transmitted to workers on swine farms. Although this is not the same strain that is now spreading in schools and locker rooms in U.S. communities, the strain can cause skin and soft tissue infections as well as pneumonia and blood poisoning in humans. (See Chapter 4 for more information on MRSA.)

A more recent example of a pathogen that jumped from pigs to humans is "swine flu." Pigs harbor flu viruses that are similar to the ones that circulate in humans. In early 2009, public health officials noticed a strain of virus that contained swine and human components. The "swine flu" virus, called H1N1, quickly spread throughout the world's human population, and just three months after detection was reported in 76 countries.

Agricultural officials deny that confined swine feeding operations contributed to the ability of this swine influenza virus to jump from pigs to humans. However, the lack of virus surveillance on pig farms may have contributed to the undetected evolution of this new pandemic strain, according to flu experts.

One strain of animal-human flu that is being watched carefully is avian flu, known as H5N1 virus. Unlike swine flu, which causes only mild symptoms in

THE FACTS

Foodborne illnesses cause an estimated 76 million cases of disease each year in the U.S., according to the CDC, and lead to roughly 325,000 hospitalizations and 5,000 deaths annually.

pigs, avian flu can cause severe disease in poultry and humans. Avian flu was able to jump from birds to humans due to close contact with animals. At present the virus does not easily cross from human to human, so it has not resulted in a pandemic, but public health officials are monitoring it closely.

ENERGY HOG Industrial animal production consumes far more energy than does traditional pasturing. Fossil fuels, industrial fertilizers, and synthetic pesticides go into the growth of corn for the diet, and industrial feedlots use more fuel moving animals to slaughter and distributing food products than would a traditional local system. These industrial facilities also use a lot of water to spray down dusty feedlots and keep animals cool.

GOING VEGETARIAN After reading this chapter, you may find beef and other animal meats less appealing. Many eco-minded people choose vegetarianism for environmental reasons, health reasons, and humane reasons. Eating plants is a more direct way to obtain your daily nutrient requirement with less impact on the ecosystem. Plants get their energy directly from the sun, so when you eat plants you are dining low on the food chain. And forgoing beef is one of the best ways that individuals can help reduce the threat of global warming.

If you decide on vegetarianism for your children, or your child has decided he or she wants to become a vegetarian, you'll want to brush up on nutrition for vegetarian children. Check booksellers for books that focus on the nutritional needs of vegetarian kids. Or consult your child's pediatrician.

Seafood

Seafood is an excellent source of protein and nutrients and most kids love tuna sandwiches. But some types of fish can contain high levels of mercury, a brain toxicant that can affect a child's mental development and performance in school. Add to that the concerns about overfishing, and seafood becomes a quandary for parents. Here's how to navigate the choppy waters.

HEALTHY HARVEST Fish are a great source of protein. Many types of fish are rich in omega-3 fatty acids, which contribute to brain development and may reduce the risk of heart disease by reducing blood pressure and reducing blood levels of certain fats called triglycerides. Perhaps more important for the children in your life, omega-3s have been shown in some studies to reduce symptoms of attention deficit/hyperactivity disorder (ADHD) and improve behavior and learning. Good sources of omega-3s are cold-water, oily fish such as salmon, herring, mackerel, anchovies, and sardines. They are found in tuna in lesser amounts.

Due to these health benefits, the EPA recommends that women of child-bearing age and young children consume two servings of fish per week. These fish should be ones that are low in mercury contamination, such as Atlantic mackerel, farmed rainbow trout, or wild Alaska salmon.

TRAWLING FOR TOXICS Many types of fish are long-lived and grow to be quite large in the open ocean. As fish grow larger by eating smaller fish, pollutants can build up so that the largest fish, including tuna and swordfish, contain the highest levels of contaminants. Other fish with high contaminant levels include bigeye tuna, tilefish, shark, king mackerel, marlin, and orange roughy. Some of the common contaminants in ocean wildlife include PCBs, dioxins, and mercury.

PCBs are industrial chemicals that were dumped into rivers and oceans. Although they are no longer manufactured in the United States today, these persistent pollutants still contaminate lakes, rivers, and streams. PCBs are probable carcinogens and can harm the immune system and brain, according to the EPA. High PCB-levels in fish may also cause cognitive birth defects in utero.[4]

Dioxins are by-products of chlorinated chemical industrial processes. They may be formed by chlorine bleaching of paper and pulp, chlorination of wastewater and drinking water, and in the production of other industrial chemicals. Dioxins may also be released into the air from waste incinerators. Dioxins are potent human carcinogens and may cause birth defects.[5]

Mercury is a naturally occurring element that can be found in coal. Coal-fired power plants emit mercury into the air. The mercury later falls into the oceans where it is converted to methylmercury and ingested by fish. Methylmercury is toxic to the developing brain. Some children born to women who ate contaminated fish while pregnant suffered from learning disabilities and had IQ scores that were lower than average.[6] The EPA recommends that women avoid eating high-mercury fish (shark, swordfish, king mackerel, tilefish) if they are planning to become pregnant, are already pregnant or are nursing. (For a list of fish low in contaminants, see Eco-Tip: Best Seafood Choices later in this chapter.)

OVER THE LIMIT The global appetite for delicious, protein-rich fish has made more than just a dent in the ocean's fish population. Many species of fish are decimated completely. Fisheries are in crisis. The ocean is unable to produce enough young fish to replace the ones fished from the sea.

About three-quarters of the fisheries in the world are either depleted, overexploited, or fully exploited and are producing catches that are at or close to their maximum sustainable limits, according to the U.N.'s Food and Agriculture Organization (FAO). Over the last 50 years, the amount of fish taken from the oceans has ballooned, from 22 million tons in 1950 to 154 million tons in 2006, according to the figures published by the FAO in 2009.

Modern fishing methods have allowed fishermen to dramatically increase their catch. But these methods are notoriously nonspecific, like trying to do eye surgery with a kitchen knife. One of the biggest problems is bycatch. Dolphins, sea turtles, seals, and even whales have been killed when trapped in nets or fishing lines. Fishermen net numerous small fish that they later discard. These fish are often dead by the time they are thrown back into the sea. About 25 percent of the fish caught are rejected as bycatch, according to the FAO.

Today's fishing practices also cause destruction of habitat. Nets that scrape the ocean floor (bottom trawlers) rake up the small crustaceans and fish that serve as food for larger fish. The activities of landlubbers are also destroying habitat. Coastal wetlands, which serve as incubators for juvenile fish, are being converted to luxury resorts. Streams deliver pesticides, fertilizers, industrial chemicals, motor oil, and sewage into the oceans.

Some of the most overfished sea creatures are the ones that grow the largest. Tuna, swordfish, and grouper grow to enormous size. An Atlantic bluefin tuna weighs on average 550 pounds, is 6 feet long, and eats about 25 percent of its body weight each day. Throughout their long lives, these top predators consume thousands of pounds of fish, which in turn consumed tens of thousands of pounds of smaller fish, says marine biologist Sylvia Earle in her book, *Sea Change: A Message of the Oceans* (1995). Eating a large predator fish, she notes, is like dining on mountain lion steak.

Consumer pressure can make a difference. The campaign to make tuna "dolphin-safe" has improved matters for dolphins. By purchasing fish captured or raised with less impact on the environment, you are sending a message to food producers that you support responsible fishing practices.

DOWN ON THE FISH FARM Fish farms produce about 47 percent of the fish that humans consume, and the farms are part of a rapidly growing industry.

Aquaculture can be an environmentally sound way to produce food. However, farmed fish may be fed unnatural diets, treated with antibiotics or given dyed food, as is done with salmon to make the meat look pink. Fish normally eat a diet made up of other marine organisms, but on farms they may be fed vegetable oils, which can alter the fat makeup of the fish and result in production of fewer omega-3 fatty acids.

Fish farming has the potential to decrease the strain on wild populations while still feeding a hungry world. It can be done in an environmentally sound fashion. However, at this time there is very little management of fish farming, and many environmental problems have occurred. The conversion of coastal land to shrimp ponds often results in destruction of mangrove swamps that act as nurseries for juvenile wild fish.

Keeping thousands of fish in crowded net pens is not only stressful for the fish, it facilitates the spread of diseases that are then treated by antibiotics, raising the possibility of creating drug-resistant bacteria. Escaped fish can spread disease and can take over habitat from wild fish.

Fish that are naturally carnivorous, such as shrimp, need to eat other fish, and this requires the farming or catching of food stocks, posing yet another drain on sea resources. Fish farms also rely on wild stocks or eggs to repopulate farms. A switch to practices that breed fish on farms could reduce this drain on wild populations.

Small farms that raise species that feed on plants rather than other fish may be the best environmental choice when it comes to fish farms. For example, tilapia is a freshwater fish that feeds on algae, aquatic plants, and small invertebrates. It can be raised on inland farms so that waste products can be processed rather than ejected into the sea.

GREEN ON A SHOESTRING

Canned wild-caught Atlantic salmon is an affordable, low-mercury alternative to canned tuna.

SEAFOOD BEST CHOICES Wild-caught, canned salmon is relatively low in mercury and PCBs, rich in omega-3s, and inexpensive. Fish farms are not allowed in Alaska waters, so any fish from Alaska is wild caught. See Eco-Tip: Best Seafood Choices for a list of fish that are low in contaminants and not overfished.

The safest form of tuna is canned light tuna because it comes from smaller, younger fish. To stay below the level of mercury that the EPA considers safe, the Natural Resources Defense Council (NRDC) recommends that you limit your child's consumption to less than 1 ounce of canned light tuna for every 12 pounds of body weight per week. A 36-pound child, for example, should not eat more than 3 ounces, or half a standard-size can, per week. Children and pregnant women should avoid albacore and white tuna because the levels of mercury are higher in these larger fish, according to the NRDC.

ECO-TIP: BEST SEAFOOD CHOICES

Here are some "best choices" for fish that have not been overfished. The ones marked with the symbol • are high in heart-healthy omega-3s and low in contaminants.

Abalone (farmed)

Barramundi (U.S.)

Catfish (U.S.)

Caviar/sturgeon (farmed)

• Char, Arctic (farmed)

Clams (farmed)

Clams, softshell

Cod, Pacific (bottom longline)

Crab, Dungeness

Crab, stone

Crawfish (U.S.)

Halibut, Pacific

Lobster, spiny (Australia, Baja, U.S.)

• Mackerel, Atlantic

Mahimahi (U.S. pole/troll)

Mullet (U.S.)

Mussels (farmed)

• Oysters (farmed)

Pollock, Alaska

• Sablefish/black cod (Alaska, Canada)

• Salmon (Alaska wild)

• Salmon, canned pink/sockeye

• Sardines (U.S.)

Scallops, bay (farmed)

Shrimp, pink (Oregon)

Shrimp (U.S. farmed)

Spot prawn (Canada)

Squid, longfin (U.S.)

Striped bass (farmed)

Tilapia (U.S.)

• Trout, rainbow (farmed)

• Tuna, albacore (Canada, U.S.)*

Tuna, skipjack (pole/troll)

Tuna, yellowfin (U.S. pole/troll)

Wreckfish

Source: Environmental Defense Fund 2009 and Seafood WATCH®. *Children and pregnant women should limit their intake of albacore and white tuna.

For a complete chart showing the best, OK, and worst seafood choices due to overfishing and contaminants, see *www.edf.org/seafood*.

Organic Produce

Organic farms provide fresh, wholesome fruits and vegetables that have never been treated with artificial pesticides, herbicides, or fertilizers. This sustainable approach to growing food is better for the health of your family, the soil, and the wider ecosystem.

Standing in the warm sun breathing the heady perfume of berry blossoms and listening to the incessant buzzing of honeybees sure beats the cool and sterile aisles of the supermarket any day. What better way to get your produce than from your own garden or a nearby farm?

Unfortunately not everyone lives near an organic farm or has space to grow a garden. We may live too far from agricultural areas or in places where the local soil is more favorable to sagebrush than strawberries. If you are lucky you can find a pot of dirt, a plot of land, or a community garden that can give you and your family the taste of fresh fruits and vegetables, if not a steady supply. For the rest, you can head to a local farmers market or the produce section of your nearby supermarket.

WHY GO ORGANIC Fresh taste, your family's health, and stewardship of the planet are the three top reasons to buy—or grow—organic produce whenever possible. If you grew up on a steady diet of iceberg lettuce and frozen or canned vegetables, you may be pleasantly surprised by the taste of fresh vegetables. Green beans make a loud crunchy sound when you bite into them. Cherry tomatoes shower your mouth with ripe fresh flavor. And sun-warmed berries delight the tongue with tart sweetness.

Several studies have found that organic fruits and vegetables are actually higher in nutrients than conventionally grown ones, according to a review article in the *Journal of Food Science* in 2006.[7] For example, one study found that organic tomatoes had higher levels of vitamin C and health-protective carotenoids and polyphenols than their conventionally grown counterparts. Future studies will determine whether organic produce is more nutritious across the board.

We think of organic farming as being all about not using pesticides, but it has the broader goal of using sustainable methods to ensure the land continues to produce its bounty for subsequent generations. Organic farming involves using practices that maintain or improve soil fertility, use renewable resources, return waste products to the earth, and do not poison the environment.

Buying organic produce doesn't have to put you in penury, although you will have to be a little creative. (See Green on a Shoestring.) By purchasing organic food you are signaling to the agricultural industry that you care about food quality. By buying from local farmers wherever possible, you are calling for the return of agricultural production to locations near urban and suburban areas instead of the massive centralized agricultural operations we have today.

THE USDA ORGANIC LABEL ensures that products have been certified by a USDA-approved independent agency to meet the following guidelines:
✓ No use of synthetic fertilizers, pesticides, fungicides, herbicides, insecticides, or other poisonous chemicals, and no sewage sludge on the land

for three years prior to certification and then continually throughout the duration of their certification.

✓ No use of genetically modified organisms and irradiation.

✓ Manufacturer uses practices that foster soil building, conservation, manure management, and crop rotation.

✓ Manufacturer provides outdoor access and pasture for livestock.

✓ Manufacturer refrains from antibiotic and hormone use in animals.

✓ Manufacturer sustains animals on 100 percent organic feed.

✓ Manufacturer avoids contamination while processing organic products.

✓ Manufacturer keeps records of all operations.

THE KILLING FIELDS Pesticides are poisons. These chemicals are designed to kill insects, fungi, and other microbes, but several of them attack the very same biological systems we humans have. Many synthetic pesticides are harmful to health, causing short-term toxicity or long-term illnesses such as cancer to workers that apply them or harvest crops.

Nor are workers the only ones that are exposed. In one study, children who ate conventionally grown produce had significant levels of pesticide metabolites in their urine. When the children switched to an organic diet for five days, the pesticide levels dropped dramatically, according to the study published in 2008 in the journal *Environmental Health Perspectives*.[8]

Studies in children have revealed links between pesticide exposure and several chronic diseases, including birth defects, childhood cancer, asthma, and problems with learning, cognitive abilities, and behavior.[9] Per pound of body weight, children eat more than adults do. Children also eat large quantities of the soft-skinned fruits, such as grapes and berries, that contain some of the highest levels of residual pesticides.

Herbicides (weed killers) can also be toxic both to wildlife and humans. The weed killer atrazine, commonly applied in the Midwest to corn, has been found to deform frogs.[10] Atrazine can also contaminate drinking-water wells and is a suspected hormone-disrupting chemical. Atrazine in drinking water is linked to an increased risk of low birth weight, preterm delivery, and small infant size, according to a 2005 study in the journal *Occupational and Environmental Medicine*.[11]

Most produce is treated with a combination of insecticides and herbicides at different points during the growing season and subsequent transport to stores. Yet the toxicity of pesticide mixtures has not been well studied. Most products also contain "inert" ingredients that may also be toxic.

Washing helps remove pesticides from the outer layer but it does not eliminate them completely. Always wash produce before eating it. Peeling

THE FACTS

Only a century ago, all foods were grown "organically," that is, without synthetic pesticides, herbicides, or fertilizers.

can eliminate pesticides from fruit skin but may eliminate valuable vitamins. To reduce your children's pesticide exposure, serve organic produce whenever possible as part of a varied diet.

RICH SOIL AT A PRICE Today's farms rely on synthetic fertilizers rather than the natural stuff that Wilbur the Pig and the other farm animals produce. These fertilizers are made using a chemical reaction that converts natural gas to ammonia, a nitrogen-rich chemical that helps spur plant growth.

Synthetic fertilizers have helped boost crop yields and have helped stave off starvation in an increasingly populated world, but at an environmental price. Synthetic fertilizers can harm aquatic life, contribute to climate change, and release harmful ammonia into the air. They do not contribute important minerals that crops deplete from the soil. By contrast, naturally occurring fertilizers such as manure, worm castings, peat, and seaweed build and retain soil health.

When synthetic fertilizers wash into streams and rivers, their high nitrogen and phosphorus levels have a devastating impact on aquatic wildlife. The nitrogen and phosphorus serve as nutrients that drive massive algal blooms. When the algae die, their decomposition consumes so much oxygen that little is available for marine organisms. This causes massive die-offs of aquatic life. Today there are about 200 of these "dead zones" in the ocean around the world, including a large one in the Gulf of Mexico.

Another risk associated with synthetic fertilizer use is increased release of greenhouse gases to the atmosphere. Researchers at the University of Notre Dame found high levels of the greenhouse gas nitrous oxide dissolved in streams that border fertilizer-treated farm fields, according to a 2009 article in the *Journal of Environmental Quality*.[12]

Organic farming uses no synthetic fertilizers so it has less of an impact on nitrogen levels in nearby water. Organic practices build up soil health by adding and retaining soil nutrients in the right amounts to recruit active communities of microorganisms and earthworms. These creatures endlessly work the soil to give it the right texture and nutrients to grow crops. Instead of using synthetic fertilizers, which are made from natural gas and other fossil fuels, farmers apply composted manure made from animal waste, food remains, mulch, and crushed leaves.

BEYOND ORGANIC: BIODYNAMIC A step beyond organic farming, biodynamic farming envisions the farm as a living organism that is self-sustaining and should be free of external and unnatural additions. Rudolf Steiner, founder of the Waldorf School, introduced the biodynamic philosophy in the 1920s.

THE FACTS

One-fifth of the petroleum products consumed in the United States goes to crop production (including the making of synthetic fertilizers) and transportation.

In addition to adhering to organic standards of not using synthetic pesticides and fertilizers, biodynamic farming includes setting aside part of the land as a wilderness to encourage biodiversity.

Biodynamic farms try to use as little as possible in the way of nonrenewable fossil fuels. Wherever possible biodynamic farmers include consideration of climate, inherent wildlife of Earth, the light and warmth from the sun and the focusing of cosmic influences through the movement of the planets. Biodynamic fans say that the produce is tastier and healthier.

ECO-TIP: TOP FOODS TO BUY ORGANIC

Pesticides more easily contaminate some fruits and vegetables than others. Here is a list compiled by the Environmental Working Group of the top 12 fruits and vegetables most contaminated by pesticides:

Peaches	Nectarines	Lettuce
Apples	Strawberries	Grapes (imported)
Sweet Bell Peppers	Cherries	Carrots
Celery	Kale	Pears

Here is a list of the top 15 fruits and vegetables least likely to be contaminated with pesticides:

Onions	Sweet Peas (frozen)	Eggplants
Avocados	Asparagus	Papayas
Sweet Corn (frozen)	Kiwis	Watermelons
Pineapples	Cabbage	Tomatoes
Mangos	Broccoli	Sweet Potatoes

Source: Environmental Working Group: www.foodnews.org updated March 2009

GET THE LOWDOWN ON FOOD LABELS It seems like every food these days bears a claim that it is healthy for you or for the environment. But not every label is backed up by an independent certifying agency. Here is a rundown of the labels certified by independent third parties:

✓ **AMERICAN GRASSFED ASSOCIATION** (AGA) Certification (Dairy, Beef, Lamb): Guarantees that animals were fed a lifetime diet of 100 percent forage, were not raised in confinement, were never treated with hormones, and were treated with antibiotics only for illness, *www.american grassfed.org.*

✓ **AMERICAN HUMANE CERTIFIED** (Beef, Pork, Eggs, Dairy): Assures humane care of livestock and no use of growth hormones or nontherapeutic antibiotics, *www.americanhumane.org.*

✓ **ANIMAL WELFARE APPROVED** (Beef, Bison, Poultry, Eggs, Goat, Pork): Animals are raised in human conditions and spend the majority of their lives on pastureland. No growth hormones or nontherapeutic antibiotics are allowed, *www.animalwelfareapproved.org.*

✓ **BIRD FRIENDLY** (Coffee): Certified by the Smithsonian Migratory Bird Center (SMBC) to be grown in a way that protects tropical habitats. (See more on this topic in Chapter 9.) *http://nationalzoo.si.edu/ConservationAnd Science/MigratoryBirds*

✓ **DEMETER BIODYNAMIC** (Fruit, Vegetables, Eggs, Cheese, Meat, Wine): Grown in harmony with planetary rhythms without pesticides, fertilizers, or near electromagnetic fields, *www.demeter-usa.org*

✓ **FAIR TRADE CERTIFIED** (Coffee, Tea, Chocolate, Tropical Fruit, Rice, Sugar, Wine): Indicates that farmers received fair prices for their crops. (See more on this topic in Chapter 9.) *www.transfairusa.org*

✓ **FOOD ALLIANCE CERTIFIED** (Milk, Frozen Food, Wheat, Meat, Produce): Assures use of sustainable farming practices, including soil and water conservation and fair treatment of workers. Cattle must be raised on pastureland without hormones or nontherapeutic antibiotics, *www .foodalliance.org.*

✓ **MARINE STEWARDSHIP COUNCIL** (Farmed Fish, Wild-caught Fish): Indicates fish are from sustainably managed fisheries, *www.msc.org.*

✓ **RAINFOREST ALLIANCE** (Coffee, Chocolate, Tea, Bananas, Pineapples, Mangos, Avocados, Guavas, and Citrus): Assures that foods were grown on farms that respect worker rights and use only pesticides approved by the EPA and European Union, *www.rainforest-alliance.org.*

ECO-TIP:
SHOPPING TIPS

When shopping for produce, bring your own reusable produce bags, plastic mesh bags, or organic cotton net produce bags. When shopping for organic produce, check for a five-digit code starting with a "9." Non-organic fruits and vegetables are marked with a four-digit code.

KITCHEN TABLE TALK

Affordable Organics

Buying the best quality food for our children can be tough to do, especially on a budget. Yet all over the country, moms and dads are finding creative ways to do it. "Our strategy is to try to go organic where it is going to make the biggest difference," says Kyndaron Reinier, a mom in Hood River, Oregon.

Last summer, her family joined a community-supported agriculture project. Each week, a box of produce arrived at their house, and three-year-old Dylan delighted in taking each vegetable out and learning its name. "It was a lot of stuff I wouldn't normally buy," says Reinier. "Dylan was learning about vegetables and getting to taste really good foods."

The family also shops at farmers markets, where prices can be lower than they are in stores. "It is fun to go there with Dylan and have him see the fresh produce," says Reinier. "He'll see the berries and eat an entire container."

Purchasing organic milk is another worthwhile expense, said Reinier, citing the potential for hormones and antibiotics in milk. "Organic milk is one thing that I can control that I know is good for him."

THE FACTS

Products made from 95 percent organic ingredients may also carry the "USDA Organic" seal. Products that contain at least 70 percent organic ingredients may use the phrase "made with organic ingredients."

✓ **USDA PROCESS VERIFIED NEVER EVER 3** (Beef): Cattle were raised without ever being given 1) antibiotics, 2) growth promotants, and 3) animal by-products, *www.ams.usda.gov.*

✓ **USDA NATURALLY RAISED BEEF** (Beef): Ensures that cattle were given no growth promotants, no antibiotics (except certain antiparasitic drugs, the use of which must be explicitly noted on the beef packaging), and were fed no animal by-products, *www.ams.usda.gov.*

✓ **USDA ORGANIC** (Fruits, Vegetables, Coffee, Meat, Various Foods): Farmers may not use synthetic chemicals or sewage sludge on crops. They must use practices that foster soil-building and may not plant genetically modified seeds nor use irradiation. They must provide outdoor access and pasture for livestock, provide 100 percent organic feed, and refrain from using antibiotics and hormones in animals, *www.ams.usda.gov*.

You can look up food labels as well as labels for wood, personal care products, and household cleaners at Consumer Reports' Greener Choices Eco-Labels Center at *www.greenerchoices.org/eco-labels*.

GREEN ON A SHOESTRING GOING ORGANIC WITHOUT GOING BROKE

Organic produce doesn't always cost more. A lot of times the price comes down to factors that have nothing to do with growing the food, such as seasonal availability and how far you live from a farming area. Here are some tips for saving money on organic foods:

✓ Join a community-supported agriculture (CSA) program. These are farms that sell shares of their harvest to nearby residents, typically for around $300 to $600 per year. In return, members get a weekly assortment of the farm's produce. Find your closest CSA at *www .localharvest.org*.

✓ Shop at farmers markets. Here you can meet the farmers and ask them about pesticide use and other practices. Some farmers don't use pesticides but haven't gone to the expense of obtaining official organic certification. Find a nearby farmers market at *www .localharvest.org*.

✓ Check your local conventional grocery stores to see what they offer—most of them have some organic produce, and they often cut prices to reduce inventory. Watch for sales and coupons.

✓ Buy organic versions of the fruits and vegetables most likely to be contaminated with pesticides. As a general rule, these include soft-sided fruits and leafy greens. See Eco-Tip: Top Foods to Buy Organic for a full list.

✓ Buy frozen organic fruits and vegetables—but check the country of origin. A lot of frozen produce, organic or otherwise, is grown in

Mexico, Ecuador, China, and elsewhere. Keep America growing by buying produce from the United States Not only is it difficult to verify organic growing standards overseas, shipping consumes fossil fuels and generates greenhouse gases.

✓ If you cannot buy organic, at least buy American. Each year the USDA tests thousands of produce samples—imported and domestic—for pesticide residues. The 2007 report found that imported produce contained residues of pesticides that the United States had phased out due to safety concerns.[13]

✓ Grow your own. A garden is a great way to teach kids about the origins of food and instill a sense of thankfulness for all the bounty that the earth provides.

✓ Compost your kitchen scraps and help your children understand the cycle of renewal that living things go through, and how we humans can choose recyclable processes over wasteful ones.

✓ Visit pick-your-own organic farms during the growing season and freeze or otherwise store foods for use later in the year. *See www .localharvest.org.* Learn how to store your organic food to keep it fresh.

Food Safety

Nothing could be more important than safety when it comes to feeding your family. Yet we routinely hear about foods contaminated with *E. coli* or other potentially deadly bacteria. Read on for tips on how to steer clear of food contaminants.

People from other countries sometimes like to mock Americans about our over-litigious society and the endless safety warnings on toys and baby items sold in the United States. But food safety is one area where our federal agencies have a mixed record of protecting us.

ECO-TIP:
AVOIDING AFLATOXIN

Don't keep nuts longer than a few months. If you must do so, store them in the refrigerator. Peanut butter manufacturers test their products for aflatoxin, but the peanut butter that you grind yourself (mainly at health food stores) may not be tested. Ask the store manager what precautions they take against aflatoxin.

The FDA and USDA lack the manpower and in many cases the regulatory capacity to police food items produced both inside the United States and imported from other countries. It is easy to criticize foreign companies for lax safety practices and cover-ups, but in fact our own U.S. companies engage in the same reckless behavior. After a major outbreak of *Salmonella* in a U.S. peanut processing plant in 2008-09, it emerged that the company knew of the contamination but shipped products from the plant anyway.

One of the easiest ways to avoid contaminated food is to stick with a back-to-basics way of eating that emphasizes whole and real foods over processed and fast ones. Eating home-cooked foods instead of going out to restaurants is an easy (and inexpensive!) way to minimize your children's exposure to foods that have traveled through many processing plants and many hands. By taking back the responsibility of preparing your children's food, you will always know that meat was cooked long enough and the produce was fresh.

Of course this strategy is not foolproof. Even fresh food can carry disease-causing illnesses if it comes in contact with animal waste or poor sanitary practices somewhere during the transport to your local market. And most of us cannot completely avoid processed and restaurant food, nor do many of us want to eat home-cooking seven days a week.

Nor should we have to. Consumers must continue to press the U.S. government for better regulation of our food supply as well as labeling that tells consumers about the safety and source of their food.

Consumer right-to-know laws are some of the most potent ways that citizens can bring about change. Food producers know this and fight the passage of these laws whenever possible. The maker of recombinant bovine somatotropin (rBST), the growth hormone given to cows to increase milk production, fought hard to prevent small dairies from labeling their products as bovine growth hormone–free. Eventually consumer sentiment won the day, however, and now it is common to see such labels. A similar food fight is going on over the labeling of meat products as tested for mad cow disease.

Consumers would also like to know exactly where their food comes from. This is getting easier with the passage of the Farm Security and Rural Investment Act of 2002, which requires "country of origin labeling" (COOL), for beef, lamb, pork, fish, produce, and peanuts. A later law added chicken, goat meat, ginseng, pecans, and macadamia nuts. Unfortunately the implementation of COOL was delayed for years for all except fish and shellfish. COOL finally became effective on March 16, 2009.

Other products have unsafe chemicals in them due to fraud. Melamine, a toxic industrial chemical, was added to milk, candy, and baby formula in China and sold to millions of consumers. Several babies died and hundreds of thousands were sickened. Melamine has also been detected in U.S.-made infant formula, but the FDA is unsure how it got there. For a list of Chinese-made melamine-contaminated products sold in the United States, see the FDA's website, *www.fda.gov.*

To ensure the highest quality of food (and the lowest environmental impact), choose foods grown as close to home as possible in the United States. Foreign-grown produce may be treated with pesticides that are not approved for use in the United States.

REDUCE THE RISK OF FOODBORNE ILLNESS:

- ✓ Keep beef, poultry, and eggs separate from the other foods in your kitchen. When preparing these foods, use separate cutting boards, plates, knives, and utensils, and then wash them thoroughly in soap and hot water or a dishwasher.
- ✓ Wash produce thoroughly. Produce can also become contaminated with pathogens, especially if produce is washed or irrigated with water contaminated by animal fecal matter.
- ✓ Cook all beef, poultry, and eggs thoroughly. Eggs should be cooked until the yolk is firm. Beef should be cooked to a minimum internal temperature of 160°F, whole chicken to 180°F.
- ✓ Prepare frozen foods according to manufacturer's instructions. Frozen foods contain raw ingredients that can harbor contamination.
- ✓ Wash your hands thoroughly after using the bathroom or changing diapers and before preparing or eating food.
- ✓ Avoid raw milk, unpasteurized dairy products, and unpasteurized juices (like fresh apple cider).

GREEN ON A SHOESTRING

If you cannot afford to buy organic milk, look for milk brands that pledge to buy their milk from dairies that do not use bovine growth hormone.

Genetically Modified Foods

Genetic modification (GM) allows food producers to add traits such as pest-resistance and other characteristics to plants. GM technology has the potential to improve food crops, but it has been implemented without much public debate about the risks.

Genetic modification of crops involves inserting a new gene or genes from another plant, insect, or organism to give the crop a new capability that it didn't have before. Bt corn, for example, contains a gene from the soil bacteria *Bacillus thuringiensis* (Bt). This gene makes a protein that kills certain insects when they bite into the plant. Since the crop naturally makes Bt, the farmer doesn't need to apply pesticides. Other GM crops include corn and soybeans that carry a gene that allows them to resist being killed by a popular herbicide called Roundup (glyphosate). Farmers can apply the herbicide without worrying that it will kill their crops along with the weeds.

Genetic engineering is a new twist on the old practice of breeding crops for certain traits, only the process is much faster, and plant researchers can more easily select desirable qualities. Genetically modified crops include corn, soybeans, canola, and cotton. Most of the corn and soybeans are made into animal feed for chickens, hogs, and cattle, although small amounts of corn can end up in human foods such as tortillas, corn muffins, and high-fructose corn syrup. GM canola oil and soy lecithin may be found in processed foods.

Since their introduction in the United States in the mid-1990s, GM crops have become commonplace in the United States, Canada, and parts of Latin and South America. Other parts of the world, including Europe and Japan, have resisted the introduction of GM crops for reasons having to do more with the sustainability of agriculture than threats to human health.

Genetically modified crops are not the dangerous "Frankenfoods" that some activists warn about. GM crops have never caused a human illness, and the processing of oil and corn syrup removes most or all of the engineered gene and protein from the food. In fact, many researchers believe that Bt cotton has helped the environment by reducing the amount of toxic pesticides applied to the crop.

Still, GM crops are of concern due to their inadequate regulation, their potential to transfer an engineered gene to other crops, economic effects on small farmers, the possible harm to "helpful" insects, the emergence of pesticide resistance, and the potential to introduce new allergens—some that could be life-threatening—into the food supply. Let's have a look at these issues.

REGULATION Regulation of GM crops is governed by a trio of federal agencies, the FDA, the USDA, and the EPA. The EPA handles crops that produce pesticides like Bt and Roundup, and the USDA and FDA handle agricultural and food products. However, few resources are given toward monitoring crops to see if negative effects are occurring over the long-term.

TRANSFER OF GENES TO OTHER CROPS Scientists know that gene transfer can happen, simply because it already happens in conventional crops that were bred the old-fashioned way. Wind and insects can carry pollen from a GM field to a non-GM field or to weeds. For example, Roundup-resistant crops could spread their genes to weeds, creating weeds incapable of being killed by the herbicide.

EFFECTS ON SMALL FARMERS The GM crops are produced by companies that have spent a lot of money investing in research and development, so GM seeds cost more than conventional seeds. Farmers caught using the seeds without paying for them are in violation of the law. Europe and Japan have been resistant to the adoption of GM crops, so U.S. farmers have a difficult time exporting their crops to these markets.

EFFECTS ON BENEFICIAL INSECTS GM crops that make Bt have been absolved of any threat to Monarch butterflies, since the amounts made by the crops are too small to make a meaningful dent in their numbers. However the potential remains for GM crops to have harmful effects on beneficial insects.

EMERGENCE OF PESTICIDE RESISTANCE Bt was sprayed on crops for years in organic farming because it is naturally occurring yet is lethal to certain pests. The adoption of Bt genes into GM crops means that Bt now is widely introduced to many more farms than just the relatively small number of organic farms. Organic farmers are concerned that pests could evolve resistance mechanisms to Bt, thereby lessening its effectiveness and depriving organic farmers of one of their most important tools.

POTENTIAL FOR ALLERGENS The potential for GM crops to introduce new allergens is real because the GM crop may produce new proteins never before found in the human food supply. Regulators *do* require testing for allergenicity. One brand of GM corn called Starlink was removed from the market because it contained a potential allergen.

THE FUTURE OF GM On the horizon are GM plants that produce vitamins, pharmaceuticals, and industrial chemicals. A type of rice that makes vitamin A (beta-carotene) could improve the nutrition of people in developing countries. Some scientists are concerned about the use of food crops such as corn to produce pharmaceuticals, since the pharmaceutical corn could breed with conventional corn and people could inadvertently consume drugs they don't need. They recommend using nonfood plants such as tobacco to produce the pharmaceuticals.

TIPS FOR AVOIDING GM CROPS:

✓ Choose certified organic produce.

✓ Buy from local farmers that you can ask about their use of GM crops.

✓ Grow your own foods.

✓ Avoid buying processed foods.

Eating Close to Home

Back in our hunter-gatherer past, all food was locally obtained. But now it is possible to buy organic broccoli from China and Chilean-grown blueberries in the dead of winter. Shipping this food around the planet generates a lot of greenhouse gas emissions. Try going local this year.

One of the ways you can reduce your impact on our planet's natural resources is by eating foods obtained from local sources rather than purchasing food grown across the country or across the planet. It sounds daunting, but it can be done through a combination of growing and gathering food during the growing season, canning and freezing as much as possible, and relying on stored foods and animal products during the cold months.

Why go to all this trouble? The average food item travels 1,500 miles from farm to table. Fossil fuels power the transit of food. A bag of frozen organic broccoli grown in China must travel a minimum 6,926 miles to get to a store in Washington, D.C. (if taking the most direct "as the crow flies" route). An airplane that travels this distance will generate 5,496 pounds of planet-warming carbon dioxide.

Eating like a locavore—a play on the word omnivore—can cut the toes off your carbon footprint. The Natural Resources Defense Council (NRDC) estimates that if all Americans cut just one quarter-pound burger from their diet per week, the greenhouse gas savings would be equivalent to taking four to six million cars off the road.

But environmental concerns are only one reason to go local. Food eaten in season tastes better. As an added benefit, you will support local farmers and help keep family-owned farms in business. You'll also build community as you meet farmers and make friends with others who are trying to live eco-consciously.

Involve your kids in the decision to take on the locavore challenge. They may be thrilled to take up the quest to find grass-fed beef from nearby farms or to pick fresh organic produce at a local farm. (Or they may want to head to the nearest fast-food chain with great haste.) Other adults in your household will probably want a say as well. If you are not ready to go 100 percent local, a viable alternative is to try to buy as many foods as possible that were grown or produced in your area whenever you can.

Drinking Water

We take clean drinking water for granted in the United States, but we only have to go back a hundred years to find epidemics of cholera and typhoid in our great cities. Although municipal water systems now provide water that is free of most pathogens, some water supplies contain impurities that can present a hazard to your family's health. Let's take a look at the issues.

GET THE LEAD OUT Lead is a potent neurotoxicant that can do irreversible damage to an infant or child's developing brain. Homes built before the 1930s often had lead pipe plumbing. Look for dull gray metal pipes that are easily scratched with a house key. Later, copper pipes with lead solder became standard. Brass fittings and faucets are still another source of lead in drinking water. These types of plumbing can leach lead into your drinking water.

Most problems with lead in drinking water come from household pipes, not the municipal water supply. Water with low pH may help dissolve lead into the water. Mineral deposits on the interior of the pipe can act as a barrier between the lead and the water, but the only way to know for sure is to test your water.

IF YOU THINK YOU HAVE LEAD IN YOUR WATER, HERE ARE SOME TIPS:

✓ Run the cold water to flush out lead from the pipes any time that the tap has not been used in the previous six hours. For example, you'll want to run the tap each morning to remove lead that may have leached out of the pipes overnight. When you feel that the water is as cold as it is going to get, you can turn off the tap (usually about 5 to 30 seconds).

✓ Use only cold tap water—not hot—for drinking, cooking, and preparing baby formula. Hot tap water contains more dissolved lead than does cold water.

✓ Have your water tested for lead. Several companies offer this test, which involves collecting some samples and mailing them off to a company. According to the EPA, it is especially important to have testing done if you live in an apartment building, since flushing does not adequately remove lead from large plumbing systems.

✓ Use a filter to remove lead. Lead can be removed by carbon filters, reverse osmosis, and distillation.

GET RID OF RADON If you live in an area with high soil radon, you may also have high levels of radon in your well water or municipal water. Radon is a known cancer-causing agent, so the best amount of it in the water is *none*. A cancer-causing agent is viewed as being able to cause cancer even in minute amounts, especially if exposure happens over a long period of time. Drinking radon in water contributes to one's risk of stomach cancer. Breathing radon gas that escapes from the water during showering can contribute to lung cancer risk. Radon can be removed by carbon filtration.

DITCH THE CHLORINE DISINFECTION BY-PRODUCTS Trihalomethanes (THMs) are disinfection by-products that form when chlorine reacts with organic matter such as treated sewage, leaves, soil, and animal waste. THMs are linked to increased cancer risk as well as toxicity to the kidneys, liver, and nervous system. They have also been linked to birth defects in some studies. THMs can be removed by carbon filtration.

ASK FOR ARSENIC-FREE Arsenic naturally occurs in soils and rocks, and it was also applied to orchards as a pesticide. Arsenic can cause lung, bladder, kidney, and skin cancer and other skin conditions. Low levels have been found to disrupt hormones. Arsenic can be removed by carbon filtration, but is best removed by reverse osmosis or distillation.

BAN THE COLIFORM BACTERIA The presence of these bacteria could indicate your water is contaminated with *Cryptosporidium,* a parasite that can be life threatening for people with compromised immune systems. Parasites can be removed by ultraviolet light treatment, reverse osmosis, and distillation.

ELIMINATE THE ATRAZINE This herbicide is commonly used on corn and has emerged as a significant water contaminant in the Midwest. Atrazine is a suspected hormone disrupter and has been linked to preterm delivery. In animal studies atrazine causes liver, kidney, and heart damage. Atrazine can be removed by carbon filtration.

SAY NO TO NITRATES Nitrates are used in fertilizers and can contaminate groundwater and surface water drinking supplies. Nitrates are converted to nitrites in the body. High levels of nitrates in drinking water can interfere with the oxygen-carrying capacity of blood in infants, causing shortness of breath and blueness of the skin as well as brain damage if not treated. Nitrates can be removed by carbon filtration, reverse osmosis, and distillation.

CHOOSING A WATER PURIFIER Before choosing a water purifier, have your water tested so that you know what contaminants you need to eliminate. The EPA recommends that private well owners test their drinking water annually for coliform bacteria and nitrates. Test more regularly if radon and pesticides are a problem in your area. Your local health department can tell you which contaminants are common where you live.

If you have municipal water, check your water company's water quality report, required by law to be sent to customers annually. To request a copy, go to your water company's website or check the EPA's website at *www.epa.gov/safewater.*

When considering installing a water purifier, it pays to do a little research. Water filters come in several different technologies (see below) and each is better at removing some contaminants than others. Reputable manufacturers will be able to provide a list of the type of contaminants as well as the level to which they are removed.

Before you buy, make sure that the device is certified by the National Sanitation Foundation (NSF), *www.nsf.org,* so that you know the filter performs as advertised. Also check whether the device is certified by the California Department of Public Health, *www.cdph.ca.gov,* which requires devices to be tested by an independent, state-approved laboratory.

CARBON FILTERS Countertop gravity carafes and faucet units use filters containing activated charcoal, a form of carbon that is extremely porous. These filters remove lead, radon, MTBE and other volatile organic compounds, THMs and other chlorine by-products, some organic chemicals, and odors and tastes. Activated charcoal filters cannot remove some pesticides, fluoride, or perchlorate. Still, for the price, these filters are extremely useful and will protect your family against many contaminants.

CERAMIC FILTERS These filters can remove bacteria and sediments, and they are often teamed with carbon filters.

DISTILLATION This water purification process removes heavy metals and minerals. It involves heating water into steam, which is then moved to a separate chamber where it is cooled and allowed to return to a liquid state. The contaminants are left behind in the original container. Distillers can be cumbersome to operate and maintain and may be overkill for most household uses.

REVERSE OSMOSIS One of the most effective water filtration methods, reverse osmosis involves pushing water through tiny pores in a membrane. Typically the water first flows through a carbon filter to remove chlorine by-products, radon, and other contaminants and then flows through the reverse osmosis membrane, which removes metals, nitrates, perchlorate, and industrial chemicals. For each gallon purified, roughly 3 to 5 gallons must be discarded, so reverse osmosis is wasteful and expensive, since homeowners have to pay for the extra water as well as the regular change of filters.

ULTRAVIOLET LIGHT This method can kill bacteria, viruses, molds, cysts, and parasites. However, it should be used as a supplemental treatment in addition to another filtration method to remove metals, chlorine, and organic chemicals.

When considering all these filters, keep in mind some basic questions:
- ✓ Does the filter remove the contaminants of concern in my water?
- ✓ Does the performance of the filter justify the cost, or are there cheaper alternatives?
- ✓ Is the system easy to maintain?
- ✓ Will the system waste water?
- ✓ Does the system take out beneficial minerals along with pollutants?

BAN THE BOTTLE Bottled water can be a temporary solution to water quality problems in your home, but you should not use bottled water for the long term. Here's why:

- ✗ Bottled water is not necessarily better or safer than tap water. In fact, regulation of bottled water is less strict than tap water regulation.

× Companies are not required to disclose the source of bottled water, the type of treatment or filtration used, or the contaminants detected. Municipal water providers must supply this information to customers annually.

× Bottled water may contain chlorination by-products, cancer-causing chemicals, trace amounts of medicines, and bacteria, according to a 2008 study by the Environmental Working Group, *www.ewg.org/reports/bottledwater*.

× Unhealthy chemicals such as bisphenol A can migrate from some types of plastic bottles to the water.

× Some bottled water *is* tap water. Some manufacturers simply pour municipal water straight into bottles despite the rural scenes depicted on the labels.

× Bottles are extremely wasteful. The plastic persists for years in landfills and contributes to a growing waste-disposal problem worldwide.

Take Action

▸ Eat beef less often. Substitute with beans, peas, nuts, and dairy foods.

▸ Choose grass-fed beef if possible.

▸ Avoid meats from animals raised using growth promoting antibiotics and hormones.

▸ Purchase lunch meats and hot dogs processed without nitrates and nitrites.

▸ Choose fish that are from well-managed fisheries and that are low in contaminants.

▸ Read labels carefully to make sure you are getting the quality foods you are paying for.

▸ Buy USDA-certified organic vegetables and fruits whenever possible.

▸ Consider planting a vegetable garden with your kids.

▸ Try to eat foods grown or raised locally as often as possible.

▸ Always wash hands prior to preparing meals. Cook all meats thoroughly.

▸ Have your well water tested regularly for contaminants. Read the water testing data sheet that your municipal water supplier sends each year.

▸ When considering installing a water purifier, check to make sure it is certified to remove the contaminants. Match the type of purifier to the type of contaminants you need removed.

▸ Use a reusable water bottle instead of buying bottled water.

▸ Get your pasteurized milk from organic producers or dairies that don't use recombinant bovine somatotropin (rBST).

THE SCIENCE BEHIND IT

Hormones in Milk

Most milk production in the United States is a highly industrialized process. Today's dairy cows produce about 6 gallons of milk per day. They eat a diet rich in cornmeal, a non-natural food for cows, and are treated with antibiotics. To stimulate additional milk production, many cows are also given recombinant bovine growth hormone (rBGH), also known as recombinant bovine somatotropin (rBST).

The practice of giving rBST to dairy cows has generated a tremendous amount of debate in the United States. Critics claim that the FDA approved rBST based on inadequate testing.

Most health agencies have found that milk from rBST-treated cows is perfectly safe for humans. The level of BST in milk from rBST-treated cows is identical to the level of BST in milk from untreated cows. What is more, BST is not active in the human body because humans lack the biological receptors for it.

Although BST is not active in humans, another hormone found in the milk *is* active. Recombinant BST stimulates cows to produce in their milk another hormone called insulin-like growth factor-1 (IGF-1). Unlike BST, which is not active in the human body, cow IGF-1 is cross-reactive with human IGF-1. Cows treated with rBST produce 25 to 74 percent more IGF-1 in their milk than do untreated cows.

IGF-1 controls normal human growth and also may contribute to increased risk of colon, prostate, and breast cancers.[14] No studies have proven that rBST causes cancer in humans. Still, many parents choose to steer clear of rBST-treated milk because of the potential for small amounts of hormones to have effects on developing fetuses and young children.

Although rBST may pose no health threat to humans, the hormone *does* pose a threat to the health of cows. Dairy cows injected with rBST are at greater risk of developing an udder infection, or mastitis. Mastitis can cause pain to the animal and cause pus to form in the milk. To prevent mastitis, cows are regularly treated with preventative antibiotics, a practice that may contribute to the development of antibiotic-resistant bacteria.

Other cow health concerns include reproductive problems, injection site reactions, and foot or leg problems, according to the product label. Owing to concerns over the health and well-being of the cows, the hormone is not approved for use in the European Union, New Zealand, Japan, Australia, or Canada.

In the United States, the company that makes rBST originally tried to stop dairies from labeling their products as "rBST-free" on the grounds that there are no significant differences between rBST-treated and untreated milk. Several court cases have found in favor of dairies to have the right to label their products. Several large supermarket chains and discount stores have pledged to stop buying milk from dairies that use rBST. The use of rBST in the dairy industry appears to be waning due to consumer opposition.

LIVING WELL

Practical Tips for Keeping Your Children Healthy

FROM FIRST AID FOR SKINNED KNEES TO DECIDING WHETHER OR not to make a midnight trip to the emergency room, parenthood is a crash course in medical education. By the time the kids head off to college, many parents feel they have earned the equivalent of a medical degree. But despite living in the information age, we parents sometimes find it difficult to locate solid advice on how to protect our children against illnesses, especially ones that have environmental causes.

Most illnesses are nothing to be worried about. Health experts believe that coming in contact with viruses and other disease-causing germs in our environment builds healthy immune systems. But some environmental exposures have been linked to more serious disorders such as asthma and allergies, learning and behavioral issues, and childhood cancers. The way in which we interact with the natural world also influences the development and spread of newer illnesses such as Lyme disease, antibiotic-resistant superbugs, and new forms of influenza.

In this chapter we'll look at ways to keep our children as healthy as possible while recognizing that sickness is a normal part of childhood. We will talk about how to treat common colds and fevers without reflexively reaching for the medicine bottle. We'll venture into the vaccination debate and address some of the concerns that have led parents to refuse lifesaving vaccines for their babies. We'll explore the "epidemics" of neurobehavioral disorders, specifically attention deficit/hyperactivity disorder (ADHD) and autism, that a growing number of scientists and parents think are related to environmental exposures. And we'll discuss emerging diseases that arise from interactions of humans with the environment. We'll investigate why asthma, allergies, and childhood cancer rates are on the rise and review the evidence for environmental triggers of these diseases. We'll round up with a treatment of dental health practices, such as the use of mercury amalgam fillings that threaten the environment and our children's health.

This chapter is not meant to substitute for professional advice, so always consult your child's pediatrician about your child's health.

Staying Healthy

A nutritious diet, regular exercise, and adequate sleep can do wonders for boosting the body's ability to fight illnesses. Help your children avoid getting colds by teaching them good hygiene practices, such as washing their hands regularly.

KEEP GERMS AT BAY The body is designed to defend against viruses and other disease-causing agents. The skin acts as a barrier to keep most pathogens out, and the immune system is standing at the ready to suppress any invaders that make it into the body through the skin, nose, mouth, and eyes.

But the immune system needs our help to keep it in good working order. Healthy food, adequate sleep, and regular exercise contribute to keeping the body, and the immune system, in peak condition. When kids stay healthy, you'll have less of a need to buy medicines that can be harmful to children's health and can damage the environment when they are discarded.

SCHOOLS AND CHILD CARE CENTERS are places where children can easily trade disease-causing germs. Here are some tips for minimizing the spread of colds and flu:

✓ Always have your children wash their hands in warm soapy water, scrubbing for 20 seconds at least, before eating and directly after going to the bathroom. (See The Science Behind It at the end of this chapter.)

✓ Avoid antibacterial soaps, which do not kill the viruses that cause colds and flu. These products often contain triclosan, a chemical that is linked to liver toxicity, is suspected of disrupting thyroid function, is harmful to aquatic life, and may contribute to the development of antibiotic-resistant strains of bacteria.[2]

THE FACTS

An increasing number of drugs are made overseas where the U.S. Food and Drug Administration (FDA) oversight is practically nonexistent. This is especially true of generic drugs.[1]

THE FACTS
Most young children have six to ten colds per year, according to the American Academy of Pediatrics.

✓ Teach your child not to share drinking cups, eating utensils, washcloths, or towels with anyone who has a cold or fever. Discourage your child from touching his mouth, nose, and eyes, which bring viruses and bacteria in contact with sensitive mucous membranes.

✓ Always have your child cough and sneeze into a disposable tissue or to-be-washed handkerchief. If none are available, tell your child to cough or sneeze "into his elbow" or "into the crook of her arm" instead of onto his or her hand.

TIME-HONORED TREATMENTS Despite our best efforts, kids will get sick. Toddlers seem to be especially prone to getting colds. The toddler years coincide with the ending of breast-feeding and the resulting lack of protective antibodies from Mom. Also at this time many young children enter preschool or child care centers and come into contact with other children with colds.

When your child is suffering, your first instinct may be to reach for a bottle of cold or cough reliever. But these medicines are not necessarily safe or effective, especially for young children. Several studies indicate that cold medicines don't work in children less than six years of age, according to the American Academy of Pediatrics. And using these medications comes with risks: More than 1,500 babies and toddlers visited emergency rooms from 2004 to 2005 and three died due to bad reactions or overdoses of cold or cough medicine, according to the Centers for Disease Control and Prevention (CDC).

COMMONSENSE REMEDIES FOR SICK KIDS:

✓ Give your child plenty of liquids to drink.

✓ Keep the room warm but not too hot.

✓ A humidifier can be used to moisten the air, which can help ease breathing.

✓ Severe stuffiness can be relieved with a few drops of nasal saline and a bulb syringe to suck out mucus.

✓ For children over one year old, a cup of weak herbal tea such as chamomile mixed with a teaspoon of honey can sooth the throat. Do not give honey to babies less than one year old.

✓ Placing pillows beneath your child's head so that he or she sleeps in a reclining position can help drain mucus from the airways and relieve coughing.

✓ If your child has a barking cough, which is a sign of croup, humidity can relieve breathing. Turn on the hot water in the shower, and take the child into the bathroom.

✓ To bring down a fever, moisten a washcloth with lukewarm water and gently wipe your child's forehead and body. The evaporation of water

ECO-TIP:
ENVIRONMENTALLY FRIENDLY TISSUES

Kids with runny noses go through a lot of tissues. Most conventional tissues are made from wood cellulose pulp from virgin trees, not recycled fibers. The average American uses 50 pounds of tissue paper per year. Look for tissues that contain a high content of postconsumer waste (PCW) recycled paper.

from the skin will help bring down the temperature. A warm bath can effectively reduce even high fevers, again because of the cooling effect of evaporation.

✓ Eighty percent of children with ear infections will get better without antibiotics, according to the American Academy of Pediatrics. Many pediatricians now recommend treating the pain and waiting two days or so to see if the infection clears up without antibiotics.

ECO-TIP: DISPOSE OF MERCURY THERMOMETERS

If you haven't done so already, dispose of any oral thermometers containing mercury. Replace mercury thermometers with digital ones. Consult your state or local health department for disposal options. Never throw a mercury thermometer in the trash. Some states have thermometer collection or exchange programs. Check the website of the U.S. Environmental Protection Agency (EPA) at *www.epa.gov/osw/hazard/tsd/mercury/collect.htm.*

THE FACTS

Pharmaceutical drugs have been found in the drinking water systems that serve at least 41 million Americans, according to an Associated Press investigation in 2008.[3] The list of medicines found includes antibiotics, birth control hormones, antidepressants, veterinary medicines, and mood stabilizers.

IF YOU NEED TO USE MEDICATION IN YOUNG CHILDREN, FOLLOW THESE GUIDELINES:

✓ Always read labels carefully and avoid overdosing by making sure you don't give two products that contain the same active ingredient.

✓ Use medications only as directed.

✓ Store medications safely out of the reach of children.

✓ Call a doctor if you are unsure of how much medication to administer.

✓ Use the measuring device (cup, dropper) that came with the medication. Never use a household spoon.

✓ Never treat a child's fever with aspirin, as it is linked to a severe disease called Reye's syndrome.

ECO-TIP: DISPOSE OF MEDICINES PROPERLY

If you have old or expired pills in your medicine cabinet, it is a good idea to dispose of them. The old advice was to dump expired pills into the toilet, but pharmaceutical products are showing up in lakes and rivers where they can pose a hazard to fish and other aquatic organisms. For example, birth control pills contain human hormones that may interfere with the hormone systems of wildlife.

HERE ARE SOME TIPS FOR PROPER DISPOSAL OF PHARMACEUTICALS:

✕ **Do not flush medications down the toilet or drain.**

✓ **Refer to the label for safety or disposal information.**

✓ **Check with your pharmacy to see if it disposes of unused or expired medications. Many pharmacies now have "take back" programs.**

✓ **Contact your municipality or local health department to locate a nearby household hazardous waste collection center.**

UNWELCOME VISITORS (LICE) Lice are a common childhood affliction. These small insects can spread from child to child in the classroom. While most parents have to deal with them at some point or other, there is no reason to use toxic pesticides to combat them. Toxic pesticides such as lindane and pyrethroids can have harmful effects on the environment and on your child.

Lindane is an acutely toxic organochlorine pesticide that easily passes through the skin. Application of lindane lotion or shampoo to the scalp has caused cases of permanent brain damage and death in children and adults who did not follow the package directions, according to the FDA. Neurological side effects can occur even in people who used the product as directed. Lindane is linked to cancer in animal studies, and it can contaminate water. Its use is banned in 52 countries and the state of California. *Never* reapply lindane because it didn't work the first time, as this is how the majority of poisonings occurred.

Other lice shampoos may contain pesticides from the pyrethroid family of chemicals. Pyrethroids may be either natural (pyrethrum, which is derived from chrysanthemums), or synthetic (permethrin). Both have potentially neurotoxic effects.[4] Malathion (an organophosphate) is also used against lice. Organophosphates have been linked to learning disorders and should be avoided (see section on learning disorders later in this chapter).

TRY THESE LICE-REMOVAL TIPS:
✓ Use a nit-removal comb to remove the nits (lice eggs).
✓ Try home remedies such as olive oil, coconut oil, essential oils such as

GREEN ON A SHOESTRING

Instead of buying tissues, save money and trees by using washable handkerchiefs. Fold the handkerchief into a 2-inch square, then unfold prior to use. After blowing, fold the hanky back up to keep viruses inside. Don't reuse the same blowing surface twice.

lavender or rosemary, castile soap, and heat from a hair dryer. If you use essential oils, dilute them according to package directions. Some essential oils can burn the skin if directly applied.

✓ Wash all bedding, towels, and affected clothing and hats in hot water.

✓ Vacuum carpets thoroughly and mop floors with hot soapy water.

✓ Check all family members to make sure the lice haven't spread.

✓ When checking family members for nits, use a louse stick (a small wooden stick, one per child) and wash hands thoroughly between checking each child.

Supplements

From herbal treatments to probiotics, dietary supplements are becoming more popular for use in children. Many parents report that herbal supplements help with the prevention and treatment of colds. If you are considering using supplements, do as much research as possible because most have not been tested for safety.

Over half of all American adults, or nearly 114 million adults, take supplements, be they vitamins, herbs, energy drinks, or products that promise weight loss, according to figures from the Government Accountability Office (GAO). Studies show that people who take supplements are indeed healthier, but these people also tend to eat better and get more exercise than the average American, so it is not clear whether the healthier status is due to supplements or other lifestyle factors.

Dietary supplements, as defined by the FDA, include vitamins, minerals, botanical products, amino acids, and substances such as enzymes, probiotics, and metabolites. In fact, many of these supplements are indeed beneficial, some do nothing, some may be dangerous, and in many cases we just don't know.

Consumers sometimes make the mistake of thinking that because these products are "natural," they must be safe. Many herbal treatments have been used in traditional medicine for centuries and have good safety and efficacy records even though they've never been rigorously tested. Others may be relatively new and have not been tested for safety, or they may be contaminated with chemicals that can be damaging to children and the environment.

In fact, many vitamin and mineral supplements are unnecessary. Public health officials recommend that children get their vitamins and minerals from a diet rich in vegetables and fruits.

USE SUPPLEMENTS SAFELY Many parents are concerned—and rightly so—about the safety of supplements. Supplements are not evaluated by the FDA the way pharmaceuticals are. Supplement manufacturers are not required to register their products with the FDA, nor do they need to get FDA approval before producing or selling products. The only course the FDA can take is to prohibit the sale of unsafe products *after* they've reached the market and *after* they've caused harm.

Many supplements are imported from countries with lax safety standards or poor oversight of manufacturing facilities. According to a January 2009 analysis by the GAO, the FDA did not conduct a single inspection of foreign supplement manufacturing facilities from mid-2000 through mid-2008.[5] The FDA did ban the importation of over 3,600 dietary supplements from mid-2002 through March 2008, and 25 percent of the bans were due to the potential presence of an unsafe substance.

Unsafe substances include metals such as lead, which is toxic to the developing brain. The FDA in 2008 tested 324 women's and children's vitamin supplements and found that all but four of the products tested contained lead. The agency determined that the amount of lead did not exceed established safety levels, but most public health officials agree than any amount of lead can be hazardous to brain development in fetuses, infants, and young children. See the website *http://vm.cfsan.fda.gov/~dms/pbvitami.html* for the list of vitamins tested.

Some popular supplements for which there is good safety information for children and at least some evidence of efficacy include vitamin C for preventing colds, echinacea for diminishing the severity of colds, evening primrose oil for relieving symptoms of eczema, omega-3 fatty acids for improving attention and cognitive function, and probiotics for treatment of irritable bowel syndrome, Crohn's disease, and other gastrointestinal issues.

GREEN ON A SHOESTRING

Sales of dietary supplements in the United States reached nearly 24 million dollars in 2007. Yet most vitamins and supplements are unnecessary if children eat a balanced diet and get plenty of rest and exercise.

TIPS FOR TAKING SUPPLEMENTS SAFELY:

✓ Before adding supplements to your child's diet, consult your pediatrician. Some supplements can interact with prescription or over-the-counter medications your child is taking.

✓ Gather as much information as you can about the supplement or vitamin you are considering. (See the section "Do Your Homework" below.)

✓ Choose reputable brands. Look for the United States Pharmacopeia symbol (USP), which ensures pharmaceutical-grade quality.

✓ Stay within the recommended daily allowances. Some supplements (including many vitamins and minerals, such as zinc) can be toxic at too high doses.

✓ Teach your child that vitamins and supplements are not candy even if they are tasty and colorful. Store all supplements out of reach of children.

✓ Beware of medical claims that sound too good to be true.

✓ Avoid kava, aristolochic acid, comfrey, androstenedione, and ephedra. A full list of FDA warnings can be found at *www.fda.gov/Food/DietarySupplements/Alerts*.

✓ If you or your child has an adverse reaction to a supplement or drug, report it to the FDA's MedWatch program at *www.fda.gov/Safety/MedWatch*.

DO YOUR HOMEWORK Lack of safety is coupled with lack of proof that the supplements actually do what manufacturers claim they do. Few supplements have been extensively studied in adults or children to find the dose that provides the maximal benefit.

LEARN MORE ABOUT SUPPLEMENTS:

- The National Institutes of Health's (NIH) Dietary Supplements Labels Database offers information about ingredients in more than 3,000 selected brands of dietary supplements at *http://dietarysupplements.nlm.nih.gov*.

- The NIH Office of Dietary Supplements (ODS) has an extensive list of dietary supplement fact sheets on everything from aloe vera to zinc at *http://ods.od.nih.gov*.

- The Institute of Medicine lists daily allowances for various populations (infants, children, pregnant women, etc.) at *www.iom.edu/Object.File/Master/7/294/0.pdf*.

- The National Center for Complementary and Alternative Medicine (NCCAM) maintains the "A to Z Index of Health Topics" with fact sheets on alternative treatments such as acupuncture, meditation, herbal supplements, and sections on alternative remedies for diseases at *http://nccam.nih.gov*.

- PubMed, the national database for all medical research, can be searched for complementary and alternative medicine and supplements at *http://nccam.nih.gov/research/camonpubmed*.

- The International Bibliographic Information on Dietary Supplements (IBIDS) database logs brief summaries of studies and is easy to use at *http://grande.nal.usda.gov/ibids*.

- USDA's Food and Nutrition Information Center (FNIC) has a section on dietary supplements with many links to more information at *http://fnic .nal.usda.gov.*
- The U.S. Pharmacopeia (USP) conducts independent testing of dietary supplement ingredients. Products with the USP Verified Dietary Supplement Mark on the label have been tested for purity, potency, and quality. See *www.usp.org.*
- The American Council on Science and Health has a website listing common drug-supplement interactions at *www.acsh.org/publications/ pubID.515/pub_detail.asp.*
- The FDA's Center for Food Safety and Nutrition maintains information on supplements at *www.fda.gov/Food/DietarySupplements.*

Vaccines

Vaccines prevent diseases. Yet today we face a controversy over the safety of vaccines. Parents and physicians alike are concerned about whether vaccines are linked to autism or health problems. We'll examine the issues.

No one wants to go back to living in a prevaccination world. Just a few hundred years ago, parents watched powerlessly as their children died from diseases that are now preventable through vaccination. Vaccines have saved countless lives and have nearly eradicated certain diseases such as small pox and, in some countries, polio.

Vaccination is successful not only because vaccinated children are protected, but also because unvaccinated children are protected through what scientists call "herd protection." When the majority of individuals in a population are vaccinated, the disease-causing pathogen cannot find nonprotected "hosts" in which to replicate and spread. But if enough parents refuse vaccinations, the pathogen could infect susceptible individuals in the population, resulting in an outbreak.

Most parents understand the rationale behind vaccination and the benefits of herd protection, but some are concerned about the ingredients in vaccines, the sheer number of vaccines, and the question of whether vaccines can cause autism or other problems. While there are many sources of information on vaccines, most parents don't have time to sift through stacks of scientific studies. Pediatricians are required to provide parents with Vaccine Information

Statements explaining the rationale for each vaccine and its potential side effects, but few doctors have the time to go over the documents with parents. In this section we'll touch on the major controversies and reveal why most parents decide to vaccinate their children.

THE PEDIATRIC VACCINES The CDC currently recommends vaccination against the following diseases:

FOR INFANTS AND YOUNG CHILDREN:
- Haemophilus Influenzae type B (HIB): A bacteria that causes potentially fatal meningitis and bloodstream infections, mainly in infants and young children.
- Pneumococcal Disease: A bacteria that causes meningitis, bloodstream infections, and pneumonia, mainly in infants and the elderly. It can be fatal.
- Diptheria: A bacteria that causes a severe throat and upper lung infection. It can be fatal. It has nearly been eradicated in the United States.
- Tetanus: A common bacteria that can thrive in deep wounds. It causes weakness and paralysis and can be fatal.
- Pertussis (Whooping Cough): A bacteria that causes severe coughing and can be fatal, mainly in infants. It is still common in the United States.
- Hepatitis A: A virus that causes diarrhea and mild liver damage. It is fairly common and seldom fatal.
- Hepatitis B: A virus that is contracted via blood transfusions or sexual activity. It causes severe liver damage and can be fatal.
- Rotavirus: A virus that causes severe diarrhea, vomiting, and dehydration in infants. It is very common and can be fatal.
- Polio: A virus that causes muscle weakness and paralysis. Vaccination campaigns have eradicated it from the United States. It can be fatal.
- Measles: A virus that causes fever and rash, can damage internal organs, and can be fatal.
- Mumps: A virus that causes fever and swelling of the salivary glands, can damage internal organs, and can lead to male infertility. It is rarely fatal.
- Rubella: A virus that causes fever and rash, and can cause birth defects in infants whose mothers were exposed to the disease during pregnancy.
- Chicken pox (Varicella): A virus that causes fever and rash. It is rarely fatal, except in elderly or immunocompromised persons.

FOR CHILDREN 6 MONTHS AND OLDER:
- Flu (Influenza): A virus that is very common and can cause fatalities in infants and elderly. Source: CDC www.cde.gov/vaccines

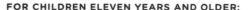

FOR CHILDREN ELEVEN YEARS AND OLDER:

- Meningococcal Disease: A bacteria that causes bloodstream infections and meningitis. It has a high fatality rate.
- Human Papillomavirus (HPV): A virus that is spread through sexual contact and causes genital warts and cervical cancer later in life. Cervical cancer can be fatal. '

VACCINE INGREDIENTS Although vaccines are thoroughly tested for safety, many parents have raised issues about the ingredients that have been used in the past or are being used today. Two of the biggest concerns are mercury, which was phased out of vaccines in the early 2000s, and aluminum, which is still used today.

Mercury: Mercury in the form of thimerosol was added to vaccines as a preservative in formulations manufactured before 2002. Mercury is a known neurotoxicant. During the 1990s, several new vaccines were added to the pediatric schedule without attention to the amount of thimerosol that babies would receive on a single day. As a result, depending on the combination of vaccines, some six-month-old babies received a cumulative dose of mercury that was 87 times greater than the EPA's safe dose, according to an article in the *Los Angeles Times*.[6] However this information did not come to light until the late 1990s, and it was then that the CDC asked pediatric vaccine makers to voluntarily stop using thimerosol.

Today's pediatric vaccines are either mercury-free or contain just a tiny amount that most health experts say presents no risk. The one exception is the influenza vaccine. Thimerosol is still commonly used as a preservative in flu shots, so ask your pediatrician if he or she stocks a mercury-free version. If not, you may want to call around until you find one.

Most studies have failed to find that thimerosol in vaccines caused or contributed to autism, according to the CDC. If thimerosol was indeed the cause of autism, we should have seen a decline in autism rates by now. But the decline has not happened, and autism rates are continuing to rise.

For a listing of thimerosol content in U.S.-licensed vaccines, go to *www .vaccinesafety.edu/thi-table*.

Aluminum: This metal is added to vaccines to improve their performance. Aluminum is normally harmless in small amounts and is found in air, soil, and food, including breast milk and infant formula. The protective mechanisms in the stomach and intestines seem capable of keeping much of this aluminum from entering the bloodstream. Yet aluminum in the blood can cause toxicity to the central nervous system. Vaccines are injected into the muscle, but few studies have looked at how much gets from the muscle into the blood.

Most of the studies of aluminum's toxicity in newborns have been conducted using intravenous (IV) infusions that premature or sick babies get in the hospital. The FDA requires that these solutions contain no more than 25 micrograms of aluminum per liter. Yet many vaccines for infants contain 200 to 300 micrograms of aluminum in a single shot, and children can get much higher amounts on a single day if the brands with the highest amounts of aluminum are used.[7]

No studies have looked to see if these high doses given on a single day cause harm. It may not be fair to directly compare intravenous administration with injection into the muscle, since intramuscularly delivered aluminum will diffuse into the body more slowly compared to intravenous infusion.

If you are concerned about aluminum or your child has a kidney impairment that would prevent him or her from eliminating aluminum, consult your pediatrician. If your pediatrician does not know how much aluminum he or she is dispensing to infants on a single day, ask for the brand names of the vaccines used at the practice, and do your own research.

A VACCINE-AUTISM CONNECTION? Many parents suspect vaccines are responsible for their child's autism. Autism is usually noticed in the toddler years around the time when children are getting routine vaccinations. Many parents can point to a specific round of vaccinations that seemed to incite fussiness and disruptive behavior. They may also have noticed regression in a child's speech and behavior.

Three different theories attempt to link autism to vaccines. One theory is that the measles-mumps-rubella (MMR) vaccine contributes to autism, and this is based on studies that found live measles virus in the gut of autistic children. A second theory is that autism is due to the presence of mercury (as the preservative thimerosol) in vaccines until 2002. A third camp says that the sheer number of vaccines, including up to five shots on a single day, are inflaming the immune system and causing damage to the brain. As evidence these researchers point to the fact that autism rates began rising in the early 1990s, around the time that the number of injections per child escalated from 10 shots in 1989 to 36 shots today.

The issue is a contentious one, with some researchers saying that today's vaccine schedule is safe and others calling for more research. A large study in Denmark, published in the 2002 *New England Journal of Medicine*, failed to find differences in autism rates between MMR-vaccinated and -unvaccinated children.[8]

Clearly more research needs to be done to reassure parents of vaccine safety. It may be that certain subpopulations of children have gene variants that make them susceptible to autism following vaccination. Some children with mitochondrial disorders, for example, have symptoms that are worsened by vaccination. Another possibility is that children with immunological problems may be more susceptible to vaccine-induced disorders.

Although public health officials stand behind the safety of vaccines and discount any connection between vaccination and autism, this subject needs further research and outreach. Parents need to be reassured that vaccines are safe. Otherwise even more parents will refuse to have their children vaccinated, raising the risk of a return of deadly diseases that are easily preventable.

ALTERNATIVE VACCINATION SCHEDULES If you are thinking about using an alternative vaccine schedule, don't go it alone. Consult with a pediatrician to find out which vaccines can be delayed or omitted without risking your child's health. Several of the vaccines received in the first year are for diseases that are only a threat in early childhood. Pertussis and rotavirus are usually serious only in the first two years of life. HIB and pneumococcus occur mainly during the first or second year. Some vaccines, like the rotavirus vaccine, need to be given early in life to be effective.

TIPS IF YOU DECIDE TO AVOID SOME OR ALL VACCINES:

✓ Raise your concerns with your child's pediatrician. The more doctors hear about concerns, the more likely public health officials will be to investigate vaccine safety.

✓ If your child is not vaccinated, you should be more vigilant about watching for symptoms like rash and fever, and take your child to the doctor soon after noticing the symptoms.

✓ Keep your child's immune system healthy.

✗ Do not send your unvaccinated young child to day care, playgroups, or other settings where he or she will be exposed to lots of children.

✓ Consider that immunization of children for rubella protects pregnant caregivers and teachers whose babies could develop birth defects if exposed.

✓ If your child has signs of an immune system abnormality, such as unusual or difficult to treat infections, or you have a family history of immune disorders, talk with your physician about vaccinating your child safely, as recommended by researchers at the M.I.N.D. Institute at the University of California, Davis.

✓ To attend public school, most children must be vaccinated or have an official exemption. Check with your state health department regarding vaccination requirements.

Some pediatricians refuse to continue to treat patients whose parents question the vaccination schedule or the need for certain vaccines. In fact, the American Academy of Pediatrics *does not* endorse the practice of "firing" patients. Nonvaccinated children will most likely need more medical care, not less, than vaccinated children.

Learning Disorders

Several chemicals are known to damage the developing brain, leaving a child with lifelong learning and/or behavioral disorders. In this section we examine the chemical exposures that are linked to learning disorders, and we talk about some of the difficulties in pinning down cause-and-effect relationships between environmental exposures and the increase in ADHD and autism rates.

The development of the brain is a complex and carefully synchronized process. The brain begins forming early in pregnancy with the creation of the neural tube, which gives rise to the brain and spinal cord. Brain formation involves an intricate rollout of different cell types that make precise connections with each other. Each neuron gets coated in an insulative protein sheath called myelin. Chemicals act as neurotransmitters that pass messages from cell to cell. Development of the brain continues through adolescence. If any one of these steps goes awry, cognitive functions can be changed forever.

Many chemicals in the environment can cause these orchestrated steps to go awry. We know this from both animal and human studies. Environmental chemicals are suspected of causing learning and cognitive impairments such as ADHD, autism, dyslexia, and intellectual disability. These first two appear to be on the rise, with rates of ADHD pegged somewhere between 3 to 8 out of every 100 children and autism reaching 1 out of every 150 children. Roughly 2 out of every 100 children are intellectually disabled. Altogether, learning and developmental disabilities affect between 5 and 15 out of every 100 children, according to the CDC.

ARE CHEMICALS TO BLAME FOR LEARNING DISORDERS? Lead and mercury are two substances for which scientists have ironclad proof of their ability to damage the developing brain. Scientists have pinpointed roughly ten chemicals (listed below) that are known to cause neurodevelopmental harm, according to a scientific consensus statement by leading researchers affiliated with the Institute for Children's Environmental Health (ICEH).[9] But the known chemicals are but drops in the bucket compared to the roughly 80,000 industrial chemicals in use today. Most of these chemicals have not been fully or even partially tested for developmental harm or neurotoxicity.

Of course, chemical exposures are not the only causes of learning and cognitive disorders. Many other factors play a role, including genes, nutritional deficits such as inadequate folate, infectious agents like viruses and bacteria, maternal stress, and parental use of recreational and medicinal drugs. These factors make it difficult to demonstrate the role of environmental chemicals in harming the developing brain.

Another reason it can be hard to demonstrate that chemicals harm the brain is that, when it comes to brain development, timing is everything. Scientists now know there are sensitive time periods during development. An exposure in the first trimester of pregnancy can have different effects than one toward the end of pregnancy. Other factors include the length of exposure, whether the chemical is rapidly excreted or prone to accumulate, the presence of combinations of chemicals, whether the chemical can cross into the brain, and whether the chemical impacts a bodily system that is sensitive to low doses of chemicals.

Yet another question is whether the chemical has different effects in genetically sensitive populations. We've learned through the Human Genome Project that we are all slightly different at the genetic level, and this discovery implies that chemicals can sicken some individuals and not others.

CHEMICALS LINKED TO DEVELOPMENTAL HARM Decades of studies have established a strong link between the following chemical exposures and learning and developmental defects in humans, according to the ICEH:

× **ALCOHOL** Prenatal exposure to alcohol causes behavioral and learning disabilities. Even low amounts of alcohol can cause damage.

× **LEAD** Lead exposure during infancy and childhood impairs memory, reduces intelligence, and causes behavioral issues. Lead is not safe even at minute exposure levels. See Chapter 1 for information about lead in paint and testing your child for lead. See Chapter 3 for lead in drinking water.

× **MERCURY** This metal causes deficits in memory, learning, and intelligence. Mercury is in the air we breathe (released from coal-fired power plants), the fish we eat (see Chapter 3 for a list of low-mercury fish), in flu vaccines, in household items like compact fluorescent bulbs (see Chapter 1), and in silver-colored dental fillings (discussed later in this chapter).

× **POLYCHLORINATED BIPHENYLS (PCBS)** These chemicals were used as insulating fluids around electrical transformers but were banned in the 1970s. However, they are extremely long-lived chemicals that accumulate in fat and can be transferred to babies in utero or during breastfeeding. PCBs can negatively affect learning and memory as well as motor skills.

× **POLYBROMINATED DIPHENYL ETHERS (PBDES)** These flame-retardant chemicals are persistent in the environment and accumulate in fat and breast milk. They are linked to poor motor skills and poor performance on learning and memory tests.

× **MANGANESE** This metal can damage the developing brain, causing impaired memory and speech. Minute amounts are needed by the body, making it an essential nutrient. Manganese is found in many dietary supplements.

× **ARSENIC** Arsenic is naturally occurring in drinking water in various parts of the world including some U.S. states. It is linked to cognitive impairment, as well as cancer and organ toxicity.

× **SOLVENTS** These chemicals are found in nail polish and hair dyes as well as in automotive shops, dry cleaners, and the household cleaning-supply closet or hobbyist's workshop. Exposure to solvents during pregnancy increases risk of developmental delays and visual deficits.

× **POLYAROMATIC HYDROCARBONS (PAHS)** PAHs are linked to lower birth weight and impaired cognitive development, among other health effects. They are made via the burning of gasoline, coal, cigarettes, and during cooking.

× **PESTICIDES** These chemicals are designed to kill insects, but they have an impact on the human nervous system as well. One class of pesticides, organophosphates, is linked to developmental disorders and deficits in

THE FACTS

Children are more susceptible to toxic substances in their environment than adults are. Per pound of body weight, children eat and breathe more than adults. Their nervous systems and organs are still forming and are susceptible to chemical interventions. Infants and toddlers spend a lot of time putting things in their mouths. Yet most studies of toxicity have been done in adults.

memory and motor skills. Exposure to pesticide mixtures is common, yet most chemical combinations go unstudied.

× **NICOTINE AND ENVIRONMENTAL TOBACCO SMOKE** Smoking while pregnant causes development delays and behavior disorders. Newer evidence indicates that breathing secondhand tobacco smoke during infancy and early childhood can also cause these disorders.

CHEMICALS SUSPECTED OF CAUSING HARM Chemicals for which the ICEH finds suggestive but not definitive evidence for a link to learning and developmental disorders include:

GREEN DICTIONARY

ENDOCRINE DISRUPTERS

Substances that act like hormones in the body to disrupt the hormonal (endocrine) processes that control the nervous system, reproduction, development, and other systems in the body. Also called hormone disrupters.

× **ENDOCRINE DISRUPTERS** (phthalates found in children's toys, dioxin contaminants in air and food, the banned pesticide DDT, perfluorinated compounds (PFCs) used to make nonstick cookware, organochlorine pesticides, bisphenol A (BPA) in plastics and the linings in food cans, and some metals): Hormone-like chemicals are involved in orchestrating brain development, so endocrine disrupters double as neurotoxicants. Researchers believe that even small amounts of these chemicals can have significant effects in the body.

× **FLUORIDE** High levels of fluoride in drinking water appear to have a detrimental effect on intelligence. (See discussion later in this chapter.)

× **FOOD ADDITIVES** Dyes and the preservative sodium benzoate have been linked to behavioral problems and hyperactivity. (See Chapter 2 for more on food dyes and additives.)

AN ENVIRONMENTAL CAUSE FOR AUTISM? Autism rates have been climbing steadily since the early 1990s. Roughly one out of every 150 children is now diagnosed as having an autism spectrum disorder, a range of disorders that spans from severe autism to milder Asperger's syndrome. Autism spectrum disorders (ASD) are characterized by a lack of social interaction, communication difficulties, and repetitive or restrictive patterns of behavior and interest.

At one time many researchers believed this increase in autism rates was due to a new diagnosis system implemented in the early 1990s, which resulted in the redistribution of children from other mental health categories into the autism category. However, researchers in California found that the seven to eight-fold increase in the number of Californian children born with autism since 1990 cannot be explained by changes in how the condition is diagnosed, according to a study published in the January 2009 issue of the journal *Epidemiology*.[10]

This finding helps settle an important question about the cause of autism. For years many researchers have insisted that autism is primarily a genetic disorder. The rapid rise in cases, however, implies that the cause is at least partly environmental because genes don't change radically over a span of two decades. The researchers in the above study suggest that chemicals and infectious microbes in the environment play a role in this complex disorder. In fact, many researchers think that the term autism encompasses several distinct disorders that have similar symptoms but different causes. Many researchers are exploring the possibility that autism disorders are caused by a combination of environmental factors and genetic susceptibility. Some of the current theories on the causes of autism are:

× **AUTOIMMUNE DISORDER** Many autistic individuals have antibodies directed against their own brain tissue. These "autoantibodies" could harm brain development and function.

× **MATERNAL INFECTION** When a pregnant mother fights off infection, the infection-fighting immune system of the mother may somehow affect the development of fetal brain anatomy or function.

× **GENETICS** A combination of genes could account for autism. This theory would explain why autism runs in families, but it wouldn't explain why the disorder is on the rise.

× **VACCINES** Most researchers do not believe vaccines cause autism, although in rare cases vaccines may worsen symptoms.

× **CHEMICALS** Prenatal or early childhood exposures to mercury, PCBs, pesticides, or other chemicals are suspected causes of autism.

× **GENETIC PREDISPOSITION AND ENVIRONMENTAL EXPOSURE** Children with certain genetic traits could be more susceptible to harm from chemicals in the environment.

ADHD Attention deficit/hyperactivity disorder is the most commonly diagnosed neuropsychiatric disorder in children. Children with ADHD have trouble sitting still, controlling their impulses, and paying attention. Researchers suspect that

ADHD is caused by the dysfunctionality of chemical neurotransmitters in the brain. Medications that reduce ADHD behaviors work by increasing the release of the neurotransmitters dopamine and norepinephrine in the brain.

Like autism, ADHD appears to run in families. Genes can explain about 45 to 90 percent of the cases of ADHD, but what about the other 10 to 55 percent of children who have no genetic risk of ADHD? Again, environmental chemicals are prime suspects.

Several persistent organic pollutants, including PCBs, are linked to ADHD-like behaviors, especially in animal studies but also in some human studies, according to a 2008 review article in the journal *Current Opinion in Pediatrics*.[11] PCBs have similar chemical structures to thyroid hormones and children with thyroid problems can exhibit ADHD-like symptoms. Prenatal exposure to tobacco smoke and lead are also linked to ADHD, according to a retrospective study of nearly 5,000 children that was published in a 2006 issue of *Environmental Health Perspectives*.[12] ADHD may be caused by a combination of genetic predisposition and environmental exposure to chemicals.

PCBs and lead are not the only chemicals that have been linked to attention and behavioral problems in children. Several studies have tied these behaviors to consumption of food additives such as dyes and preservatives. (See Chapter 2 for more information.) The timing of the rise of ADHD coincides with the increase in food additives in the food supply, according to proponents of this theory. A natural diet devoid of artificial ingredients may reduce symptoms in children with ADHD, several studies have found.

In fact, there is nothing revolutionary about eating a diet rich in healthy, whole foods. The American Academy of Pediatrics now recognizes a preservative-free, food coloring–free diet as being a reasonable intervention for the treatment of ADHD symptoms.

GREEN ON A SHOESTRING

Eating foods without preservatives and dyes can actually be cheaper because you avoid having to load up on pricey prepackaged snacks. You'll also benefit the environment by keeping packaging out of landfills.

Emerging Infectious Diseases

Some diseases are related to how we humans interact with our environment.

In this section we look at the environmental factors that fueled the development

or spread of emerging infectious diseases, including bird and swine flu, Lyme

disease, and methicillin-resistant *Staphylococcus aureus* (MRSA).

We humans are changing our environment at a breakneck pace. Natural resources are being harvested and shipped around the globe, people are moving into territories that formerly supported only sparse human habitation, and we are introducing new medicines that spur the evolution of disease-causing organisms.

Our increasingly mobile world population is bringing faraway diseases closer to home. One example of a recently imported disease is West Nile virus. A mosquito-borne disease, West Nile virus arrived in North America in 1999, possibly on a transatlantic airline flight. Since then it has marched (or rather flown) across the United States from east to west, causing mostly mild cases of fever but occasionally causing fatalities among the elderly and medically fragile.

Another disease headed our way is avian influenza virus (bird flu or H5N1). This virus has been spreading across Europe along the flight patterns of migratory birds. At least 400 cases have been reported since 2003 and several children in Asia have died from bird flu acquired from livestock. If the disease becomes readily transmissible from human to human, a dangerous pandemic could result.

Yet another type of influenza virus that has recently emerged is "swine flu," also called H1N1 virus. This virus was identified in the spring of 2009 as being a pig virus that acquired the ability to infect humans. The virus is extremely contagious from human to human, prompting the World Health Organization to declare a global pandemic. Although to date most people have recovered without medical intervention, medically fragile individuals, pregnant women, and young children may be at higher risk of severe illness.

LYME DISEASE While some new diseases have resulted from our penchant for global travel, or from contact between animals and humans, others are spreading due to destruction of natural habitats and decreased biodiversity. The spread of Lyme disease, a tick-borne illness that can cause permanent neurological damage, is due at least in part to changes in land-use patterns that have brought humans in greater contact with animal carriers of the disease, increased the number of these animal carriers, and decreased the amount of land that these animals occupy.

Over the last two decades, Lyme disease rates have more than doubled, from 10,000 cases in 1992 to more than 25,000 cases in 2007, according to the CDC. As woodland and farming areas are increasingly turned into subdivisions, the number of humans coming in contact with infected wildlife is increasing. In turn, deer populations are being hemmed in by housing tracts and their numbers are expanding since they have no predators. Human habitation also crowds out a variety of small mammals that don't carry Lyme bacteria, and as a result the ticks feed increasingly on the white-footed mouse, a known Lyme-carrier, and less often on other small mammals that don't harbor the spirochete, according to a 2003 article in the *Proceedings of the National Academy of Sciences.*[13]

Some of the most common places to encounter deer ticks are the grassy areas bordering tracts of forest. These places include backyards, public parks, and sports fields. Lyme disease rates spike in children ages 5 to 14 and later in mid-adulthood, suggesting that the risk of disease correlates with the amount of time people spend outdoors playing or doing yard work.

Lyme-carrying ticks are no bigger than the period at the end of this sentence. When the tick bites a person, it transfers a spiral-shaped bacterium, or spirochete, into the person's body. In active children who spend a lot of time outdoors, the biting ticks can easily go unnoticed. They are most likely to transmit the disease during the spring, summer, or early fall. Deer ticks do not jump onto people but rather climb on, often to the ankles or feet, and then start crawling upward to find available skin. The ticks need to be attached for 36 to 48 hours to transmit the disease.

In the first few days or weeks following infection, the Lyme spirochete can cause flu-like symptoms, such as fever, muscle aches, headache, fatigue, and an overall feeling of poor health. A rash shaped like a bull's eye is considered one of the hallmarks of Lyme disease, yet not all infected people get the rash, and it doesn't have to look like a bull's eye. Nor does it have to be centered on the tick bite.

Unless you live in an endemic area, your pediatrician may be reluctant to test your child for Lyme disease. If possible, take a picture of the rash. A picture can be worth a thousand words.

When antibiotics are given during the first few weeks or months following the bite, children and adults nearly always recover and have no further symptoms. However, if the disease goes untreated, the spirochete can spread in the body and cause joint pain, arthritis, heart problems, extreme fatigue, memory loss, and depression. Since these symptoms can be caused by many other ailments, it can be extremely difficult for practitioners to diagnose Lyme disease.

Lyme disease is found all over the world but is most common in Northern Europe and North America. In the United States, it is most common in the Northeast, the upper Midwest, and the Pacific Northwest from California to Washington. However, it has been found in nearly every state. You can find out how prevalent it is in your state by going to the CDC's website at *www.cdc.gov/ lyme* and clicking on "Statistics."

TIPS FOR LYME DISEASE PREVENTION:

✓ Dress your family in light-colored long pants and long-sleeve shirts whenever gardening, hiking, or exploring wooded areas.

✓ Tuck shirts into pants and pants into socks and wear closed shoes.

✓ Wear a snug-fitting cap with hair tucked inside or braided.

✓ Stay on the middle of trails and don't take shortcuts through the tall grasses and brush.

✓ During activities outdoors, frequently check for ticks and inspect your companions.

✗ Avoid sitting on the ground or on stone walls, which are havens for ticks.

✓ At the end of the day, remove all clothes, and check your family members for ticks (and make sure they check you).

✓ Get familiar with your kids' skin so that you can easily find ticks among freckles and moles. Ticks prefer warm areas like the naval, groin, armpits, head, and hairline. Also check behind the knees and ears.

✓ Teach your children to recognize ticks. Although tick bites don't usually hurt, they can produce a fleeting irritating feeling or itch. Teach your children to recognize that feeling, and tell them that if they find any unusual bumps, they should show them to you, a camp counselor, school nurse, or other caregiver immediately.

✗ Prevent pets from coming in contact with ticks. Ticks may jump from the family pet to your child.

✓ Washing clothes in hot water *does not* kill ticks, so don't rely on this method. Drying clothes for one hour in a hot dryer should kill them, however.

✓ Some people erect fencing to keep deer off property. You can also landscape your yard to reduce deer ticks by removing leaf litter, tall grass, and brush, and keeping play areas away from wooded areas.

✓ If you must use tick repellent, DEET (N,N-diethyl-meta-toluamide) is effective but has potential environmental and health effects. Avoid spraying near the eyes, nose, mouth, and hands (since children put their hands in their mouths). Never use DEET products on pets or on children younger than two months old. See Chapter 10 for more information on insect repellent.

Source: American Lyme Disease Foundation and *http://HealthVermont.gov*

ECO-TIP: SHOULD YOU USE PESTICIDES TO KILL TICKS?

One method of preventing Lyme disease is to kill the ticks in your yard using a synthetic pesticide. However, if you live next to woods or if your neighbors don't also spray with pesticides, it is likely that new ticks will repopulate the area as soon as the pesticides wash away, in about six weeks.

Although studies show that insecticides can reduce tick populations by 60 to 100 percent, the chemicals can be potentially toxic to children, pets, and wildlife. Pesticides commonly used are carbaryl (a carbamate) and members of the pyrethroid family (cyfluthrin, bifenthrin, deltamethrin, cyhalothrin, permethrin, and pyrethrin). Carbaryl is a neurotoxicant that is linked to cancer in laboratory animals, according to the EPA. Pyrethroid pesticides are also neurotoxicants but are considered less toxic than carbamates. Many are suspected to be endocrine disrupters. Some animal studies point to the potential for pyrethroids to harm the developing brain, according to the EPA. Pyrethroids can be toxic to cats.

METHICILLIN-RESISTANT *STAPHYLOCOCCUS AUREUS* (MRSA)

Just ten years ago this superbug was considered a danger only to hospitalized patients. But the last decade has seen the emergence of a strain of MRSA that can be passed among toddlers in child care programs, schoolchildren, and high school and college athletes. Another strain is spreading among pigs crowded into factory farms and to farmers and their families.

MRSA is a drug-resistant form of *Staphylococcus aureus* (often just called "staph"), a type of bacteria that causes skin infections. Staph infections, whether drug-resistant or not, usually appear as an enlarged pimple, bump, or "boil" that is red, swollen, painful, warm to the touch, full of pus, and can be accompanied by a fever. About 25 to 30 percent of the population carries staph bacteria in their nose where it presents no danger whatsoever. About one percent of people are infected with MRSA, according to the CDC.

If your child has a bump or skin lesion, or complains of a spider bite or a mosquito bite that doesn't go away, contact your health care professional, especially if your child has a fever. Your pediatrician can take a sample of the pus and send it to the laboratory for evaluation.

If your child is diagnosed with MRSA, take precautions to prevent the spread of disease. At home, clean every surface, especially door knobs and toilet facilities. Place alcohol-based hand sanitizer in the bathroom (out of reach of young children) and make sure that your family members use it often. Wash any sheets, towels, and clothes that come in contact with the infected area in warm water and laundry detergent. Use a dryer (or the hot sun if you line dry) to make sure that clothes are completely dry. For more information, see *www.cdc.gov/mrsa*.

MRSA skin infections can go away without treatment with antibiotics, but occasionally they can develop into more severe infections. Physicians are now reporting an increase in MRSA among ear, nose, and throat infections in children, according to a 2009 study in the *Archives of Otolaryngology—Head & Neck Surgery*.[14] If bacteria spread into the blood through an open cut or wound, these microbes can launch a dangerous and potentially deadly infection.

TIPS FOR PREVENTING MRSA:
- ✓ Wash hands thoroughly after using the toilet and before eating.
- ✗ Avoid contact with toilet seats.
- ✓ Tell your children never to touch other children's sores.
- ✓ Keep cuts and scrapes clean and covered with a bandage.
- ✓ Warn older children not to share personal hygiene items and to cover shared workout equipment with a clean towel. Repeated rubbing of skin against contaminated equipment can work the bacteria into the skin.

TIPS FOR TREATING MRSA Your pediatrician may drain the infection and possibly prescribe an antibiotic. Do not drain the infection yourself since you risk spreading it to yourself and other family members. Securely tape a sterile bandage over the infected area so that draining pus cannot escape the bandage. Always wash your hands after changing a dressing. Make sure your child takes the medication as directed. Contact your child's day care or school to find out if they have a policy about how long to keep a child home.

OVERUSE OF ANTIBIOTICS AND THE RISE OF SUPERBUGS The overuse of antibiotics in livestock production, pediatrician's offices, and in hand soaps and other consumer products may be contributing to the development of superbugs such as MRSA.

Antibacterials are now showing up in everything from soaps to high chairs. But studies have failed to show that these products prevent disease transmission. A 2008 review in the *American Journal of Public Health* found that people who wash their hands with antimicrobial soaps get sick just as often as people who use regular soap.[15] What is more, the antibacterial soap users have just as much bacteria on their hands after washing as people who use regular soaps. (See The Science Behind It.)

The overuse of antibacterials in consumer products could help MRSA and other superbugs evolve to become resistant to the very drugs we need when we become infected. These antibacterials kill off the weaker bacteria and leave the stronger ones to survive and reproduce. The more often MRSA encounters an antibacterial drug, the more likely it is to evolve defenses to that drug.

Hand sanitizers are alcohol-based cleansers that can be used when you don't have access to a sink, soap, and warm water. They are proven to kill bacteria and while they do not necessarily kill viruses, they make it difficult for viruses to stay on the hands. Most studies have found that hand sanitizers *do not* contribute to antibiotic resistance.

Never hand over your bottle of hand sanitizer to a young child. Hand sanitizers are more than 60 percent alcohol, a substance that if swallowed can damage the developing brain and cause fatalities. Just a few squirts can boost a child's blood alcohol limit into the legally drunk range.

Asthma and Allergies

Asthma and allergy rates have increased dramatically and are continuing to climb in the United States and other industrialized countries. Environmental factors clearly play a role in the rise of these conditions.

Asthma rates in children under the age of five increased more than 160 percent from 1980 to 1994, according to the American Academy of Allergy, Asthma & Immunology (AAAAI), and asthma now affects about 35 million Americans. Allergies ranging from hay fever to food allergies are also on the rise, and afflict about 40 to 50 million Americans, according to the AAAAI.

Asthma and allergies have similar triggers, and about 70 percent of asthmatics also suffer from allergies. Although asthma and allergies have strong genetic components, family history alone cannot explain the rise in rates.

Food allergies are also on the rise, having increased 18 percent from 1997 to 2007. They now affect roughly 6 percent of children under the age of three. Every parent now knows not to send peanut butter in their child's lunch if the child will be sitting with children with peanut allergies. Many schools and day care centers have banned all nuts, and some prohibit parents from sending home-baked goods due to the risk of peanut contamination.

BREATHING ROOM Many children who suffer from asthma are unable to play sports, have furry pets, or live without fear of having an attack. The feeling of not being able to breathe is extremely frightening. In 2005, asthma was responsible for more than 3,000 deaths (adults and children combined) in the United States, according to the AAAAI.

Some of the environmental triggers that are linked to asthma are pollen, mold, pet dander, dust mites, cockroach droppings, industrial pollutants, and environmental tobacco smoke (secondhand smoke). (See Chapter 1 for more information on eliminating these allergens safely.) New evidence suggests that household cleaners, often used to rid the house of the asthma and allergy triggers, also contribute to asthma risk. A multicountry study published in a 2007 issue of the *American Journal of Respiratory and Critical Care Medicine* found that adults who used cleaning products were more likely to develop asthma.[16] Air fresheners and glass cleaners are two of the biggest culprits.

Another possible trigger of asthma is lack of vitamin D, according to a 2007 study in the *Journal of Allergy and Clinical Immunology*.[17] Children spend less time outdoors than ever before, and during the winter vitamin D is deficient in many people who live in northern latitudes.

ALLERGIES: NOTHING TO SNEEZE AT Global climate change is one factor suspected of driving the increase in asthma and allergy incidence, according to an article published in a 2005 issue of the journal *Environmental Health Perspectives*.[18] Several studies suggest that warming temperatures and higher carbon dioxide levels are extending the growing season of plant species that produce pollen. The plants start making pollen earlier in the year than usual and make greater quantities than they used to do. It also appears that the pollen produced under these warmer conditions is more potent at triggering asthma and allergies.

Our changing land-use patterns are also contributing to the increase in allergies such as hay fever. One often overlooked reason for the rise of asthma and allergies is the steady expansion of allergen-producing plant species throughout the world. Ragweed, for example, is one of the major pollen-producing plants associated with seasonal hay fever. It was relatively confined to the northeastern sections of the United States when Europeans first arrived, but with the building of the railroads, the weed, which thrives in the disturbed soils alongside the tracks, began spreading throughout the country.

As people move to new areas, they tend to bring vegetation with them. Wealthy individuals who used to escape to allergy-free vacation spots such as Tucson, Arizona, found their havens destroyed because people moving to the area brought pollen-producing ornamental trees and shrubs from the Northeast.

For more information about what you can do to reduce asthma triggers around the home, see Chapter 1.

Cancer

Cancer is the fourth leading cause of death among children, behind injuries, homicides, and suicides. About 10,000 new cases are diagnosed every year in the United States in children under the age of 14. Each baby that is born today has a roughly 1 in 300 chance of developing cancer during childhood, according to the U.S. National Cancer Institute.

The good news is that more children than ever are surviving cancer thanks to new treatments. The bad news is that childhood cancer rates continue to rise, according to the U.S. National Cancer Institute.

Cancer is not a single disease but rather behaves differently depending on the type of tumor, location in the body, genetics, and many other factors. As such, cancer can have multiple causes that probably reflect a combination of genetic factors and environmental exposures. Some associations are well known, such as smoking and lung cancer, but most causes of cancer are still under investigation. This is especially true in children, who have relatively fewer risk factors than adults.

A number of toxic substances that children are exposed to during childhood can increase their cancer risk later in life. Examples of these exposures are radon, environmental tobacco smoke, and sun exposure.

In addition to these known culprits, several environmental causes of cancer are under investigation. A few of the more controversial ones are electric and magnetic fields (EMFs), cell phones, and pesticides.

ELECTRIC AND MAGNETIC FIELDS (EMFs) Power lines and electrical appliances generate invisible electric and magnetic fields. The electric fields fall off quickly, but magnetic fields can travel farther from the source and are not blocked by walls or clothing. A number of studies have investigated whether living near power lines contributes to an increased risk of childhood leukemia, brain tumors, or other cancers. Some studies found a connection while others did not.

Due to the uncertainty about the connection between EMFs and cancer, it is better to play it safe and avoid living near power lines. When you are choosing a place to live, look for a home that is at least 100 yards (one football field) away from power lines. At this distance the EMFs will have weakened to the point where they are not a hazard.

Electric and magnetic fields are generated any time an electrical appliance is turned on. Household appliances that give off EMFs include hair dryers, computers, televisions, electric blankets, and heated waterbeds. Keep your child away from these items while they are turned on. Also avoid electric blankets and heated waterbeds while pregnant, since a Canadian study found an association between prenatal exposure to high magnetic fields and childhood leukemia.[19]

CELL PHONES AND OTHER WIRELESS DEVICES Cell phones use radio frequency (RF) waves to send signals to and from cell phone towers. Other gadgets that send signals via radio frequencies include cordless phones, wireless headsets, baby monitors, and wireless computer networks.

Kids love cell phones because they are a status symbol and parents like the idea that they can easily contact their child at any moment. But many parents wonder, can these devices cause brain cancer in their child?

The short answer is that researchers don't know whether prolonged cell phone use causes cancer. Most studies have found no association between brain cancer and cell phone use, but a few studies have found that cell phone use increases the risk of certain types of brain tumors. A 2008 study in the *American Journal of Epidemiology* found that cell phone use is linked to an increased risk of tumors of the parotid gland, which is located near the ear and jaw.[20] A 2009 multicountry study in Europe indicated that cell phones used for ten years or more may be linked to brain cancer, according to a study in the journal *Pathophysiology*.[21]

No studies have looked specifically at cell phone use and cancer in children. Children may be more susceptible to cell phone–induced cancer because they will use the phones for decades and because their brains are still developing through adolescence.

Radio frequency signals can heat bodily tissues, which may suggest a mechanism for how they cause cancer. There are also nonheat-related biological effects but most scientists discount the ability of these to cause cancer.

The part of the cell phone that sends out the radio waves is the antenna, so this is the part of the phone to keep as far from the body as possible. Hands-free devices for cell phones also use radio frequency signals but at very low power. Household wireless networks are another source of radio frequency signals, but they operate at very low power and most researchers think they are unlikely to increase the risk of cancer.

TIPS FOR KIDS (AND PARENTS) WITH CELL PHONES:
- ✓ Use a (preferably wired) hands-free device.
- ✓ Hold the phone away from the body while talking.
- ✓ Limit the use of the phone to short conversations.

MORE ADVICE FOR AVOIDING EMF AND RADIO FREQUENCY ENERGY:
- ✗ Do not live within 100 yards of power lines or electrical transformers.
- ✓ Place electrical appliances such as clocks and baby monitors across the room from the baby's crib.
- ✓ Stay at least 3 feet from televisions, microwave ovens, and other appliances while they are turned on.
- ✗ Do not use electric blankets while pregnant and do not use them with young children.

> **GREEN ON A SHOESTRING**
>
> An affordable way to provide pesticide-free produce and save money at the same time is to grow your own vegetables. If you don't have a yard, you may be able to plant tomatoes and peppers in pots on a terrace. Or check to see if your area has a community garden.

PESTICIDES AND CANCER Many studies have pointed to pesticides as increasing the risk of childhood cancer. The types of cancer consistently linked to pesticides are childhood leukemia, brain cancer, neuroblastoma, non-Hodgkin's lymphoma, Wilms' tumor, Ewing's sarcoma, and colorectal cancer.[22]

Agricultural pesticides may predispose children to cancer, according to many studies. Children living in U.S. counties with moderate to high levels of agricultural activity were at greater risk of developing a variety of childhood cancers, according to a 2008 study published in *Environmental Health Perspectives*.[23]

Home use of pesticides has also been tied to an increased risk of developing cancer. A 2007 study in the journal *Environmental Health Perspectives* found that children had roughly twice the risk of developing acute leukemia or non-Hodgkin's lymphoma if the mother used insecticides in the home while pregnant.[24] A 2009 study in the same journal found a link between residential herbicides and brain cancer in children.[25]

Farms and backyards alike are sprayed with a combination of pesticides throughout the year. Yet few studies have looked at the risk of cancer associated with pesticide mixtures.

INTEGRATED PEST MANAGEMENT (IPM)

A pest control strategy that focuses on prevention and intervention rather than using synthetic pesticides as a first line of defense. For example, IPM in the home or school could mean blocking pest entry and removing food sources. In the garden, IPM could mean planting native, naturally pest-resistant varieties of plants or co-planting food crops with plants that naturally discourage pests.

In addition to agricultural and home use, pesticides are found in small quantities in fruits, vegetables, and drinking water. However, children usually encounter the highest concentrations in their own homes, apartment complexes, yards, schools, and parks. Homeowners and housing managers often overapply pesticides and fail to keep kids and pets from treading on recently treated areas. Kids and pets can track pesticides into the house or apartment where they settle on carpets and continue to expose the children for months.

TIPS FOR REDUCING YOUR CHILD'S EXPOSURE TO PESTICIDES:

✓ Eliminate use of household pesticides (see Chapter 1 for suggestions on preventing pests from entering the home). If you must use pesticides indoors, use traps, baits, or gels instead of sprays or foggers.

✓ Serve organic produce to your children.

✓ Outdoors, remove weeds by hand and use prevention and intervention rather than chemicals to eliminate pests in the yard and garden. If you've tried everything and must apply pesticides, read the label and follow it to the letter. The EPA approves pesticides based on their proper use, not on the assumption that any amount is safe.

✓ Advocate in your child's school and your town for the use of a no-pesticide or integrated pest management (IPM) approach, where natural methods are tried before resorting to pesticides.

Dental Health

Preventing and treating cavities is important for both healthy children and a healthy planet. Read on to find out what fluoride, mercury, and bisphenol A are doing in your child's mouth and in the environment.

THE FUSS ABOUT FLUORIDE Check the label on your toothpaste tube, and you'll find warnings such as "Keep out of reach of children under six years of age" and "If more than used for brushing is swallowed, get medical help or contact a Poison Control Center right away." If fluoride is so good for children, why do toothpastes bear such dire labels?

Fluoride is effective in preventing cavities, but ingesting too much can cause teeth to acquire a permanent mottled brown stain, a condition called fluorosis. Infants and young children are especially susceptible to getting fluorosis because their teeth—and their bodies—are still growing and developing. Severe fluorosis, however, weakens tooth structure and leads to more cavities.

Fluoride appears to prevent cavities by stopping calcium and phosphate minerals from being stripped away by acids at the tooth surface that help to restore those minerals and by inhibiting bacterial activity.

Although fluoride is a naturally occurring substance found in nearly all soil and water at varying levels, many municipalities add fluoride to public water supplies. The U.S. Public Health Service recommends maintaining fluoride concentrations at 0.7 to 1.2 parts per million (ppm). The CDC hails fluoridation of drinking water as one of the major public health accomplishments of the 20th century.

Fluoride's critics say that water fluoridation is toxic to both humans and the environment. Some studies, mostly conducted at levels much higher than are used to prevent cavities, found that fluoridated water can harm fish and aquatic life. Fluoridated water may also be unnecessary. The critics claim that the chemical's cavity-fighting effect is due to direct application on teeth, not ingestion and delivery to pre-eruption teeth under the gums.

SO IS FLUORIDE BAD FOR YOU OR NOT? A handful of studies have linked fluoride to neurological damage to children, according to a major review published in 2006 by the U.S. National Research Council (NRC).[26] According to the review, fluoride in drinking water has been shown to lower thyroid hormone levels, which in pregnant women can harm the developing fetal brain. A few studies conducted in China suggest that fluoride exposure to 1.5 to 2 ppm fluoridated water in infancy is linked to lower IQ. Studies in animals indicate that high amounts of fluoride may have hormone-like effects, leading to possible effects on fertility and timing of sexual maturity.

Fluoride has also been suspected of causing skeletal fluorosis, bone fracture, chronic kidney disease, and bone cancer. The NRC report found that drinking water levels in the United States were unlikely to cause skeletal fluorosis. However, the report found evidence that lifetime consumption of 4 ppm fluoride in water (the maximum the EPA allows) was linked to increased bone fracture risk. The report found no increased risk of chronic kidney disease or other organ disease, and the authors noted that the evidence for bone cancer was "tentative and mixed." However a study published later that year by Harvard University researchers found that young males under age 20 living in fluoridated areas had a slightly increased risk of a rare form of bone cancer called osteosarcoma.[27]

Federal health agencies recommend that parents limit fluoride exposure in infants and young children. Depending on the level of fluoride in your water, you may want to purchase fluoride-free water when reconstituting infant formula. According to CDC estimates, up to 33 percent of children get too much fluoride through all sources, from drinking water to swallowing toothpaste, combined.

In light of the uncertainty surrounding how much fluoride infants and children are getting from public water supplies, private well water, fruit juices, toothpaste and other sources, it seems wise to limit your child's ingestion of fluoride while still allowing it to be applied to the teeth during brushing.

TIPS FOR GETTING THE RIGHT AMOUNT OF FLUORIDE:

✓ Use nonfluoridated water to reconstitute baby formula.

✓ Consider using nonfluoridated toothpaste until your child is old enough to spit it out (especially if your child is getting fluoride from other sources).

✓ Check with your water supplier to find out how much fluoride is in your water. You may be able to find the information on the CDC's My Water's Fluoride website at *http://apps.nccd.cdc.gov/MWF.*

✓ If you use well water, test for fluoride.

✓ If the level in your water is above 2 ppm, the CDC recommends using an alternate source for children under the age of eight.

✓ If your child has good brushing habits, eats a healthy diet, and hasn't had a cavity for the last three years, consider skipping fluoride gels and varnishes given at the dentist office. Evidence shows that these are of little benefit in children who are already at low risk of getting cavities.[28]

RISK FACTORS FOR GETTING CAVITIES:

× Having cavity-causing strains of bacteria in the mouth

× Eating a diet high in sugar

× Poor oral hygiene

× Prolonged bottle use or nursing

TIPS: BABY STEPS FOR CAVITY PREVENTION

✓ Hold your baby during feedings—don't prop up bottles. Remove the bottle when your baby falls asleep.

✓ Put water in your child's sippy cup for between meal drinks.

✓ Wipe baby's teeth and gums with a damp washcloth or small toothbrush after baby is done eating.

✓ When your child is old enough to brush, use only a pea-size dab of fluoride toothpaste.

KITCHEN TABLE TALK

Happy Mouths

A child's first tooth shows up around six months of age, but decay prevention needs to start at birth. Yet many parents unwittingly expose their infants and toddlers to millions of tooth decay risk factors every day.

What are these risk factors? Bacteria. The real culprits behind cavities are the bacteria living in our mouths. They feed on the sugars that are left behind on our teeth after eating. These sugars come from sweets as well as from healthy foods like milk, fruits, rice, and pasta. Bacteria consume the sugar and make acid, which eats away at the minerals on tooth surfaces, carving out depressions we call cavities.

Many parents are surprised to learn that babies are born without any bacteria whatsoever in their mouths. In fact, dental cavities are a *communicable* disease. We parents infect our babies and children with decay-causing bacteria every time we share spoons over a jar of baby food or clean off a pacifier by putting it in our mouths.

The first line of prevention, long before limiting sweets or nagging kids to brush twice a day, is to keep cavity-causing bacteria out of your child's mouth for as long as possible. As your children get older, advise them never to share cups with friends. Make sure they wash their hands frequently and discourage habits like thumb-sucking and nail-biting that lead their hands to their mouths.

Along with keeping bacteria out, parents also need to limit the amount of sugar they let their kids eat. Juice seems like a healthy alternative to sodas and other adult beverages, but in fact one 8-ounce cup of 100 percent apple juice has the same amount of sugar—26 grams—as an 8-ounce cup of soda. Help your child avoid developing a preference for sugary drinks. Serve juice diluted in water and limit the total amount of juice to six ounces per day. (For more recommendations on healthy eating, see Chapter 2.)

OTHER TIPS FOR AVOIDING THE DENTIST DRILL:

× Avoid letting your child snack all day, especially on sweets. When it comes to preventing cavities, it is better to allow kids to eat several pieces of candy followed by brushing rather than eating candy throughout the day. Aim to limit the amount of time that sugar sits on the teeth.

✓ Xylitol is a natural sugar that bacteria cannot digest, so it doesn't promote tooth decay. It is available in gums, as sugar packets, and in large quantities for baking and cooking. If buying gums, look for xylitol as the first ingredient.

SEAL OF APPROVAL Sealants are plastic resins that can protect teeth from decay. They are usually applied to the chewing surfaces of permanent molars that come in around age six or seven. If your dentist suggests sealants for your child, ask whether the dentist offers a bisphenol-A-free brand of sealant. Bisphenol A (BPA) is a potentially toxic hormone-like chemical that has been linked in animal studies to prostate and breast cancer, early onset of puberty, hyperactivity, lowered sperm count, miscarriage, and diabetes.[29] Several BPA-free sealants exist, but not all dentists are aware of the options, so you might want to call dentists in your area to enquire.

TOOTH TROUBLE If that dreaded day comes and despite all your best efforts your child gets a cavity, what is the best type of filling to use? Although there are many materials that are used as fillings, the choice usually boils down to amalgam versus composite.

AMALGAM These silver-colored fillings are made of a combination of about 50 percent mercury metal along with silver, tin, copper, and possibly other metals. Mercury is a known neurotoxicant that is especially harmful to the developing brain. The dental industry maintains that mercury-amalgam fillings are safe for children because the mercury is bound up with the other metals. However studies have shown that the mercury vaporizes in the mouth during chewing and can be inhaled and reach the brain.[30]

Exposure to mercury during fetal development and early childhood can harm the developing brain, according to the EPA. Some pregnant women exposed to mass accidental mercury poisonings gave birth to children with learning and cognitive difficulties. Infants and young children who were exposed also went on to develop learning and cognitive deficits.

Yet the dental industry defends amalgam as safe. A pair of studies published in 2006 in the *Journal of the American Medical Association* followed 1,000 children who were randomly assigned to receive either amalgams or composites.[31] The studies found no significant differences in IQ and other cognitive measures. However the children were only studied for five to seven years and it may take longer for effects to show up. Also, individuals vary in their ability to metabolize mercury, and 25 percent of the U.S. population has a gene variant that makes them more sensitive to mercury, according to an editorial that accompanied the study.[32]

The continual use of mercury in dental fillings stands out as incongruous with the fact that nearly every other mercury-containing device—from thermometers to lightbulbs—is either being phased out or bears numerous warning labels. Yet many parents were unaware until recently that amalgam fillings contain mercury because of industry-imposed "gag rules" that prohibited licensed dentists from discussing the toxicity concerns with patients or advertising that they were "mercury-free" dental practices.

Court cases across the nation in the mid-2000s put an end to the gag rules. The FDA now seems set to make new rules regarding the regulation of mercury in dental fillings. In 2008, a successful lawsuit brought by advocacy groups against the FDA forced the agency to make new guidelines for the regulation of mercury in dental amalgam by June 2009.

Human health concerns are not the only problem. Mercury is toxic to fish and wildlife. Many states now regulate the collection and proper disposal of mercury that would otherwise be washed down the drain at dentist offices. However, the EPA does not require dentists to install mercury collection traps, and the American Dental Association (ADA) only began recommending that dentists install the traps in 2007.

Mercury in dental fillings is also an environmental justice issue. With the rising awareness of the health and environmental consequences, people who can afford to change are switching to other options. The poor and underserved children are getting stuck with a mouthful of mercury.

COMPOSITES A dental composite is a compound of acrylic resin and powdered glasslike particles that is white in color and blends in with the surrounding teeth. According to the ADA, composite fillings can wear out more quickly than amalgam fillings so they need to be replaced more often. Some brands can contain BPA, but the ADA says it is rarely added as an ingredient but may be left over as a contaminant. BPA has been found in the saliva of people undergoing composite filling installation. If you are considering composite fillings for your child, ask your dentist for a BPA-free formulation.

PREVENT MERCURY EXPOSURE FROM FILLINGS:

✓ Keep your child's teeth healthy so that he or she doesn't get cavities.

✓ Choose composite fillings.

✓ If your child already has amalgam fillings, leave them in place until they wear out, since mercury can be dispersed into the mouth during removal.

Take Action

▸ Stop the spread of colds and flu by teaching your children good hand-washing techniques.

▸ Avoid antibacterial products that contain triclosan or triclocarban, which are harmful to the environment.

▸ Build a healthy immune system by making sure your child gets plenty of rest, eats a healthy diet, and exercises daily.

▸ Dispose of medicines properly by contacting your pharmacy or municipality's household hazardous waste collection center.

▸ Use environmentally friendly recycled tissues or washable cotton handkerchiefs.

▸ Do your own research before giving your child supplements. Most are not tested for safety in children.

▸ Protect your child from life-threatening diseases by having him or her vaccinated.

▸ Demand a mercury-free flu shot. Question your pediatrician about the amount of aluminum in the vaccine brands used by your child's pediatric practice.

▸ Eliminate toxic chemicals around your home that are linked to learning and behavioral disorders.

▸ Protect your child from tick-borne and mosquito-borne diseases by covering him or her with light cotton, long-sleeve clothing when outdoors, and tucking pants into socks and shirts into pants.

▸ Cover large skin sores with a bandage and tape before sending your child to school. Teach your child to never touch other children's sores.

▸ Limit the amount of fluoride that your child ingests by using nonfluoridated water to mix baby formula, using nonfluoridated toothpaste until your child can spit it out, and testing your water if there are concerns about fluoride in your area.

▸ Choose composite fillings over ones made from mercury-containing amalgam.

THE SCIENCE BEHIND IT

The How and Why of Hand Washing

What do hand washing and playing piano have in common? Both need to be taught and practiced over and over again. Start early and repeat often, and your child will have the skills he or she needs to stay healthy in a germ-infested world.

The best time to start teaching your child to wash his hands is when he is old enough to stand at the sink. Around this age, he won't be very good at it, so you'll have to help him pull up his sleeves, turn on the tap to get warm water, and reach the soap. After he's done his best to put soap on his hands and spread it around, you can step in and finish the job.

Hand washing needs to be retaught over and over as your child acquires better motor skills. Your four-year-old should be able to do a better job at it than your two-year-old. By first grade, your child should be washing his or her hands like a professional surgeon.

Why is hand washing so important? It is one of the best things you can do to prevent disease. Every time a child touches his eyes, nose, or mouth he is potentially bringing bacteria, viruses, or other disease-causing agents into his body.

The skin, though an excellent barrier, is susceptible to infections as well. Boils from staph infections, impetigo (a contagious skin infection), and fungal infections are just some of the skin diseases that children may acquire. Hand washing can, however, prevent the transmission of these diseases.

How do we know that hand washing is so good at preventing disease? Scientists have studied the matter. In the early half of the 2000s, scientists from the CDC conducted a test of hand washing in squatter settlements around Karachi, Pakistan. They wanted to know if regular hand washing could reduce the incidence of diarrhea and pneumonia in children under age five. Globally these two diseases kill about 3.5 million children a year, mainly in developing countries.

The researchers randomly assigned about 300 households to a hand-washing promotion program and another 300 households to no intervention. The hand-washing program consisted of weekly visits from fieldworkers to teach family members to wash hands and review how to do it. The fieldworkers also noted any disease symptoms in both the hand-washing and nonhand-washing families.

The results were striking. Compared to the nonhand-washing children, the hand-washing children younger than five years had a 50 percent lower incidence of diarrhea and pneumonia and a 34 percent lower incidence of the skin infection impetigo.[33] The study, published in the journal *Lancet* in 2005, also found that antibacterial soap containing 1.2 percent triclocarban did not work any better against preventing disease than did plain old ordinary soap.

When Should Kids Wash Their Hands?

- ✓ After using the bathroom
- ✓ Before meals and snacks
- ✓ After playing on playground equipment
- ✓ After blowing the nose, sneezing, or coughing

When Should Adults Wash Their Hands?

All of the above, plus:

- ✓ After changing diapers
- ✓ Before and after caring for a sick child
- ✓ Before preparing food
- ✓ After touching animals or animal waste
- ✓ After taking out the garbage
- ✓ Before and after giving first aid

Source: www.cdc.gov/cleanhands/

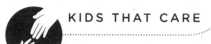

KIDS THAT CARE

Raising Kids for Lifelong Green Living

TODAY'S CHILDREN ARE MORE REMOVED FROM NATURE THAN EVER. Food comes in sanitized, disposable wrappers. Vacations are spent strolling in synthetic wildernesses or floating down artificial rivers inside the walls of theme parks rather than hiking a trail or canoeing in the great outdoors. Our experience of nature has largely been replaced by watching it, either through the windshield of a car or on a flat panel TV screen.

Yet most children have an almost innate affinity for nature. Young children thrive in outdoor areas where they can let go of a parent's hand and run fast, get lost, dig in dirt, and enjoy the primitive side of human nature that we adults spend a lot of time trying to suppress. Children find joy lying in a field of tall grass and looking up at clouds in a wide swath of blue sky, or rolling down a grassy hillside.

Childhood is the perfect time to teach children to respect and protect planet Earth. These habits are much easier to impart than the many others we try to instill in our children, such as brushing teeth and putting away toys. It is much more pleasant to take a walk in the woods or down a tree-lined lane, smelling flowers and listening to birds chirp.

Enjoying nature is a good prelude to teaching kids how to live in ways that protect nature. You may not have a national park just down the road, but you can find living and growing things in sidewalk cracks and front yards, or watch a lizard scurry across a warm rock. Whether you live in a high-rise apartment or a suburban tract home, your child is likely to be at least a little curious about what lies beyond where the sidewalk ends.

When children enjoy the outdoors, it is a logical next step to explain why it is important to make lifestyle choices that ensure the protection of clean water, fresh air, and wildlands for animals to make their homes in and for people to explore. Kids will get these lessons in school, typically around Earth Day, but these instructions won't lead to lifestyle changes unless they are followed by practice in everyday life. It is one thing to learn in the classroom that we should cut our carbon emissions by using our bikes for errands. But if you never take your children on bike trips to the library or corner store, they are unlikely to take these lessons to heart.

To raise children to become the next generation of Earth's caretakers, we need to move the message about living green out of the classroom and into children's daily experiences. We need not just to celebrate Earth Day once a year but rather every day. We need to raise a generation of children who care about natural places, protection of resources, and putting an end to pollution.

Up to now, this book has discussed what you can do for the health of your family and the planet. This chapter covers what *your kids* can do, with your help, to make their world—be it their neighborhood, school, or town—a better place. This chapter breaks "living green" down into age groups. These are only rough guides. Children mature at different ages and have different exposures to ideas and resources. You know your child best, and you can use the suggestions in this chapter to help your child develop his or her own plans about how to save the planet.

The First Years

Your child is beginning to show an awareness of the world and is increasingly curious about his or her natural surroundings. Help your child develop an appreciation for nature through neighborhood walks, visits to parks, and nature-based crafts.

Your child's first years are spent just learning the basics—walking and talking, for example—but that doesn't mean he or she is too young to absorb lessons about how to be a caretaker of the planet. Your eco-friendly lifestyle will rub off on your child, and so-called green activities will seem like business as usual. Simple activities such as recycling, picking up trash in the park, and bringing reusable bags to the grocery store will set the stage for lifelong green habits.

As your baby gets older, take her or him with you on long outdoor walks in the baby carrier or stroller. Baby backpacks are great for babies old enough to support their head because the little ones get an adult's-eye view of their surroundings. Fresh air and sunlight are your baby's first exposure to the great outdoors. Be sure to dress for the weather and bring along a sun hat (see Chapter 6 for suggestions on sun protection for babies).

At home, avoid "containerizing" your kid in a car seat or high chair. Instead put your baby down on a blanket in a childproofed room and see where he or she will roam. As your child grows into a toddler, resist grabbing the stroller for every outing. Take your child by the hand and allow him or her to walk whenever possible. These walks will build muscles that will serve your child for a lifetime.

WHAT TO TALK ABOUT Talk to your baby in an animated fashion to encourage him to develop speech. You don't have to use words like "ecology" and "carbon dioxide" to help him grow into a budding naturalist. As your child becomes more aware of the surrounding world, point out the names of things on your walks and outings.

As your child gets older, and you encounter pets or squirrels, start to explain the concept of a habitat. Everyone needs somewhere to live. Your child's habitat might be his room, his house, his street, or his neighborhood. Explain the importance of leaving some areas in a natural state so that animals can have a place to live. Talk about what sorts of things we need to survive. Humans need food, clean water, air to breathe, and shelter. What do animals need? Talk about how we get our food, versus how pets get their food, and how wild animals get their food.

Read to your child beginning early in life. Include books about nature, trees, and animals. Or head to the Internet for a paper-free experience. You and your child can read conservation-themed books such as *Manny Manatee and the Mystery of the Murky Water* online at the Rainforest Alliance website: *www .rainforest-alliance.org.*

TRIPS AND ACTIVITIES Your first trips and activities will probably be low-key walks in the neighborhood and crafts at the kitchen table. Take short walks at first. You don't want your child's memories of nature to be of you nagging him or her to keep walking. Wherever possible encourage your child's natural curiosity.

NATURE WALK Take a nature walk around your neighborhood. If your child is learning colors, ask him or her to point out things that are yellow, green, etc. If she is learning to count, have her count flower petals or trees in the park. Help her sort items into categories of things that are natural (trees, flowers) and man-made (cars, buildings). Talk about the seasons. After the walk, have your child draw a picture of something he saw on the walk.

✓ **MAKE A NATURE COLLAGE** Collect leaves, sticks, seeds, grass, and other natural items and glue them onto a piece of paper. Make leaf rubbings.

✓ **PICK-YOUR-OWN BERRIES** Take your child berry-picking or apple-picking at a pick-your-own farm. Or visit a community garden project.

✓ **GO TO A FARMERS MARKET** At the farmers market, point out different kinds of vegetables and fruits. Bring your own reusable bags.

✓ **EXPLORE THE STORE** Turn grocery shopping into lessons about where our food comes from. In the grocery store's produce aisle, ask: Where do apples grow? On trees, bushes, or vines? What about blueberries? Strawberries? Visit the fish counter to look for fish that still look like fish (with heads, tails, and scales, intact). Where did these fish live? How did they get from the ocean to the store?

✓ **GO CAMPING** The toddler age is a good age to start camping. (Many people take babies camping, too. Read more about camping vacations in Chapter 10.)

✓ **PLANT SEEDS** Preschool-age children will delight in planting a seed and watching it germinate, then transferring it to an outdoor pot or garden.

✓ **GO FOR A RAMBLE** When on walks, let your child be the leader. Let him run ahead and have that independent feeling while keeping him in view. Let him decide where to go next.

✓ **ASK QUESTIONS** Where do you think that ant is going? Where does he live? Why is that squirrel scurrying about so much? Model curiosity about nature for your child.

THE FACTS

Containers and packaging made up 31 percent, or 78 metric tons, of the garbage generated by businesses and consumers in 2007. Roughly half (39 tons) was recycled, according to the U.S. Environmental Protection Agency (EPA).

✓ **EXPLORE ANIMALS** Help your child look for the similarities between humans and animals. How do animals use sound to communicate? Listen to the back-and-forth calls of birds.

✓ **HAVE FUN WITH WATER** Playing in the sprinklers is a time-honored tradition, but it is very wasteful. Find ways you can enjoy water with less waste. Does your town have a municipal sprinkler park or pool you can visit? Could you fill up a kiddie pool, making sure to cover it at night to keep the water free of leaves and debris? Can you fold sprinkler play into your lawn-watering regimen?

✓ **READ** Subscribe to a childrens' wildlife magazine. Seeing the photographs and reading about animals can inspire kids to want to protect natural resources.

GREEN ON A SHOESTRING

The old cliché about children starving in (insert country of your choice) is, well, old. As a way to get kids to finish the food on their plates, it never really worked anyway. A better tactic is to teach your children to load their plate only with the amount of food they'll eat. Recycle the leftover pasta and vegetables into a casserole and top it with tomato sauce and cheese. You'll save money at the grocery store and toss less food into landfills.

SKILLS TO TEACH The early years are a great time to establish lifelong habits because many children are less apt to question the natural order of the world. This is a great time to establish bedtime and tooth brushing rituals, for example. Here are a few lifelong eco-conscious habits you can teach:

✓ **TURN OFF LIGHTS** Teach your kids to turn off lights when they are tall enough to reach the switch. Before then, you can say, "We are leaving the room. Time to turn off the light."

✓ **SAVE WATER** Don't leave the water running during hand washing and tooth brushing.

✓ **NEW IS NOT NECESSARILY BETTER** Use these early years to help kids understand that we don't always need brand-new items to make us happy. Emphasize that it is nicer to have a few well-loved toys rather than a roomful of junk.

✓ **HOUSE HELPER** Teach your child that helping around the house is a natural part of life. Picking up after oneself, making beds, and putting dishes away are normal, daily activities. Start these habits when your children are very young, and patiently help your toddler do the best that he can with these activities. He won't do as good a job as you do, but he will develop the sense of responsibility that is needed later in life.

✓ **ECO-JOBS** Your child can hand you the clothespins while you hang laundry or help you water the garden. Yes, you can get these jobs done much faster without your little helper, but think how much easier life will be when you find you have raised a helpful older child or young adult.

ECO-TIP: DON'T FEED THE DUCKS

Tossing breadcrumbs at ducks is a time-honored childhood pastime, but it is not good for the ducks. Bread lacks the nutrition that birds need and can lead birds to forget how to find their own food. Uneaten bread can quickly develop mold or bacterial growth that can poison and kill ducks. An outbreak of a feeding-related disease can spread among ducks and kill the entire population at a pond.

Feeding bread to ducks also encourages crowding at the lake or pond where birds will compete for other scarce resources when the bread tossers have gone home. Crowding can also lead to an increase in duck droppings, promoting the spread of disease among the ducks and creating unsanitary conditions for humans. The sure supply of food leads birds to delay migration, raising the risk that they will overwinter in areas that are too cold for them.

Avoid feeding geese, especially. These birds tend to be more aggressive than ducks and can frighten or injure small children. Teach your children that respecting wild animals means not feeding them.

PROJECTS TO DO At this tender age your child is still developing motor skills, so parents must do a lot of guiding and helping. The goal is simply to get your child involved in projects to help the planet, so that he or she gains the early knowledge that the natural environment is worth protecting.

✓ **COMMUNITY SERVICE** Pick up trash in the park. Join a neighborhood cleanup activity. Bring gloves and garbage bags.

✓ **YARD CLEANUP** Rake leaves as a family. Young children can use toy rakes. Dump the leaves in the compost pile if you have one.

✓ **COMPOST** Have your child help you figure out which kitchen scraps can go into the compost bin and which items need to go in the trash.

✓ **RECYCLE** Let your child sort recycled items such as paper, plastics, and glass. Separating out the types of plastic using the small numbers stamped on the bottom is fun for older toddlers and preschoolers.

✓ **MAKE GREEN CRAFTS** Use odds and ends from around the house that normally would have ended up in the garbage. Take old socks and make them into puppets. Turn clothing they've grown out of into stuffed toys.

✓ **MAKE A PET ROCK** Take care of it. What sort of habitat does it live in? What food does it eat?

✓ **RAISE BRINE SHRIMP** Children love to watch the shrimp larvae swim about in a small tank.

✓ **ADOPT A WILD ANIMAL** Several zoos and wildlife organizations have "adopt an animal" programs. In exchange for your donation of $25 or so, your child will receive an adoption certificate and picture of the animal. It can be a fun way to donate funds to an important cause, and it is a good gift for the child who already has all the toys and clothes he needs.

GREEN ON A SHOESTRING

Toys don't have to dent your budget. Depending on where you live, you may be able to get them for free just by keeping an eye on what other people put in their garbage. Sadly, many Americans don't even bother to donate high-quality, gently used toys to charities. They just put them out on the curb. Some cities have a robust informal swap system where people routinely pick up items off the curb. But in most suburbs, once beloved toys sit in the burning sun or get ruined by rain until a garbage truck comes to swallow them up. Keep your eyes open and you will find bicycles, dollhouses, dolls, picnic sets, and many other items that you can save from the landfill. Also check garage sales, consignment stores, thrift stores, and online sites such as *freecycle.org* and *craigslist.org*.

It's Elementary

As your child heads to school, he or she will start becoming more aware of the world. Your child will learn to read, which offers a limitless new way of learning. At school, science classes for this age group usually focus on the natural world, including the study of rocks, plants, and insects. Guide your children in ways that they can apply these lessons to real-life problems and solve them.

WHAT TO TALK ABOUT Kids in this age group are starting to gain greater self-awareness. This is the age for dinosaurs, volcanoes, predator-prey interactions, and space exploration. Children love using the tools that bring our natural world into closer view. These tools include magnifying glasses, microscopes, binoculars, and telescopes. A lot of children at this age develop a love of collecting rocks, learning the names of birds, and of course learning the names of dinosaurs. At this magical age children often combine facts about the natural world with their imaginative play. Stuffed animals, toy dinosaurs, and endangered animals made from carved wood are excellent toys for stimulating a child's fertile imagination.

ENDANGERED SPECIES Polar bear cubs and baby pandas are some of the cutest animals around. The affinity that children feel for baby animals can help excite their interest in saving endangered species. Help your child form the questions about why animals become endangered. Help him come to his own conclusions about what people can do to prevent animals from becoming endangered and restore endangered populations. Emphasize that species don't just become endangered or extinct in far-away countries, but that many animals have already gone extinct right in your child's own state or region.

RAIN FOREST DESTRUCTION With army ants patrolling the forest floor, pythons hanging from tree branches, and monkeys swinging from vine to vine, the rain forest is a wonderful playground for a child's imagination. Yet these forests are being cut down at an alarming rate. Help your child understand why people cut down rain forests, and how we can help protect them. Ask how our individual actions can reduce the destruction of rain forests. For example, we could refuse to buy wood products that originated from old-growth rain forests.

THE FOOD WEB Animals depend on other animals and plants for their survival. Kids love to figure out what eats what. They admire the skill and power of the lioness that catches and consumes the gazelle. And what does the gazelle eat? Where does the grass get its energy?

HOW OUR CAR CAUSES AIR POLLUTION The driving we do everyday contributes to air pollution and global climate change. How do our personal choices about using the car to get to school, lessons, playdates, and parks affect the environment around us? Can we walk, bike, or take a bus instead? If not, why not?

GLOBAL CLIMATE CHANGE Climate change is an abstract concept even for many adults. However, most children can understand that global warming can make life tough for polar bears and emperor penguins. Since children are also fascinated by natural disasters such as hurricanes and tornadoes, you can discuss the fact that many experts have found that global climate change is worsening severe weather events.

PLUMBING This sounds like a funny topic, but lots of kids grow up these days never knowing where clean water comes from or where it goes when it disappears down the drain. Lots of kids this age get a kick out of thinking about where their human waste goes once they flush the toilet. Talk about how we get our water, how we make sure it is clean, and how we clean up wastewater.

WHERE DO THINGS COME FROM Many children may not have thought about where their toys come from. The sweet notions of elves building Christmas toys up at the North Pole couldn't be farther from today's reality of sweatshops in China. You don't have to destroy all your child's illusions, but you could talk about what toys are made of. How is metal different from plastic? How can you tell whether a toy is made to last versus break easily? Look around for any toys you may have saved from your childhood, and pass them on to your son or daughter. Help your children choose toys that are durable. Maybe some day *their* children will play with them.

ECO-TIP: TAKE A CHANCE ON WALKING

One of the main reasons that parents cite for driving their kids everywhere is safety. If they drive their child to school, the child won't have to cross dangerous intersections. If they drive their child to a playdate with another child, they will know that their child arrived safely at the friend's house. Safety is important, but fears need not paralyze us. Why not ride your bike with your child to the playdate? Take your child by the hand when crossing the street. If your town's major intersections lack pedestrian signs and lights, lobby for them at the next town council meeting.

TRIPS AND ACTIVITIES School-age children are a pleasure to take on outings. Not only are children able to carry their own lunches, water bottles, and sweatshirts, they are also a lot more engaged in learning about animals and the natural environment.

ZOOS, WILDLIFE REFUGES, AQUARIUMS Animal parks are already the only way most people can see certain endangered species. In addition to seeing rare animals, your children can learn about the lives and habits of more common animals from near and far. One criticism of zoos is that many of them lack plaques or signs that tell where the animal is from, what it eats, etc. Bring along a wildlife book when you visit the zoo. Your child is sure to have plenty of questions, and you'll be able to help her or him look up the answers.

TIDE POOLS, MARSHES, AND COASTAL SAND DUNES Strolling a sandy beach is a marvelous way to get close to nature. Go off-season before the sun worshippers show up. Watch for sand crabs burrowing into the sand as waves retreat. Watch sandpipers run up and down the beach as they hunt for crabs. Tide pools are a magical world for children. Look for sea anemones and snails and the occasional sea star or urchin. Marshes and sand dunes are wonderful places to explore, but these are fragile ecosystems. Look for parks that have boardwalks over the dunes and through marshes. Don't wander on your own through these sensitive areas.

YOUR HOME Take your child on a tour of the systems in your house. Show him or her where the water comes into the house, where the electrical wires come in, and where sewage pipes go out. Show your child your utility bills so that he understands that there is a cost for these services and a need for conservation.

CAMPING This is an excellent age to take kids camping. Teach your child to be a respectful camper. Store human food where wildlife cannot reach it and leave the site cleaner than when you found it.

PLAYGROUND GAMES Work environmental themes into your playground games. Play tag or hide-and-seek using a predator and prey theme. Get more ideas from Joseph Cornell's *Sharing Nature with Children* (Dawn Publications, 1979).

MAKE CRAFTS Make molds of animal tracks out of nontoxic clay (see Chapter 7 for nontoxic clays). Turn a pinecone into a turkey by adding feathers, a beak, and eyes cut from construction paper.

VACATION JOURNAL Keep a journal about travel and nature experiences.

COMMUNITY SERVICE Select gently used toys and clothing to donate to a charity in the community or help out at a trail cleanup.

READING Subscribe to a nature magazine such as *National Geographic Kids* (ages 6 to 14).

SKILLS TO TEACH Take advantage of your children's imagination to introduce fun skills that will get them off the couch and into the backyard. Some of these skills will stick with them for a lifetime, while others are childhood games that they'll look back on fondly for years to come.

HOW TO IDENTIFY ANIMAL TRACKS It doesn't matter if you don't know a dog print from a deer track. You can find books and websites to help you. Visit a natural area with your book and look for tracks. Or hunt around your house or at the local park. In cities you can look for tracks of squirrels, cats, and dogs.

HOW TO BE A WATER DETECTIVE Do you know how many gallons can fill your bathtub? How many gallons does your toilet use per flush? Kids can use their budding math skills to calculate how much water your family uses every day in bathing, flushing, washing dishes, and washing clothes. Then they can help you think of ways to reduce your family's water use.

HOW TO GARDEN Most kids love to get dirty, and the garden is a great place to do it guilt-free. Get your children involved in the planning aspects, such as choosing in what part of the yard to put the garden, designing the soil beds, and deciding which vegetables and flowers to plant. Your kids will love watching seeds sprout into seedlings indoors while waiting for the weather to warm up. Once it is warm enough, your children can plant seeds directly in the garden. Or make it easy by buying seedlings at the garden center or farmers market.

HOW TO DISPOSE OF GARBAGE It is surprising how many children and adults think nothing of tossing garbage out a car window or onto the ground. Most good habits need to be taught, so don't miss out on teaching your child to always use garbage cans. Better yet, teach them to generate less garbage in the first place by using reusable water bottles and packaging.

DO YOU REALLY NEED IT? In the three Rs of environmentalism, we often forget that the first R is for "reduce." As in, reduce the amount of unnecessary stuff you buy. Question your child about his or her need to have the latest toy or boots that everyone else is wearing. Teach your child to ask himself, "Do I really need that?" and "Will it make me happy?"

HOW TO BE A SAVVY TV WATCHER If you've managed to keep your kids from becoming TV addicts, more power to you. But if your child spends a lot of time watching TV, let him in on the big secret of commercials: Those kids are *actors*. Yes, those children enjoying that new toy are *being paid* to act as if it is fun. Those children who are eating that sugary cereal are paid to pretend it tastes good. You never see commercials showing those kids at the dentist getting their cavities filled, now do you? (See Chapter 7 for more suggestions on savvy TV watching.)

HOW TO TAKE CARE OF A PET If at all possible, opt for a pet from a shelter. If you are adopting a shelter dog or cat, do your best to learn about its disposition around children. Over time, have your child take increasing responsibility for pet care.

PROJECTS TO DO At this age kids can do a lot to help the planet and their local community, but they'll need adult guidance to carry through a project. That means you, a teacher, or another adult may have to make some phone calls, write letters, or talk to community leaders. Wherever possible let your kids take the lead and provide help when they ask for it. One option is to join a group that does community service and environment-oriented projects. For example, find an ecologically minded scouting troop or a church youth group. Consider creating such a group if none exists in your area.

RECYCLING AT SCHOOL Does the school have a program, and are kids participating in it?

CELEBRATE ARBOR DAY Have your child plant a tree, either on your property or at a park. Many cities have tree-planting programs.

HAVE A BIRTHDAY FUND-RAISER Your child may choose to ask his or her friends for charitable gifts to a wildlife preservation fund in lieu of birthday party gifts. (See Chapter 9 for more birthday ideas.)

CRAFTS Make an animal habitat using a shoebox. Take a nature walk and have your children collect leaves, acorns, and dirt. Create a diorama for

THE FACTS
In 2007 the United States recycled and composted 85 million tons of municipal waste, equivalent to eliminating the greenhouse gas emissions of 35 million passenger cars, according to the EPA.

a woodland creature such as a beaver, deer, or squirrel. Draw in a stream with blue marker. Ask your child, what will happen if one part of the habitat has been spoiled by pollution? How will that change the animal's habitat? How will the animal respond?

DO AN ECO-MAKEOVER Have your children do an eco-makeover on your house. Have them inspect cabinets looking for disposable products that can be replaced by reusable ones. Replace paper plates with washable picnic plates. Replace paper napkins with cloth ones. Replace disposable cups for brushing teeth with reusable ones.

RAIN BARREL Set up a rain barrel (it can be as simple as a plastic bucket) and encourage the kids to use the rainwater to help Mom or Dad water the grass and yard.

The Green Preteen

During the preteen years, children are developing their critical thinking skills and becoming more independent. At school they are gaining abilities in math and reading that can help them understand environmental issues and calculate the impacts of their lifestyles on the planet. In science classes they are learning to collect and analyze data and draw conclusions. Help them apply these lessons to understanding the impacts of water and air pollution on people and the environment.

WHAT TO TALK ABOUT This is an excellent time to talk about big-picture concepts like protecting the planet and conserving resources. Help your child identify wasteful practices at home or around her school or community, and teach her that *she* can make a difference.

ROLE MODELS Talk about people who have devoted their life to preserving nature and protecting the environment. You could mention writers like Henry Thoreau, photographers like Ansel Adams, or people who campaigned for protection of wild spaces, like President Theodore

Roosevelt. Or find some modern-day celebrities, such as actor Leonardo DiCaprio and actress Julia Roberts, who have lent their star status to environmental causes.

SENSE OF SELF Help your child develop the courage to have different opinions than his or her friends. Encourage your child to do what is right for the environment and for his or her own health.

SHARING WAYS TO HELP THE EARTH Not all your children's friends will be eco-minded. Share with your child ways to talk to friends about how to protect Earth.

RECYCLING Ask your child to imagine a pile of soda cans in the backyard. That could fill a landfill quickly unless you recycle. What does recycled aluminum get turned into? Try to find out.

ENVIRONMENTAL JUSTICE Why is it that power plants and sewage treatment plants are clustered in poorer neighborhoods? Why do some people live in neighborhoods that lack supermarkets and other places to buy healthy foods? How can we help overburdened communities?

CLIMATE SCIENCE How do scientists know that the climate is warming? Share with your child the evidence for climate change. Discuss the environmental and health impacts for future generations.

CLIMATE CHANGE AND HEALTH How will warming global temperatures affect food production, the spread of infectious diseases, and children's health?

DEFORESTATION What does cutting down trees have to do with climate change? What happens to the climate when people burn forests to clear land for agriculture? Why are trees beneficial to global carbon dioxide levels?

TRIPS AND ACTIVITIES Keep your kids busy outdoors as much as possible. Some parents choose to limit access to TV, computers, and video games to give children the opportunity to play outdoors. Kids may resist being pushed out the door to play in the yard when their favorite TV show or video game is available, so try to find some structured sports or activities that they really enjoy.

GREEN DICTIONARY

BIODEGRADABLE
Biodegradable items are capable of being broken down by microscopic life-forms such as bacteria and fungi. Fruit peels take a few weeks to biodegrade, whereas cotton clothing takes a few years. Plastics do not biodegrade at all.

One option if you can afford it is to enroll your children in after-school or summer-time nature-center enrichment programs.

BUILD A TREE HOUSE Kids at this age spend time reading and may crave a quiet place where they can escape into their own worlds. Building a tree house is a great family project that can involve designing the house, incorporating recycled materials, using basic tools, and the joy of conceiving and completing a project.

CAMPING Outdoor trips will be longer and more involved. In addition to pitching your state-of-the-art tent and popping open the gas-powered camp stove, use your camping outings to teach your children some survival skills. How could you make a shelter if you were caught out on a trail in bad weather? Are there any edible berries or other plants you can eat?

BACKPACKING If your child is physically fit and emotionally ready, try a backcountry trip. Far away from cars and buildings, your family can enjoy the feeling that you have escaped into the wilderness.

PLAY ELECTRICITY DETECTIVE Have your child make a list of all the environmentally harmful things your family does around the house, from leaving the TV on when no one is watching, to leaving windows open when the air conditioner is on.

THE FACTS

Each U.S. resident generates 4.5 pounds of garbage per day; 1.5 pounds of this is recycled or composted while the rest gets sent to a landfill, according to the EPA.

TRAIL CLEARING Moving branches and raking leaves needs to be done on a regular basis in most parks. Work with a park ranger to organize a trail-clearing day for your child and his friends. Then grab some gloves, rakes, and maybe a small saw (used by an adult, of course) and head out onto the trail.

DO ERRANDS BY BICYCLE Take your children on weekly trips to the library by bike. Or ride to the park or a nearby ice cream shop. Whenever possible, substitute a bike trip for a car outing. Your children may balk at doing errands with you in the car, but they will probably love going by bike.

WALK OR BIKE TO SCHOOL Many people have good reasons for driving their kids to school, including busy schedules, the need to drop the child on the way to work, and severe weather. But if you can spare the extra time, try walking or biking. Your child probably would enjoy the novelty, and it may become a lasting habit.

VISIT THE PAST Have your family spend one week living like people did in the past (best done in the summer when the kids don't have to go to school). Go to bed when the sun goes down. Don't use any electrical appliances. What was life like back then?

HAVE A "REUSE EVERYTHING" WEEK Wait, don't throw out that junk mail envelope—you can use it the next time you write a letter to Grandma. Spend an entire week trying not to throw anything away and reusing everything you can. After the week is over, keep some of the habits going.

CRAFTS Kids can make notepads out of used computer paper that has printing only on the back.

SKILLS TO TEACH Keep the lines of communication open as your children grow up. Good parenting involves talking regularly to kids about the pressures they face at school and with friends. You can apply the same sort of thinking to your child's views of protecting the planet. Check in with your kids to see what they are doing to help protect the environment. Offer suggestions. Help them get their friends involved.

HOW TO MAKE ECO-FRIENDLY GIFTS AND WRAPPINGS When your child goes to a party where gifts are expected, help her select a gift that protects natural resources. You could recommend an organic cotton T-shirt or a bath-and-body set made from organic ingredients. Help your child find a creative way to wrap the gift, using either a reusable tote bag or a bag made from items that were destined for disposal, such as fabric scraps or newspaper.

HOW TO BUY FASHIONS THAT DON'T COME FROM SWEATSHOPS Most consumer goods are made overseas because companies can pay laborers less. But these companies or their subsidiaries routinely cut corners on environmental regulations, too. They use toxic chemicals that have been banned in the United States. Help your child learn to check labels to find out where clothing is made and what material it is made from. One label to look for is the UNITE union label, which guarantees clothing was not made in sweatshops.

NATURAL BEAUTY MAKEOVER Conduct research into the products in cosmetics, lotions, shampoos, and deodorants, and see if there are alternative brands available without chemical hazards. The same can be done with household cleaners.

HOW TO READ LABELS Help your children learn how to decipher the nutrient facts on food packages. Talk about the nutrients in food. Look at the ingredients. Are most of them recognizable or are many of them chemical additives? Discuss the difference between 100-calorie packages of cookies and the 100 calories found in an apple. Which is better for you?

PROJECTS TO DO Kids are bursting with ideas and plans at this age. Capture that enthusiasm and direct it toward a project that will help the planet while showing your child that it *is* possible for a kid to make meaningful change in the world. Here are some ideas:

ORGANIZE A RECYCLING DRIVE Help your child collect used goods from households and sell them at a garage sale, then donate the proceeds to an ecology-minded charity.

START A LETTER-WRITING CAMPAIGN Is there a cause that your child feels passionate about? It could be drilling in the Arctic National Wildlife Refuge or a planned housing development that will destroy a wooded lot in your town. Help your child craft a letter and guide him on soliciting the involvement of his friends and schoolmates.

REVAMP HER SCHOOL LUNCH Have your child take a look in her lunch sack. Is she using reusable containers, or does she routinely toss out plastic bags and snack wrappers? Help her design an eco-friendly lunch.

CONDUCT AN ECO-AUDIT AT HOME OR AT SCHOOL Identify ways to reduce toxic exposure. Assess the school for environmental health concerns.

TRACK YOUR TRASH Has your child ever wondered how much trash his or her classroom generates each day? With permission from the child's teacher and the school custodian, your child and his classmates can log the amount of trash generated each day (in units of full trash bags). After the week, the kids can see how much they generated and brainstorm ways to reduce what they throw away. Could more items go into recycling? Could the students reuse paper scraps?

GROW A WORM COLONY Several online stores sell worm farms. Kids will enjoy watching the worms tunnel through the soil. Talk with your child about how worms do wonders for soil. When your child is done watching worms, have her release them into your garden or flowerbed.

SWITCH TO REUSABLE BATTERIES Rechargeable batteries are available in most stores. Although they cost more at first, they can save a lot of money over the lifetime of a device. Have your child run her handheld games and other toys off rechargeable batteries.

HOMEMADE GIFTS Why give the teacher a store-bought candle or other knickknack when what she really wants is a way to remember your child? Help your son or daughter create gifts for teachers and other adults in his or her life. Throughout the year, collect glass and plastic containers that your recycling program won't take. Decorate the salvaged containers with glued on bits of colored paper and decorations. Use them as containers for homemade cookies.

PASS IT ON When your child gets a new toy or clothing item, help her figure out what to do with one of her existing toys or clothing. Help your child develop the habit of passing on used items instead of tossing them into the garbage.

PLANT A BUTTERFLY GARDEN Convert a patch of your yard or grow flowers in a pot on your patio. Choose nectar-bearing flowers such as butterfly bush, butterfly weed, common milkweed, globe amaranth, heliotrope, marigold, and zinnia. Choose flowers and plants that are native to your area.

EXPERIMENT Bury both degradable and biodegradable objects (papers, plastic, a discarded toy, etc.) in a dirt pile, and check back over the course of the next few months to see what items have degraded and which have not.

SURVEY YOUR FELLOW STUDENTS' ECO-HABITS Do they walk or ride a bike to school? Do they use reusable bottles? Just taking the survey could help students think about changing their habits. Post the results in the student newspaper.

GREEN DICTIONARY

WORM CASTINGS
Worms create castings (or poop, as your child might call it) that enrich the soil and help plants grow.

Teen Power

Teens have loads of energy and enthusiasm—they just need a little bit of help to harness it. We parents and teachers can help them gain the skills they need to write letters, organize groups, and approach the decision-makers in our community.

Teens often look back on their adolescent years and can point to a single teacher who inspired them, or an activity that changed their direction in life. A dedication to protecting the planet can be the anchor a teen needs to survive the choppy seas of adolescence. Keeping teens busy with service projects, sports, homework, and hobbies is a good way to keep these young people from dabbling in drugs and other self-destructive behavior.

WHAT TO TALK ABOUT Kids handle the teen years in different ways. Some become very introverted while others run for class leadership positions. Some spend weekends in front of the TV while others play multiple sports. Parents need to nurture teen interests and help kids find activities that stimulate their minds and broaden their horizons.

DIFFERENT IS GOOD Teens love their independence, yet they sometimes follow trends like sheep. Help your child realize that being different is a good thing. Help her express her artistic creativity through her style of dress and her choice of hobbies. Extend the idea of individuality to her choice of what she buys. Does she have to buy the same style boots that everyone else has? Or could she choose a pair from a thrift shop and create her own unique look?

WHO IS BEHIND THIS? One way to get kids thinking about being different is to help them question why certain styles are popular. Is there a TV actress that everyone is dressing like? Why should we all try to look like her? What type of lifestyle is she selling? (If it is a green lifestyle, is she marketing green products that you don't need, or is she giving advice that is truly Earth-friendly, like reducing the amount of stuff we buy?)

WHAT ARE THE UNDERLYING ISSUES? Many times in the course of history, health and environmental scientists have sounded the alarm over the use of a dangerous chemical or product, only to be silenced or ignored.

Leaded gasoline and cigarettes are two products that were known to be harmful long before the government began to ban or regulate them. Help your child understand these issues and discuss the incentives that industry and government had for delaying taking action.

MAN VERSUS NATURE The reintroduction of wolves into Yellowstone National Park has resulted in the return of a predator that kills not only wild elk and bison but also livestock on nearby cattle ranches. Help your child discuss the struggle between environmental preservation and the need to have livelihoods. Discuss America's frontier mentality and how it is has led to a different regulatory environment than found in, for example, Europe.

WHO SHOULD PAY FOR CLIMATE CHANGE Why are nations refusing to reduce their greenhouse gas emissions? Which nations would be hurt the most by reducing their emissions? Should developing countries have to make the same reductions that industrialized nations do? This is a great topic for a family dinner discussion and a school project or paper.

HOW POLITICS AFFECT SCIENCE Why did it take so long for the U.S. population to accept the scientific consensus that human activities contribute to global climate change? Why didn't the media do more to report the story?

TRIPS AND ACTIVITIES By now your child is able to handle longer camping trips and hikes, some of them without you tagging along. Try to keep your child involved in organized outdoor activities like scouting or a high school wilderness club. Here are some outings and activities to consider:

WATER TREATMENT PLANT Does your local sewage treatment plant give tours? Many will allow student groups or scouting groups to take a tour. Help your child to organize a trip or suggest the idea to a science teacher or other school advisor.

VISIT A FARM If you live not far from agricultural areas, your teen and his friends can learn a lot about where food comes from by taking field trips to local farms. The teens can compare the differences in farming methods, the cost of the meat or produce, and the environmental impact of each method.

GET RID OF "VAMPIRES" All those cell phone rechargers and computer monitors that your family leaves plugged in draw power even when they are not in use. Suggest that your teen inventory the house and put power-sucking devices on a power strip so they can be turned off and on easily without always having to plug and unplug them.

USE AN ONLINE ENVIRONMENTAL ASSESSMENT TOOL Your child can learn about the health connections to exposures at school and home with an online environmental assessment tool. See the National Center for Healthy Housing, *www.nchh.org*, and the EPA's Healthy School Environments Assessment Tool (HealthySEAT), *www.epa.gov/schools/healthyseat*.

WRITE YOUR OWN ENVIRONMENTAL IMPACT STATEMENT (EIS) An environmental impact statement is often required before breaking ground on a new building. Your teen can construct her own EIS. How much electricity does she use, and how much water and food? Once she has calculated these figures, she can work backward to figure out the amount of natural resources that must be used to support her lifestyle. How much coal is used to generate the electricity? How many gallons of fuel went into producing that food? She can get some of the information she'll need at the Energy Information Administration website, *www.eia.doe.gov*.

JOIN THE DEBATE CLUB Your teen will gain valuable speaking skills on the debate team. What is more, he or she can introduce environmental topics that are sure to fire up some excellent verbal exchanges. Questions include: How certain are we about climate change predictions? Why should we save endangered species when their habitats are being destroyed? Who should pay to clean up toxic waste sites?

WALK OR RIDE BIKES TO FRIENDS' HOUSES If your teen is always pestering you for a ride here or there, suggest he or she take a bike. Make sure the route is a safe one, away from major thoroughfares, and make sure your teen wears a helmet.

FIGHT JUNK MAIL Suggest that your son or daughter help reduce the number of catalogs arriving on any given day by visiting *www.catalogchoice.org*.

GREEN DICTIONARY

VAMPIRE
An electrical appliance that draws power even when in "off" mode. Examples include TVs, DVD players, and cell phone chargers.

KITCHEN TABLE TALK

Teens That Took Charge to Help Save the Planet

Today's teens know a lot about the environmental challenges we humans have created. Television programs and school curricula have pretty well covered topics like global warming and plastics in the ocean. You can't blame these teens for wondering, "How did our adults get us into this mess, and how are they going to get us out of it?"

A lot of these questioning teens aren't waiting for adults to solve environmental problems. They are doing it themselves. A New York City teen started a program to distribute energy-saving compact fluorescent lights to low-income people. A 12-year-old from Arizona raised money to help build clean water wells in India. An Alaska teen who loved to ski converted his car to run on electricity because he could see the everyday effects of global warming on the disappearing snow on the ski slopes. These are just some of the inspirational stories featured in the book *The Green Teen* (New Society Publishers, 2009), by Jenn Savedge. "These teens were so excited to be part of the solution," says Savedge.

The greatest challenge these teens faced, not surprisingly, was being taken seriously, says Savedge. Adults were skeptical that young people could pull off what they set out to do. But these teens didn't get discouraged when officials didn't return phone calls or e-mails. They kept on trying to reach out to their fellow teens, the media, and government officials, as well as donors looking for good causes to fund.

Many of these teens found that in the end, their youth was an advantage, says Savedge. Once a project gets rolling, adults become interested in helping motivated young people. Many teens find that rather than calling officials and being ignored, the officials and the media are calling *them.*

Savedge's book is full of practical information on how teens can identify a worthwhile cause and organize a project. She reminds us that there are all sorts of ways for teens to use the skills they have—no special environmental education is required. For example, teens who are computer savvy could help a nonprofit group build a website or enter information into a database. Teens who are very social could help organize their friends to come to a park for a clean up day.

To parents, Savedge gives the advice not to nag your teens into helping the environment. Otherwise helping the environment becomes one more chore, like cleaning their room or completing that college entry essay. Rather, she suggests guiding kids on ways to apply their passions— whether it be strumming a guitar or playing video games—to helping the environment. Maybe your teen could play music at a fund-raiser, or hold a fund-raising video game "play-a-thon." When teens can work their favorite activity into a worthwhile cause, the environment is the winner.

SKILLS TO TEACH One of the most useful skills you can teach your child is how to feel comfortable dealing with adults. Good communication skills can help your teen do everything from making small talk with relatives to offering services as a babysitter. These skills can help your child make a good first impression when interviewed by prospective colleges or when applying for his or her first job.

HOW TO TALK TO ADULTS Grown-ups appreciate good grammar, proper pronunciation, and the absence of the ubiquitous filler "like." Help your child achieve his or her goals by ensuring that he or she can talk in a language that the adult world can understand.

HOW TO ORGANIZE A SERVICE PROJECT Kids need guidance on how to identify a need (lack of curbside recycling); how to reach out to like-minded friends and fellow students (contact friends via e-mail or social networks); drum up support for the cause (organize an informational meeting or rally); and approach the people who can change the policy (speak at a city council meeting or initiate a letter-writing campaign).

HOW TO WRITE A LETTER Good writing can not only help your child's letter about the destruction of a local wetland get noticed by a newspaper editor, it can also help her get into college and have a successful career. Offer to proofread your child's letters and offer suggestions on how to get ideas across simply and powerfully. Create a list of government representatives, from local to national, that your teen can write to

GREEN ON A SHOESTRING
Encourage your teen to look for diversions that don't cost money, instead of shopping at the mall. Take her (and her friends) on a thrift shop expedition. They may be surprised at the bargains they find!

on behalf of her cause. Encourage her to involve her friends in the letter-writing campaign.

HOW TO ATTEND A PLANNING MEETING AT THE CITY COUNCIL Help your child understand what the city council does and how he or she can approach the council with concerns. The first step may be to simply attend a meeting to see what goes on.

HOW TO LEARN ABOUT VOTING RECORDS Help your child learn about his or her local representatives and their voting records on environmental issues. Several organizations maintain voting records on environmental issues. A good one is the League of Conservation Voters' National Environmental Scorecard at *www.lcv.org.*

HOW TO GET PUBLICITY Help your child learn the basics of writing a press release. Have her practice calling local newspapers and other media outlets.

ECO-TIP: GET A BEAUTY ROUTINE MAKEOVER

Encourage your teen to look her best with as little environmental impact as possible. She could take shorter showers, turn off lights when leaving the bathroom, unplug appliances when not in use, and use cosmetics that don't contain harmful chemicals.

PROJECTS TO DO Many teens view service projects as one of the many hurdles they must leap over on their way to completing that all-important document, the college application. Help your child take a less cynical attitude by finding a cause that resonates with your child's personality and interests. If your teen loves surfing, suggest a project that involves improving ocean water quality. If your teen plays in a rock band, how about putting on a benefit concert for an environmental cause? Some projects may be personal, like trying to eat only from local sources, whereas others may benefit thousands of people, like lobbying the state to preserve farmland and keep local produce flowing to farmers markets.

EAT LIKE A "LOCAVORE" Eat foods only from farms and ranches within a radius of 100 miles (or so, given your area). Obviously this is easiest to do during the growing season, but if your teen is feeling ambitious, he or she may try to extend it into winter by planning ahead and doing some freezing and canning.

GET YOUR SCHOOL TO GO PAPERLESS Schools send reams of paper home in the form of parent notifications. Yet most parents these days have access to e-mail. Support your child in his or her drive to get the school to go paperless.

START A GREEN CLUB Your teen may want to start a club to raise awareness about global deforestation or a committee to preserve a tract of town land by turning it into a woodland park. He or she will have to find a teacher or other adult sponsor, advertise the club, sign up members, and vote on the issues that the club wants to tackle.

START AN ORGANIC LAWN SERVICE Many homeowners would like to move away from using synthetic fertilizers and pesticides, but don't know how. Few green lawn services exist. If your teen wants to earn money, this is a great business for a teen.

HOST A STUFF SWAP Find out if your town has a free stuff swap (also called an open-air mall) where people can take used items to exchange them for others. If not, your teen may want to start one.

RAISE CHICKENS A good small business for a teen is raising chickens and selling the cage-free eggs. Some people even raise chickens in cities, depending on zoning regulations. Teens can start an egg cooperative and deliver eggs to neighbors on a regular basis.

GIVE THE SCHOOL AN ENVIRONMENTAL AUDIT Your teen could work with his or her friends (and the blessing of the principal) to audit the school for wasteful practices. Does the lunchroom use polystyrene containers and other nonrecyclable items? Does the school recycle? Help your teen work with school officials to come up with alternatives. If major fast-food chains can switch to recyclable packaging, the school lunchroom surely can.

BRING "LOCAVORISM" TO SCHOOL Your teen can do some detective work to find out where the cafeteria food comes from. Does any of it come

GREEN DICTIONARY

LOCAVORE

A person who eats only foods gathered, raised, or grown in their local area.

from local farms? If not, your teen can work to bring local produce into schools. (See Chapter 8 for more farm-to-school ideas.)

STOP FOOD WASTE What happens to food that is about to expire at your local market? Is it donated to a food pantry? Maybe your teen might organize a program to reduce food waste and keep people from going hungry.

WALK, WALK, WALK EVERYWHERE Can your teen get to school for a week without going in a vehicle? Can he do it for a month?

USE PUBLIC TRANSPORTATION Does your town have a bus? Encourage your teen to try for one week to go everywhere by public transportation. One bus can carry the same number of people as 40 cars.

GO WITHOUT For fun, your teen could try to live without using anything made of plastic for a week. Can he last a month? A year?

START A COMMUNITY GARDEN Lots of communities offer a central location where people can claim a small plot of land and grow their own vegetables. If your town lacks a community garden, your teen might want to organize one. Help him to contact city leaders, scout a good location for the garden, and drum up interest from the local community.

GET A GREEN-COLLAR JOB Your teen will at some point want to get a job or take a volunteer position. Why not make it a green job? Your teen could apply at a nature preserve, a summer camp, or at a recycling center.

CARPOOL When your teen gets his or her license, encourage him or her to carpool when possible.

Take Action

▸ Raise kids to appreciate nature by taking them on walks starting at a young age.

▸ Help your children choose healthy foods.

▸ Read books with environmental themes to your toddlers and preschoolers.

▸ Let your toddler help with green tasks, such as sorting recycling and hanging clothes out to dry.

▸ Send your child to school with reusable water bottles, lunch bags, and snack containers.

▸ Have your child use the backside of junk mail and computer paper for her drawings.

▸ Make crafts out of plastic yogurt containers and other items that would have ended up in the garbage.

▸ Take your kids on trips to the zoo, aquarium, or wildlife center. Bring along a book about animals so that the kids can learn while they are there.

▸ Work with your child on how to write a letter to the mayor or other government official.

▸ Talk with your child about staying true to his or her own values and not going along with the crowd.

▸ Help your child think of ways to persuade her friends to join her in working to make the environment a better place.

▸ Encourage your child to conceive of an environmental project, gather the necessary resources, and carry out the project.

▸ Present positive role models, including movie stars, who work toward improving the environment.

▸ Introduce your child to the concept of environmental justice, and how we can work to make sure that everyone has access to clean air and a healthy environment.

▸ Plant a garden.

▸ Support your teen in his or her efforts to start a small business that helps the environment, such as a green lawn service.

▸ Provide the tools and supervision for a trail-clearing project.

▸ Suggest that your child enlist schoolmates and her teacher in devising an ecology-based project for the classroom.

▸ Help your child get a "green job" by assisting him or her in Internet searches and other job-seeking techniques.

THE SCIENCE BEHIND IT

Getting Rid of Witches' Knickers

Our children have never known a world without the ubiquitous plastic grocery bag. The Irish call bags caught in the branches of trees "witches' knickers." People in Africa collect them and weave them into baskets, handbags, and bowls. Far too many of the bags wind up in the ocean where they are responsible for the deaths of tens of thousands of turtles, whales, dolphins, and other creatures.

A mere 150 years have passed since Alexander Parkes put the first plastics on display at the Great International Exhibition in London in 1862. The ensuing decades saw many inventions by chemists including the invention of viscose (Rayon) and polyvinyl chloride (PVC). The first true plastics came along in 1909 when Leo Hendrik Baekeland used coal tar as the basis for his Bakelite plastic.

Roughly 50 years would go by before plastic could be made flexible enough for use in bags. The key innovation was the use of petroleum rather than coal as the source for plastic's building blocks. Today, oil and natural gas serve as the starting ingredients for most plastics. Plastic lunch bags for sandwiches and snacks gained popularity in the 1950s and plastic trash bags started appearing on curbs by the late 1960s.

Plastic shopping bags, however, took even longer to become widely adopted. It wasn't until the late 1970s that grocery stores began switching from bagging groceries in paper bags to offering consumers a choice: paper or plastic. Since then many stores have dropped paper bags altogether. Today, about 100 billion plastic bags are used each year in the United States, according to Worldwatch Institute, an environmental research organization.

All these bags are creating a huge waste-disposal problem. Petroleum-based plastics never actually biodegrade but rather break into very small parts. No one knows how long it takes for the typical grocery store bag to break down because the items haven't been around long enough. Estimates range from 400 to 1,000 years.

Although many supermarkets and big box stores collect plastic bags for recycling into plastic lumber and containers, only about 12 percent of all bags, wraps, and sacks are recycled, according to the EPA. Over four million tons of plastic bags, sacks and wraps were discarded in the United States in 2007. Given the cost and energy inputs involved in recycling, it may be better for the planet to just not use plastic bags in the first place.

Luckily today there are well-designed, inexpensive reusable bags for sale at nearly every supermarket. We lived without plastic bags in the not-too-distant past, and we can do so again. With reusable bags costing just a fraction of the typical grocery bill, most of us can afford to pick one up even when we've left our stash of reusable bags in the car. For quick trips we can carry purchased items out in our hands (receipt prominently displayed, of course). By helping to spread the word about the environmental impact of plastic bags we can help limit demand for disposable bags and get rid of the witches' knickers once and for all.

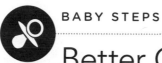

BABY STEPS

Better Choices for Your Baby's First Year

HUMAN BEINGS NEED CONSTANT CARE IN THE FIRST YEAR OF LIFE. A newborn foal learns to walk within hours after birth, but a human child lives a full year before he takes his first faltering steps. Human infants are utterly dependent on parents and caregivers for food, shelter, and protection.

Food, shelter, and protection seem like simple requirements, yet we humans love to make things complicated. First-time parents experience not only feelings of joy but also less enjoyable emotions ranging from inadequacy to anxiety. Suddenly there are numerous decisions to be made. Who will change the diapers? Which kind, cloth or disposable? What kind of feeding, breast or bottle?

An eco-friendly and health-oriented mindset can help answer all these questions. Eco-friendly baby care is better not just for the babies and their caregivers but also for the mother of us all, planet Earth. When it comes to purchasing baby supplies, the choices seem endless, and sorting out the claims of manufacturers and consumer reports becomes a daunting task. It helps simplify matters to think in terms of a back-to-basics approach that emphasizes natural baby care items over synthetic ones, tried and true practices over unproven theories, and needs over consumerism.

Providing healthy food means providing the highest quality food, including breast milk if possible, high-quality formula if not. Sheltering baby means providing a safe place to grow and clothes that are gentle to the skin. Protection means protecting baby not only against falls and accidents but also from infusions of industrial chemicals that come in via food (including breast milk and formula), items placed on the skin, and the air that your baby breathes.

Whether you are new to environmentally conscious living or you are looking to update your knowledge with the latest science, this chapter will provide you with a practical guide to healthy baby care that dovetails with best practices for the planet.

We'll delve into diapering decisions, gain insight on infant attire, lay bare the breast-feeding versus formula debate, discover topless baby sunbathing, and geek out over baby gear.

Bottoms Up

Today's diapers are feats of waste disposal engineering. New materials and designs have led to diapers that leak less often and are easy to use. Today's parents have to balance eco-friendly sensibilities with other considerations like practicality and requirements from day care centers.

THE TIDY (THROWAWAY) DI'DY An entire generation of parents has now been raised in disposable diapers, which first gained popularity in the late 1970s. Since those early days, the design and construction of the disposable diaper has been improved considerably. Today's diapers are nearly leakproof, keep babies feeling dry, and take only seconds to whip off, toss into the garbage, and replace with a new disposable diaper.

The secret to the diaper's success is a superabsorbent polymer (SAP) in the form of a gel or granules tucked deep into the innards of the diaper. This wonder chemical can soak up about 200 times its weight in water. A special plastic fabric on the inside of the diaper wicks moisture away from the baby's skin. Soft fluff pulp serves as padding. The plastic outer layer and fitted leg cuffs keep leaks to a minimum.

Yet all this convenience comes at a cost to the environment. Producing disposable diapers requires numerous resources. Trees are the source of cellulose pulp, which is usually bleached snowy white before use. Petroleum products are used to make plastic. Acrylic acid, a toxic chemical that can kill fish if improperly disposed of, is used to make SAP.

GREEN DICTIONARY

SUPERABSORBENT POLYMERS (SAPS)

Chemicals used in diapers that can soak up massive amounts of liquids. Most diapers contain a SAP called sodium polyacrylate.

All these products create one whopper of a waste disposal problem. A typical baby wears several thousand disposable diapers by the time he or she potty trains, usually somewhere around age three.

Once in the landfill, disposable diapers take roughly 500 years to break down. Although cellulose pulp can biodegrade rather quickly given adequate air and light, landfills usually feature densely packed heaps of garbage. The plastic lining will shred into bits but will take years to degrade further. The SAP eventually migrates into soil and groundwater. SAP is not acutely toxic, however, and is even used in houseplant soil to retain water around roots.

The superabsorbent core and wicking paper keep babies feeling dry long after they wet the diaper—even multiple times. This is great for caregivers but has a downside: Caregivers may change the baby less often, creating ideal conditions for diaper rash. If babies are not changed promptly, the superabsorbent gel can absorb so much urine that it bursts through the diaper lining and comes in contact with baby's skin. Some babies can develop rashes from SAP, although a safety study by diaper company scientists that appeared in a 2008 issue of *Regulatory Toxicology and Pharmacology* states that SAP is nontoxic even if swallowed.[1]

Other studies have found that disposable diapers contain toxic chemicals such as dioxins (leftover from bleaching) and other toxic chemicals associated with the manufacture of plastic—styrene, for example—as well as chemicals from the glues used to hold the diaper together.

These chemicals may not be toxic, but babies can develop sensitivities to them. The dyes in disposable diapers, with names like Disperse Yellow 3, Disperse Orange 3, Disperse Blue 124, and Disperse Blue 106, can cause skin rashes that parents may mistake for diaper rash, according to a study published in the journal *Pediatrics* in 2005.[2] Glues and rubberizing agents can also cause skin irritation, the study found.

In recent years, a number of eco-friendly disposable diapers have come on the market. Most brands contain SAP but use chlorine-free, perfume-free, and dye-free materials. Some use cornstarch-based linings instead of plastic. A few brands can be composted, and one features a flushable or compostable insert.

Composting your diapers sounds like a good idea, but you may encounter some practical hurdles. Your backyard compost pile is unlikely to be able to process the 40 or more diapers per week that your baby goes through. You may be able to find a commercial composting facility that will take them.

If you go with disposable, be sure to dump your baby's waste into the toilet before you toss the diaper. When human waste ends up in a landfill, it can eventually pollute water and soil.

Speaking of trash, you'll want to use a secure trash can or diaper pail that crawling babies can't knock over. But think twice before buying a diaper disposal system that locks you in to buying a specific brand of plastic liner—and spending money buying nonreusable plastic products. Chances are you have a few grocery store plastic bags that could stand to be reused.

Many day care centers require disposables because they can be neatly wrapped and tossed, and they are potentially—but not necessarily—more sanitary than cloth.

A final note: You may have read that disposable diapers lead to male infertility because they trap heat in the groin area. In fact, a cloth diaper covered with a plastic cover could do the same thing. Newer disposables have breathable linings that let heat out.

COTTONING ON TO CLOTH DIAPERS Cloth diapers have undergone a number of product redesigns over the years. Velcro fasteners have replaced cumbersome pins, eliminating the risk of painful pricks. Cloth diapers fit inside neat snug plastic pants that help reduce leaks. Some have replaceable inserts for quick changes on the go.

Like their disposable cousins, cloth diapers also require resources to produce. Cotton is one of the most chemical-dependent and water-intensive crops. Seventy percent of the cotton grown in the U.S. is genetically modified, according to the U.S. Department of Agriculture (USDA). Cotton is usually bleached and then dyed prior to being woven into fabric. If poor disposal practices are used, bleach and dyes can harm aquatic life in streams.

Like their disposable cousins, cloth diapers will also eventually settle in landfills, but most get there after a long life of service, first as diapers for multiple children and then as household cleanup rags. Caregivers can either launder the cloth diapers at home or send them out to a diaper service, which picks up soiled diapers and drops off a fresh pile of snowy white cloth diapers in their place. Diaper services can cost roughly the same amount monthly as buying disposable diapers, depending on where you live.

Here is a brushup on the current terminology for cloth diapers:

PREFOLD DIAPER A large rectangle of fabric folded and stitched into three panels, two outer panels and a thick center panel. Separate waterproof pants are put on over the diaper.

FITTED DIAPER A diaper tailored to fit baby, secured by Velcro or snap closures. Fits inside separate waterproof pants or wraps.

ALL-IN-ONE Shaped, fitted diapers inside a waterproof cover, secured with Velcro or snap closures.

POCKET DIAPER A diaper cover containing a pocket into which you place a prefolded diaper or specially designed insert.

If choosing cloth, look for ones made of unbleached, undyed, organic cotton. Other alternatives include hemp or bamboo fabrics.

THE GREAT DIAPER DEBATE You may have read that both types of diapers are equally bad for the environment. Disposable diapers consume vast amounts of resources from wood pulp and petroleum-based plastics that take several hundred years to decompose. Cloth diapers are reusable but require cleaning with harsh detergents, chlorine bleach, and several thousand gallons of water over the two to three years your child wears them.

Yet most studies compare disposable diapers to *commercial cloth diaper services*, not cloth diapers laundered at home. If you launder cloth diapers at home only once or twice a week and *dry them on a clothesline*, you can reduce the environmental impact of cloth diapers, according to a 2008 Environment Agency study in the United Kingdom,[3] whereas disposables will still remain a single-use, unsustainable item.

In other words, the environmental impact of the cloth diaper is highly dependent on how it is laundered, according to the analysis conducted by the Environment Agency. Washing cloth diapers in full loads, always drying them on a clothesline, and reusing the diapers on a second child lowers the global warming impact by 40 percent as compared to average washer and drier use. Over a two-and-a-half year period, taking these steps would prevent the production of the amount of global warming gases equivalent to driving your car 620 miles, according to the Environment Agency study.

Laundering cloth diapers at home can save you money, too. Cloth diapers are usually cheaper than buying disposables, although washing them is time-consuming. Nor is home laundering and line drying feasible for many apartment dwellers.

If you have the right facilities, however, laundering diapers can be done relatively easily. Cloth diaper devotees recommend three steps: dump solid wastes into the toilet, soak diapers in a mild detergent, and then launder in water that is at least 140°F to kill pathogens. Chlorine bleach should be avoided because it is harmful to the environment and it degrades fabrics.

Although cloth diapers have many benefits, washing them does consume a lot of water. If you live in an area where water shortages are common, but

ECO-TIP:
GREEN DIAPERS

When buying green diapers, check not only what they are made of but also where they are made. Some brands, marketed as being ecologically sound, ship from manufacturers as far away as Israel and Vietnam. Factor the energy that goes into shipping before you decide they are a green choice.

landfill space is plentiful, you might find paper diapers a more environmentally sound choice.

Last to weigh in on the diaper debates are the babies themselves. No baby likes a wet nappy, but as long as cloth diapers are changed quickly, this is not an issue. The only way to know which diaper works best for your baby is to try a few of them out and then listen to his or her reaction.

DIAPER RASH REHASH As to which sort of diaper—cloth or disposable—is more likely to cause diaper rash, the studies are mixed. The wicking action of disposables is a definite advantage, but the synthetic materials can act as a skin irritant. Of course, the detergents used to wash cloth diapers can irritate as well.

Whatever type of diaper you use, you can help prevent diaper rash by changing baby promptly. If a rash crops up, wash the diaper area gently with a warm moist washcloth. Keep the diaper area open to the air as long as possible. Most diaper creams contain unnecessary and potentially harmful fragrances and preservatives such as boric acid, which is irritating to the skin. Instead try zinc oxide cream, which acts as a barrier to keep moisture and microbes out.

Avoid baby powders, as the fine particles can be inhaled and damage the sensitive lining of the lungs. Cornstarch is sometimes recommended as an alternative to talc because it is not as fine, but many pediatricians recommend giving up powder altogether. Also, cornstarch can be food for yeast infections.

Severe diaper rash can be caused by yeast growing on the baby's skin. Yeast infections are more common in babies that are taking antibiotics, since these drugs kill off not only disease-causing bacteria but also ones that help keep yeast growth in check. If your baby is on antibiotics, watch for diaper rash and consult your pediatrician if it develops. Interestingly, infants who are breast-fed develop diaper rash less often, according to the American Academy of Pediatrics (AAP).

GREEN ON A SHOESTRING

Some parents and caregivers have skipped the diaper wars altogether in favor of going diaperless. You can reduce your family's impact on the environment and save money at the same time.

In diaperless parenting, parents learn to interpret the subtle clues that babies give before they urinate or defecate, a process called "elimination communication." The parents respond by placing

the child in an area of the house or yard where they can do their business without ruining carpets or furniture. Diaperless babies tend to potty train far earlier than diapered babies.

ELIMINATION COMMUNICATION

A diaperless approach where parents learn to read the signals that babies give before pottying.

WIPE OUT THE WIPES Diaper wipes are another nursery staple that deserve scrutiny. These premoistened wipes are certainly convenient but, like disposable diapers, are used once and then sent to the landfill along with (often wrapped up in) diapers. Most brands are made from cotton or wood pulp that has been bleached with chlorine. The diapers are treated with perfumes to make baby smell good, preservatives to keep items from spoiling on the shelf, and antiseptics to kill microbes found in human waste. These perfumes and preservatives are simply unnecessary for babies and could be harmful.

Fortunately several baby-friendly and Earth-friendly brands are now on the market. Most of these do not contain harmful chemicals and are made from unbleached pulp. Before using a new brand of diaper wipes on a baby with diaper rash, make sure the wipe is nonirritating. A good test is to try the diaper wipe on your skin where you have a paper cut or chapped hands. You may be surprised to find out how many diaper wipe brands sting.

One eco-friendly choice is to use a very soft wet washcloth. Keep plenty of freshly laundered washcloths on hand. Keep a squirt bottle handy filled with room-temperature water. Just prior to changing the baby, wet the washcloth and wipe. If you need extra cleansing power, place a dilute solution of natural baby soap mixed with water on the washcloth. (See the baby bath section later in this chapter for suggestions on finding natural baby soaps.)

Most babies get on just fine without wipe warmers, the electrical appliances that keep baby wipes warm at all times so they are at the ready when baby needs changing. Yes, babies probably prefer a warm wipe (wouldn't we all?), but they get used to room temperature ones fairly quickly.

ECO-TIP: BABY SHOWERS

If you have a large family and group of friends, or if this is a long-awaited grandchild/cousin/younger sibling, you may be inundated with baby gifts. Don't feel you need to register for every conceivable piece of baby gear, especially if you are committed to reducing your consumption of hard-to-recycle plastics and nonsustainably harvested wood. Spread the word that you prefer organic cottons and that you don't need cases of baby shampoo. Suggest that in lieu of buying an item the giver make a monetary contribution to a fund set up for the purchase of items you'll need in the near future, such as clothes in larger sizes, or shoes when your child learns to walk. Other options are gift cards for grocery stores or a personal gift, such as favorite books or songs from the giver's childhood.

Clothing not Chemicals

Babies have delicate skin, so you'll want to take care when buying baby's first clothes. Cottons and other natural fibers are the obvious choice because they are softer and less scratchy than synthetic fabrics like polyester. They also breathe better. Read on to find out what clothing works best for baby and the environment.

Natural fibers are generally better for the environment than synthetics, which are often made from petroleum products and require processing with toxic chemicals. Polyester is made from petroleum products. The manufacture of rayon, often touted as coming from natural wood fiber, involves highly toxic chemicals. Many rayon factories are located in regions of the world where industrial hygiene (a fancy name for protecting workers from workplace hazards) and industrial ecology (which includes the practice of ensuring the proper disposal of chemicals rather than dumping them into the nearest river) are not widely practiced.

Of course, no clothing choice is without environmental impact. The growing of cotton consumes fossil fuels for making synthetic fertilizers, running farm equipment, and transporting harvested cotton and products. Conventional cotton is one of the crops most heavily treated with pesticides. During processing, chlorine bleach is used to turn cotton fibers snowy white before they are dyed with chemical dyes. The dyes can be hazardous to the environment, and some can irritate the skin in the final product.

Whenever possible choose organic cottons, preferably those that were grown and milled close to home. Organic cotton is grown without synthetic fertilizers using only naturally occurring pesticides. Choose clothes that are made with natural dyes made from berries, flowers, barks, and other plant materials.

Another Earth-friendly option is to buy used clothing. Shop thrift stores, consignment shops, garage sales, and Internet sites. The clothes you find will likely have been washed several times, reducing any chemical residues they may have harbored when new.

SAFE AND SOUND SLEEPWEAR Who can resist the picture of a crib decked in matching sheets, blankets, quilt, and crib bumper? Yet experts agree that infants should sleep in a close-fitting pajama outfit rather than snuggled among blankets. Babies who sleep with blankets are at higher risk of sudden infant death syndrome (SIDS) and suffocation. About one-quarter of all deaths involving cribs are due to suffocation from quilts, pillows, and blankets, according to the U.S. Consumer Product Safety Commission (CPSC).

Another reason to choose close-fitting sleepwear is fire safety. All baby and child sleepwear for babies older than nine months sold in the United States must either be made of flame-resistant fabric, be treated with flame-retardant chemicals, or be "tight-fitting," according to CPSC regulations. Flame-resistant fabrics are usually synthetic fabrics made with flame-resistant fibers. Flame-retardant chemicals come in many varieties, and it is not always easy to find out which chemicals have been used on a garment you are planning to purchase. These chemicals cause concern because they may turn up in consumer products before they've been adequately tested. In the 1970s the CPSC had to recall children's pajamas after it was found that the flame retardant brominated Tris caused cancer in animals and could cross from the fabric to skin and into children's bodies.

Flame-retardant chemicals include brominated flame retardants, chlorinated flame retardants, inorganic flame retardants, and phosphate-based compounds. Manufacturers have phased out several varieties of polybrominated diphenyl ethers (PBDEs), which may disrupt thyroid hormone balance and contribute to neurological and developmental problems.[4]

A common flame retardant used on cotton is tetrakis(hydroxymethyl)phosphonium chloride, or THPC. Studies show THPC doesn't migrate from fabric to skin and does not cause cancer or other harm, although it does cause allergic reactions in some individuals.[5]

The best choice is snug-fitting garments made of natural fabrics. The close fit between fabric and skin means fabric is not easily ignited, and if it does catch fire, there is often not enough oxygen between the skin and the cloth to support the flame. When shopping, don't assume that just because pajamas are made from cotton that they are retardant-free. Many manufacturers treat their 100 percent cotton close-fitted pajamas with flame retardants, so check the label. Look for a brand that advertises it is chemical-free.

Avoid screen prints. These can contain lead and other toxic metals such as cadmium. Plastic appliqués may contain phthalates, which are hormone-disrupting chemicals that may be toxic to young children.

AIRING THE LAUNDRY Once you've stocked up on organic cotton onesies, you'll want to keep them in good shape. Wash them in mild detergents and use chlorine bleach only when absolutely necessary. As babies get older, it seems they are constantly dribbling food on their clothes or crawling through that part of the kitchen you forgot to mop. Unfortunately, few products remove stains without using strong chemicals, so here is a tip: At the first site of a stain, be ready to whip the clothing off the child, rub the stain with detergent and toss it in the hamper for the next load. Quick stain treatment is the secret to keeping clothes clean without having to resort to bleach or other chemicals.

Avoiding harsh chemicals is important, not only because they are harmful to the environment but also because household chemicals are a leading cause of child poisonings. Careful parents will have baby-proofed the house by putting all cleaning products on high shelves (and in locked cabinets, depending on your bundle of joy's climbing abilities). Don't depend on locking ground-level cabinets because all too often someone forgets to lock the cabinet.

Eco-friendly laundry detergents are a good step toward doing right by the planet. But there is a lot more you can do. Washing clothes is one of the most energy intensive activities in the average household. Washing machines rely on natural gas or electricity to heat water. Reduce your consumption by washing on the coolest temperature possible. One tip is to use warm water at the start of the cycle but rinse in cold. Use a cold-water wash whenever the items are not heavily soiled.

Skip fabric softener and dryer sheets. Both dryer sheets and fabric softeners coat fabrics with a layer of synthetic chemicals that can cause skin irritation and potentially reduce the absorbency of cloth diapers. The label of one brand of dryer sheet notes that the product should not be used on children's sleepwear because it can "reduce flame resistance." That seems to imply that it makes your child's pajamas more flammable.

Some dryer sheets come with the warning to "keep out of reach of children," so do you really want these chemicals on your child's clothes? Although companies

GREEN ON A SHOESTRING

Dryers are one of the most energy-hogging appliances in your house, according to the U.S. Department of Energy. Yet one of the best clothes-drying appliances is available for free: the sun.

do not list the chemicals in their products, you can learn more about the health effects of dryer sheets by checking the U.S. Department of Health and Human Services Household Products Database at *www.householdproducts.nlm.nih.gov.*

BABY FASHIONS Babies are cute just as they are, but some parents and grandparents like them to also be fashionable. Unfortunately, clothing designers (many of whom, it is obvious, have never taken care of a baby) sometimes go to extremes. When choosing baby clothes, think practicality first, style second. Mini-skirts in a size six months look downright uncomfortable. Knitted hoodies with a large pom-pom hanging down the back are impractical for babies that cannot even sit up yet. Avoid hoods and sweaters with drawstrings—they are a strangulation hazard.

BIRTHDAY SUIT: SUITABLE FOR (ALMOST) ALL OCCASIONS If climate permits, many parents prefer to let baby go bare, with only a diaper (or sometimes without—see Green on a Shoestring: Go Diaperless). Many parenting experts believe that skin-to-skin contact with Mom, Dad, or caregiver is ideal for promoting the attachment that serves as the foundation for emotional security throughout life. Going bare is easy during the summer or in climates that are warm year-round, but you are not doing the environment any favors if you have to turn up the thermostat. On chilly days, snuggle with your baby under the covers rather than heating a whole room just for baby. Space heaters and young children don't mix: Babies may touch hot surfaces or use them to pull themselves up, so they are best avoided until children are older.

Soul Food

To the casual observer, the breast versus bottle debate may appear tedious. But to new moms and public health officials, no issue could be more important. Breast milk is clearly nutritionally superior to formula for the majority of babies, according to the Centers for Disease Control and Prevention (CDC). Mother's milk contains the right mix of fats, proteins, vitamins, and protective factors for newborns and babies. The protective factors include antibodies passed from the mother that ward off infections as long as the infant continues to nurse and beyond.

The AAP and numerous other public health organizations recommend that most infants breast-feed exclusively for the first year. The first few days of life are especially important because the early milk, or colostrum, is especially rich in nutrients and antibodies. At around six months, a parent can begin to add solid foods to the baby's diet, and the need for nursing diminishes, but, as long as nursing continues, the beneficial nutrients and antibodies continue to benefit the child.

THE MARVELS OF MOTHERS' MILK Breast-feeding transfers numerous health-promoting factors to babies, including antibodies and disease-fighting white blood cells (leukocytes) that help the infant fend off harmful bacteria, viruses, and parasites. Formula-fed infants do not have this advantage. Breast-fed children have stronger immune responses when they encounter pathogens. They even respond with better protection after vaccination.

Breast-feeding can reduce the incidence or severity of ear infections, respiratory infections, invasive bacterial infections, urinary tract infections, and diarrhea. Breast-feeding reduces national health care costs because breast-fed infants require fewer sick visits, prescriptions, and hospitalizations. Numerous moms have related that as soon as they weaned their babies, their child developed ear infections or colds.

Some studies suggest that breast-feeding protects against chronic diseases such as type 1 and type 2 diabetes; blood cancers such as leukemia; high cholesterol; celiac disease; and inflammatory bowel disease. Other studies have suggested a link between breast-feeding and lower rates of sudden infant death syndrome (SIDS) in the first year of life.[6]

It is also thought that breast-feeding reduces a child's risk of eczema, asthma, and food allergies. A January 2008 review paper by AAP scientists reports evidence that "breast-feeding for at least four months, compared with feeding formula made with intact cow's milk protein, prevents or delays the occurrence of atopic dermatitis (eczema), cow's milk allergy, and wheezing in early childhood."[7]

Studies conflict on the question of whether lactating women should avoid peanuts and other common allergens, but in the January 2008 paper, scientists found that there is no convincing evidence to suggest that avoiding these allergens will reduce your child's risk of developing food allergies or eczema.

IS BREAST MILK BETTER FOR PREVENTING OBESITY? Is breast milk better than formula at reducing the risk that your baby will become an overweight or obese child? Nutritionally, human milk is superior to formula because it contains the right mix of fats, proteins, carbohydrates, enzymes, and other nutrients. Breast-fed babies tend to be leaner than formula-fed babies, which is perfectly normal and in fact recommended. Infants with high body weights are at greater risk of becoming obese later in life. One study found that the longer a child was breast-fed, the less likely he or she was to become obese, according to the AAP.

Some research has indicated that infant formula can contribute to obesity later in life by "teaching" the body to respond differently to the food it encounters.[8] These studies have found that formula-fed infants have hormonal responses to feeding that are different from breast-fed infants. These hormonal responses include greater insulin release, potentially leading to early fat deposition. Formula contains more protein than breast milk, and one study suggests that this high protein intake can reprogram glucose metabolism to encourage fat deposition.

The beneficial nutrients in breast milk are numerous. Omega-3 fatty acids such as docosahexaenoic acid (DHA) and eicosapentaenoic acid (EPA) are essential for learning, mental development, and visual acuity. Formula manufacturers now routinely add these fatty acids to their formulations, but some nutritionists suspect that maternally produced varieties are better absorbed. Premature infants who were breast-fed fared better in tests of overall intelligence than did similar infants who were formula-fed.[9]

BREAST MILK A BONUS FOR MOMS, TOO Nursing has many advantages not only for babies but for mothers, too. Women who breast-feed may be at lower risk of developing breast and ovarian cancers, according to a report by the U.S. Surgeon General. Breast-feeding can also protect against heart disease and diabetes later in life. In a large study featuring nearly 140,000 women, those who had breast-fed for at least one year were 9 percent less likely to have had a heart attack or stroke later in life than were women who had never breast-fed. Women who had breast-fed were also 20 percent less likely to have diabetes, 12 percent less likely to have hypertension, and 19 percent less likely to have high cholesterol than women who had not breast-fed. Women who breast-fed for just 7 to 12 months had a decreased risk of developing heart disease.

Another selling point for breast-feeding is that it can help women shed weight they gained during pregnancy. It also helps the uterus regain its shape after delivery and can reduce postpartum bleeding. Lactating women experience a natural form of birth control, although as the daily feedings drop women become more likely to get pregnant again, so the method shouldn't be relied upon.[10]

Breast-feeding is far more convenient than formula, at least in the first few months of life. There is no need to measure and mix formula, or warm a refrigerated bottle in the middle of the night. Nursing provides important bonding time between mother and child. Studies suggest that infant cuddling and holding promotes emotional security in adulthood. Because breast-fed infants have fewer infections, women can stay productive rather than making endless trips to the pediatrician.

How long to nurse is a personal decision, but keep in mind that the longer you nurse, the more protection your baby will have against sickness. The human immune system is not fully developed until the child is two years old. Some committed parents nurse until well into the toddler years, while others begin to wean their children at about a year. Weaning can be done to cow's milk in a bottle after the first year, or directly to a cup, thus eliminating the need to purchase bottles and nipples.

TOXICS IN BREAST MILK Breast milk can contain toxic substances that have negative consequences to developing babies, leaving some of us to wonder if breast milk could be harming the cognitive development of babies. All of the chemicals listed below have been found in breast milk and are known to cause cognitive deficits (measurable in lower IQ scores, for example).

These contaminants are no reason to choose formula, however. Health officials say the health benefits of nursing far outweigh the risks from these chemicals, and formula can contain some of the same contaminants, depending on how it was manufactured. A 2008 review published in the journal *Breastfeeding Medicine* looked at three studies of breast-feeding women previously exposed to dioxin and found that their breast-fed infants suffered no problems with growth or development as compared to infants whose mothers had not been exposed to dioxin.[11] One study actually found that the breast-fed infants scored better on developmental tests than their nonbreast-fed counterparts.

Some of the chemicals that can be passed via breast milk are:

× **PERSISTENT ORGANIC POLLUTANTS (POPS)** POPs include the industrial chemicals known as polychlorinated biphenyls (PCBs), industrial by-products known as dioxins, organochlorine pesticides such as DDT, and flame retardants known as polybrominated diphenyl ethers (PBDEs). PCBs and DDT have been banned for years, but they accumulate in the body and persist for decades.

× **ORGANIC SOLVENTS** Found in household and industrial products, organic solvents can be passed from mother to her nursing child. These do not accumulate in the body over time the way the POPs do, so the best way to protect your infant is by avoiding solvents.

× **LEAD** This toxic metal is stored in the bones and can be released during lactation if nursing moms are deficient in calcium.

× **OTHER POTENTIAL CONTAMINANTS** Breast milk has also been found to contain perchlorate, a water contaminant from the manufacture of rocket fuel; hormone-bending chemicals called phthalates, which are found in plastics and personal care products such as shampoos and cosmetics; and methylmercury from contaminated seafood.

× **NONENVIRONMENTAL CONTAMINANTS** Nursing can also pass pharmaceutical drugs, illicit drugs, chemicals from cigarette smoke, and alcohol.

The best way to reduce the risk of these chemicals being excreted is to maintain a healthy calorie intake so that your body does not begin to mobilize its fat stores for energy. A nursing mother's diet should contain adequate amounts of nutrients for both her own needs and the needs of her baby. Nursing mothers often report being ravenously hungry and being able to eat anything they want without gaining weight. Make sure that the foods are nutritious with plenty of whole grains, fruits and vegetables, protein, and the healthy fats found in foods such as olive oil and avocados. Eat calcium-rich, low-fat dairy foods, or check with your doctor about taking a calcium supplement. Avoid fish that are likely to be high in PCBs and mercury. (See Chapter 3 for safer seafood suggestions.)

As a rule of thumb, avoid chemicals with strong smells, such as paints, paint thinners, strong household cleaners, nail polish and remover, strong glues and hobby materials. Avoid recently dry-cleaned clothes and have a friend gas up your car. Do not apply pesticides around the home or yard, or to your pet.

BREAST IN SHOW Although public health officials are strong supporters of breast-feeding, studies show that the public at large is not completely on board. Many surveys have found that people are uncomfortable seeing a mother breast-feed in public. Studies show that most women breast-feed only about six months at most. Although three-quarters of women start out breast-feeding, by the end of the first six months only 36 percent of babies receive *any* breast milk, according to a study published in a 2008 issue of the

Journal of Lactation.[12] (Only 12 percent were being breast-fed exclusively at six months of age, according to the CDC.) Moms cite reasons such as having to go back to work, having to take care of siblings, and lack of support from family members and peers.

Not all doctors and nurses have caught up with the times, and discouragement of breast-feeding can start before a first-time mother has even left the hospital. Family members may not be up on the latest baby care advice and can pressure a new mom to give up too easily on what for many women is a struggle that pays off in the end.

Check with the hospital where you plan to deliver to find out what its breast-feeding attitude is, or better yet, check with other moms who have delivered there to find out how supportive the staff was. The World Health Organization (WHO) and the United Nations Children's Fund (UNICEF) maintain a list of "baby-friendly" hospitals that adhere to the WHO's set of ten recommendations to support breast-feeding. The hospitals offer breast-feeding education, provide assistance to new mothers, and prohibit pacifiers and bottles from being offered to baby. You can check the list of hospitals and get more information at *www.babyfriendlyusa.org.*

SOOTHING SORENESS Sore nipples are common, but think twice before applying a conventional nipple cream. Your baby will ingest the chemicals the next time he or she nurses. Instead, try placing a few drops of freshly expressed milk on the nipple to aid healing and provide antibacterial protection. Or try a 100 percent anhydrous modified lanolin, endorsed by La Leche League International, a breast-feeding support organization.

BREAST PUMP BLUES A breast pump is a highly personal item—you hardly want one falling out of your purse during a business meeting. However, there is another way in which they are personal and should not be shared. Breast milk contains bacteria and viruses that can lodge in the internal workings of the pump. When the pump is turned on, these microbes can be thrust back out of the pump and into the bottle or bag where you are collecting your breast milk. Pumps available for rental at hospitals are designed for multiple users and feature a one-way barrier against microbes, so they are appropriate for multiple users. Few personal-use breast pumps have this feature. If you are thinking of buying a used pump, check with the manufacturer first.

When shopping for a breast pump, choose a brand that uses tubing, shields, and storage jars that are free of the hormone-bending chemicals bisphenol A (BPA) and phthalates. La Leche League International recommends

KITCHEN TABLE TALK

Breast-feeding Against the Odds

The first thing my just-born twins' pediatrician said to me was, "You plan to nurse with twins? You probably will have to supplement with formula." He said it when I was still in the hospital, reeling from postcesarean painkillers and not in my best frame of mind. And he said it right in front of my husband, who was new to this whole breast-feeding thing.

But I knew that the public health establishment backed breast-feeding, and I knew feeding twins was possible, because I'd read lots of online postings from moms who had done it. But at that moment in the hospital, I never anticipated how difficult it would be.

It was difficult because my daughter was immediately sent to the neonatal ICU for a breathing problem, and she would remain there for ten days. It was difficult because her twin brother would fall asleep after 30 seconds of nursing, and I had to dig my fingernails into his heels to wake him up. It was difficult because some family members couldn't understand my compulsion to nurse, and I was so sleep-deprived that I couldn't muster the intellectual acumen to argue my case.

But I kept at it. I visited my daughter in the NICU to nurse her. Once she came home, I developed a routine where I would nurse the two infants, then give them each a bottle of formula, then apply a breast pump to help stimulate milk production. I tried everything I could to increase my milk supply—special teas and so forth—but nothing seemed to work. At times I despaired because my entire day was devoted to feeding them, with maybe a diaper change or two here and there.

At wit's end, I turned to drinking—water, that is, and lots of it. I forced myself to down a 12-ounce bottle every hour. And that turned out to be the trick to ramping up my milk supply. At four months after their birth, I was finally able to go formula-free.

After that turning point, nursing became easy and convenient. I never had to wash bottles, mix formula, or pack bottles for day outings. And I felt good knowing I was giving my children the best nutrition possible.

Today I look back on that experience and feel glad that I stuck it out. Many women give up breast-feeding because it is too hard, and they lack support from family members. But my experience taught me that if you keep trying, it can really pay off.

storing breast milk in hard-sided containers made of glass or plastic that does not leach BPA. Plastic bags designed specifically for storing breast milk are usually made of polyethylene, which does not leach chemicals into the milk. An excellent option is heavy-duty glass canning jars. These hold up to temperature extremes—such as the transfer from the cold freezer to warm water for thawing. Do not use plastic bottle liners or other plastic bags—they are not sturdy enough for the job and may be made from plastics that can leach chemicals.

Formula One

Many moms rely on formula for either the baby's entire diet, to supplement now and then, or in a pinch. When choosing a formula, look for ones with adequate nutrition and a good safety record.

Though breast milk is best, today's parents have to weigh the benefits of breast-feeding with the reality that it is extremely time-consuming at first and may be incompatible with today's dual-income way of life. Most mothers will turn to infant formula at some point for some or all of their baby's needs.

A woman's decision to use formula hinges not only on her own needs but also on the infant's circumstances. Some infants spend long stints in the neonatal intensive care unit and have little opportunity to nurse and so develop a preference for the bottle that can be difficult to shake later. Some infants don't take quickly to nursing, even under ideal conditions.

Reputable formula companies have entire scientific teams devoted to optimizing the nutrition in these formulas, so rest assured that they are adequate. Formula is usually milk-based and supplemented with vitamins, minerals, fats, and other nutrients. Most brands use cow's milk but you'll also encounter soy-based formula.

GOT COW'S MILK? Formula made with cow's milk is the most common type on the market. Whenever possible choose organic formula, made from milk from cows not treated with bovine growth hormone (also called recombinant bovine somatotropin, or rBST), which is given to cows to increase their milk production. (See Chapter 3 for more information on rBST.) While the U.S. Food and Drug Administration (FDA) maintains that bovine growth hormone is safe, European regulatory agencies have refused to approve it, not because of human health concerns but because it worsens the health of the cows.

Cows treated with rBST are more likely to develop an udder infection called mastitis, requiring treatment with antibiotics. Steer clear of rBST, and you'll steer your baby clear of both added hormones and antibiotics. In the U.S., several large supermarket chains have pledged not to sell milk produced using rBST. Check the selections at your area supermarkets or buy USDA-certified organic milk, which is not allowed by law to be from hormone-treated cows.

Another reason to buy organic milk is to support an Earth-friendly approach to agriculture. In this approach, cows graze on their natural diets of grass and grains rather than corn flakes and additives. Cow feed is grown with natural fertilizers (produced, incidentally, by cows) and naturally occurring pesticides, rather than industrial agrochemicals.

Although infant formula is based on cow's milk, many of the fats come from soybean oil. Soy also shows up in infant foods from teething biscuits to arrowroot cookies to numerous other prepackaged baby "snacks" marketed to busy moms. Nearly 90 percent of the soy grown in the U.S. is genetically modified, according to the USDA. Only a small percentage of the nation's soy crop is grown organically.

SOY FORMULA Soy has a reputation of being a health food, but it takes some creative chemistry to make soy into a suitable source of nutrients for babies. Soy formula is rich in protein but contains other compounds that restrict the ability of the body to digest those proteins. These compounds must be removed by applying heat during the processing of soy beans into hydrolyzed soy protein isolate, the powder from which formula is made. This processing involves caustic chemicals and energy inputs.

Another problem with soy is that it contains natural plant acids that block the uptake of minerals such as calcium, phosphorous, iron, and zinc, so these must be added to the formula. And here's yet another strike against soy formulas: They contain table sugar or corn syrup to make up for the cow's milk sugar (lactose) that gives babies energy and makes milk taste good.

Perhaps of greatest concern is the fact that soy contains compounds that bear an uncanny resemblance to the female hormone estrogen. These naturally

THE FACTS

By age three months, about 70 percent of U.S. babies will have consumed at least some formula, according to the CDC.

GREEN ON A SHOESTRING

Parents who rely on formula for all their baby's bottle feedings will spend $1,500 to $4,000 on formula in the first year of life, according to *Consumer Reports.* Breast-feeding is an eco-friendly practice, far more so than using formula. It is the ultimate "locavore" diet, requiring no food miles traveled, and no packaging.

occurring plant estrogens, or phytoestrogens, are suspected of causing endocrine-disrupting effects, such as early onset of puberty, premature breast development, cancers of reproductive organs, and changes in menstruation cycles in females. They may potentially have feminizing effects in males. A review of all the available studies on this topic, conducted by the U.S. National Toxicology Program, found that there is insufficient evidence to link soy infant formula to adverse developmental or reproductive outcomes and called for further research.[13]

In other studies, rats fed soy protein isolate developed hyperactivity of liver enzymes that detoxify toxic chemicals and metabolize drugs. This finding could explain why soy appears to have a beneficial preventative effect against prostate cancer, but also could result in too-rapid metabolization of medically important drugs.

Few studies in humans have followed the growth and development of soy versus cow's milk formula-fed infants. One such study is ongoing now and is sponsored by the USDA Agricultural Research Service's Arkansas Children's Nutrition Center (ACNC) The researchers reported in 2009 that, five years into the study, all children—whether fed milk from soy, cow, or breast—are growing and developing normally.[14]

Some parents choose soy formula on the assumption that it is good for babies who have milk allergies. For babies who lack the enzymes to digest lactose, soy formula is certainly one alternative, but there are lactose-free cow's milk formulas available. If the baby is allergic to cow's milk protein, however, soy may not solve the problem. About 5 to 30 percent of babies allergic to cow's milk proteins are also allergic to soy proteins.

Nor does evidence support the theory that soy formula prevents allergies, asthma, or eczema. A scientific review published in the journal *Cochrane Database of Systematic Reviews* in 2006 failed to find evidence that soy formula prevents allergies, asthma, or eczema in children who are at risk of developing these conditions based on family history.[15]

While soy formula does not prevent allergies, another specialized type of formula just may do so, according to another *Cochrane* review published the same year.[16] These formulas contain hydrolyzed cow's milk protein. In this type of formula, the two cow's milk proteins, casein and whey, are broken down into smaller pieces that don't induce an allergic reaction. The review found "limited evidence" to suggest that prolonged use of hydrolyzed cow's milk protein formula may reduce allergies, including allergies to milk proteins, and eczema in babies who are at risk. However, the hydrolyzed formula did not prevent allergies better than did breast milk.

IT'S IN THE CAN Formula comes in cans as either ready-to-consume liquid or as a powder that must be reconstituted with water prior to feeding. Most of these cans are lined on the inside with a plastic resin made with bisphenol A (BPA). This suspected hormone-disrupter can leach into the formula. Formula-fed infants who get 100 percent of their diet from formula ingest the largest concentration of BPA of any age group. Separate studies by the Environmental Working Group and the FDA found BPA in liquid formula at levels on average of 5 parts per billion with some samples testing as high as 17 parts per billion.[17] These levels sound low, but scientists are concerned that even low levels of BPA put infants at risk.

Cans containing powder can also leach BPA, although at levels 8 to 20 times lower than the level that canned liquids do, according to the analysis by the Environmental Working Group. In fact plastics are so ubiquitous in our lifestyles that 9 out of 10 of us have BPA in our blood at this moment, according to a representative survey by the CDC. The survey did not include children under six years old, but given infants' exposure through bottles and formula, it is likely that many infants also have BPA in their blood. In the same study, BPA was found in breast milk collected from American women. It has also been found in umbilical cord blood and amniotic fluid, suggesting exposure even before birth.

Some companies have started replacing BPA in can liners with other resins. However, it is unclear whether these replacements contain other toxic chemicals.

FORMULA FRAUD Melamine caused a nationwide pet food recall when it was found to have sickened and killed hundreds of animals. The industrial chemical was purposely substituted for protein in shipments of wheat gluten from China. In 2008, melamine was also detected in U.S. infant formula by FDA inspectors.[18] It is unclear how the melamine got into the formula, although some research suggests the chemical may be a breakdown product of pesticides used in growing cow feed and soybeans. Although the FDA states that the level of melamine was too low to cause toxicity, melamine is of concern because it causes kidney malfunction. Use a reputable brand of infant formula. If you are concerned about melamine, call the consumer hotline number on the formula can and ask what the company is doing about melamine.

Another chemical that shows up in infant formula is perchlorate. In 2009, scientists at the CDC reported detecting this chemical, which is a component of rocket fuel and aerial firework shows, in several brands of powdered infant formula—both cow and soy versions.[19] Perchlorate alters thyroid function, which controls growth and many other systems in the body. Again, when choosing a formula brand, call the manufacturer to see if the company is testing for this

GREEN DICTIONARY

PHYTOESTROGENS
Plant estrogens that may be capable of acting like hormones in the human body.

chemical and what they are doing about perchlorate contamination. If reconstituting formula with tap water, check your state environmental health department to see if perchlorate water contamination is a problem in your area.

JUST ADD WATER When reconstituting formula, use filtered tap water. Municipal tap water is thoroughly tested and treated to ensure the water doesn't contain disease-causing microorganisms. However, you may want to test your water for certain contaminants, such as lead, which can leach from older pipes in your home. See Chapter 3 for more information on water contaminants and a discussion on the types of filters available.

A common set of contaminants in municipal water are chlorination by-products called trihalomethanes, including chloroform, that are known to increase the risk of cancer. A carbon filter that sits in a countertop carafe is plenty adequate to remove chlorination by-products. You can view your area's tap water report at www.epa.gov/safewater/ccr/whereyoulive.html.

If you have a private well, consider that well water is not tested regularly the way municipal water is. Radon and arsenic are two naturally occurring contaminants that are known to cause cancer. If you live near farms or orchards, you may have high levels of pesticide chemicals or nitrates from fertilizers in your water. Nitrates are especially harmful to newborns under three months of age because they can cause methemoglobinemia, a dangerous blood condition that limits oxygen in the circulation. It is sometimes called blue baby syndrome because baby's skin acquires a bluish tinge. Wells located near gas stations may be contaminated with petroleum products. In some areas, perchlorate contamination is a problem.

A complete water test costs in the neighborhood of $200 and is a wise investment in your infant's future health. The EPA recommends using a state-certified water-testing lab. You can find a water tester by calling the Safe Drinking Water Hotline at 800-426-4791 or visiting www.epa.gov/safewater/labs.

Many municipal drinking water supplies are fluoridated to reduce the risk of tooth decay. However, fluoridated water can contribute to a brown mottling of the teeth called fluorosis. Find out if you have fluoridated municipal water or naturally high levels of fluoride in your water by contacting your local utility. If you use well water and live in an area naturally high in fluoride, have your water tested. Consider reconstituting infant formula with a nonfluoridated variety of bottled water. (See more about water fluoridation in Chapter 4.) Carafe-style filters do not remove fluoride. Ready-to-feed formula contains little fluoride.

Bottled water is a less than-eco-friendly option, but if you have to go with bottled water to avoid high levels of fluoride, you should know that manufacturers are not required to list fluoride levels on the bottle. Some fluoride-free brands are now being marketed. Alternatively look for water labeled as purified, distilled, deionized, demineralized, or produced through reverse osmosis.

BOTTLE BLUES If you are choosing formula, you'll also have to choose bottles and nipples. Bottles are usually made of plastic or glass. Today's plastics are safer than ever, and glass bottles are making a comeback.

PLASTIC BOTTLES Plastic bottles are lightweight and shatter-resistant, making them the preferred choice for the past 30 years. However, concerns have surfaced that the chemicals in some kinds of plastics can leach into formula or milk. Frequent use and washing in dishwashers can cause the plastic to degrade, increasing the chances that chemicals can migrate into the milk. Not all plastics are created equal, however, and some are more prone to leaching than others.

Best avoided are bottles made from polycarbonate, labeled either with the letters PC or with a #7 on the triangular resin identification symbol found on most plastic items. Polycarbonate is a hard, clear plastic made using a softening agent called bisphenol A, a hormone-like chemical linked to increased risk of numerous health problems later in life. (See The Science Behind It.)

Most studies that detected BPA leaching from plastic into the baby bottle contents tested plastic polycarbonate bottles repeatedly washed at high dishwasher temperatures (175°F or higher). If you have polycarbonate bottles, wash them by hand in warm soapy water rather than in the dishwasher, or replace them with glass or another kind of plastic.

The growing public concern has led some manufacturers to phase out the use of BPA in their product lines. Some major retailers have taken BPA-containing bottles off their shelves. It is now easier than ever to find BPA-free plastic baby bottles. However, the safety of some of the BPA replacements has not been tested, so many people opt for glass (see below).

If you are sold on plastics, safer ones include high-density polyethylene (#2), used in milk and juice bottles, low-density polyethylene (# 4), and polypropylene (#5). Another plastic is polyethersulphone, or PES, which does not leach BPA or phthalates, but contains other chemicals that have not been fully tested for safety. PES may be labeled with a #7, which is a category for "other" plastics. If you see a #7 and aren't sure if it's PES, PC, or something else, call the manufacturer before using it. Avoid breast milk storage bags made of polyvinylchloride, or PVC (#3).

PVC can release phthalates and other chemicals known to be hazardous in laboratory animals.

Whenever possible, bring filtered tap water from home in a reusable container rather than purchasing disposable plastic water bottles. The discarded bottles are filling up landfills where they take hundreds of years to decompose. In terms of recyclability, plastic types #1 and #2 are the most commonly recycled.

GLASS BOTTLES Glass bottles are making a comeback as consumers steer clear of bisphenol A and other chemicals that can leach from plastics. However, they have their own pros and cons. The pros include that they can be washed in the dishwater and sterilized in hot water without worry that the material will degrade or break down.

The cons are that they are more expensive than plastic bottles, and they can break when exposed to temperature extremes, like taking the bottle out of the freezer and placing it directly into warm water. They can also break during use, potentially harming the child in the process. Some child care centers do not allow them. With infants, breakage should not be much of an issue, but as the baby starts to hold his own bottle, limit the use of glass bottles to carpeted areas and other safe surfaces. A sturdy bottle may survive being dropped on a linoleum floor but is likely to shatter against a tile floor. New products are addressing the safety issue with the introduction of baby bottle sheaths made from neoprene or silicone.

NIPPLES Nipples can be made of silicone or latex rubber. Silicone is the preferred choice because some babies fed with latex rubber may be at higher risk of developing allergies to latex. Latex rubber may contain harmful impurities that can increase baby's risk of developing cancer later in life. Discontinue use of nipples when they become cracked, hardened, discolored, or ripped.

WASHING Whether glass or plastic, nipples, pacifiers, breast shields, pump tubing, and containers should all be sterilized by soaking in boiling water for several minutes prior to first use. After that, regular washing in hot soapy water and air-drying will keep germs at bay.

BOTTLE WARMERS Some baby innovations really do improve the lives of babies and their caregivers, whereas others may only provide a minor improvement. In the case of many newer items on the market, ask yourself, "Do I need this item?" and "Is this item harmful in some way to the environment?" Bottle warmers consume electricity and may be one of those baby care inventions you decide you don't need. If you are reconstituting powdered formula, use filtered room temperature tap water and serve directly. For refrigerated formula or breast milk, warm the bottles in a pan of warm water. Do not put the bottle directly into the microwave oven because the milk heats unevenly and hot spots can scald sensitive infant tongues. Microwaves may also enhance the leaching of chemicals from plastic. Chilled milk directly from the refrigerator is often perfectly acceptable to older babies.

SWITCHING TO SOLIDS Around six months, your baby will be ready to start adding solid foods to his or her diet. A common first food is rice cereal. It is convenient to buy rice cereal made especially for babies, but if you have the time you can cook rice and puree it in a food processor. Make sure it is made from organic whole grain rice instead of processed white rice, which has been stripped of its vitamin-rich brown layer and then refortified with the very same vitamins.

Rice cereal in a bottle was a popular practice in older generations, but today's pediatricians don't recommend it. For one thing, some babies do not swallow the cereal well and end up choking or breathing it into their lungs, causing serious complications. And some researchers suspect it contributes to obesity later in life because babies consume a lot of high-caloric-density rice very quickly and don't learn how to stop eating when they are full. Feeding your baby spoonful by spoonful will help him learn lifelong healthy eating habits.

When planning baby's first meals, think organic. Since babies eat far more than adults in terms of grams of food per pound of body weight, it pays to give your baby the healthiest food possible. A number of pesticides have been detected in baby food, according to a 2008 study published in the journal *Environmental Health Perspectives*.[20] Choose organic beets, carrots, and sweet potatoes. Other good high-nutrient foods are broccoli, avocados, and blueberries. Organic meats are also important. Grass-fed beef cattle are raised on a natural diet of grasses and don't require extra antibiotics to treat infections that arise due to the high stomach acidity produced by an unnatural diet of cornflakes. Grass-fed beef tends to be higher in beneficial omega-3 fatty acids and lower in fat, too.

Several eco-friendly and health-friendly brands of baby food are available. Large supermarket chains usually carry at least one organic line in most regions of the country. Read labels carefully to avoid giving too much of the same food. You may be surprised how many baby food jars list as the first ingredient carrots even though the label says "beef and vegetables." You may want to introduce new foods one at a time so that you can monitor your baby for allergies.

One way to know what is in your child's food is by making it at home using a food processor or special baby food grinder. When you make your own baby food, you have a greater choice of organic food items to choose from rather than being limited by what the store offers. And, you cut down on your consumption of glass baby food jars, which, after your child's five-minute encounter with them, go directly to a landfill or, in some areas, a glass recycling facility.

For better prices and more variety, shop for baby foods such as applesauce outside the baby aisle. Products don't need to be labeled "baby" to be OK for baby. Buying larger containers (of applesauce, for example) cuts down on packaging waste and is cheaper, too.

Making your own baby food doesn't have to be an extra chore. Cook your meats and vegetables until they are tender and then mash them with a fork. Home-cooking may actually be easier for busy families because you won't have to make special food for the youngest member of the family.

ORAL FIXATION: TEETHERS AND PACIFIERS Babies use their mouths to explore their environments. They start putting items into their mouth shortly after birth, so it pays to provide a safe and nontoxic environment for these motor mouths. (See Chapter 1 for creating a safe home environment for babies and Chapter 7 for safer baby toys.) Choose teethers made of organic cloth or unfinished wood from trees grown without pesticides.

Bathing Beauties

Our modern concept of baby care includes never having to encounter a noxious smell, at least, if advertisements are to be believed. Each member of the family should remind us of an alpine meadow rather than having the good old-fashioned human smell.

Unfortunately most of those enticing floral smells are created not by real flowers but by chemicals, many of which are either harmful or not adequately tested for toxicity. Fragrances are often created using phthalates, chemicals that are linked to endocrine disruption, according to the U.S. National Research Council.

When you bathe your baby with one of these sweet-smelling shampoos you are sending phthalates into the wastewater stream and eventually into a river, lake, or ocean. Personal care manufacturers usually don't put the word "phthalate" in the ingredients list, opting for the vague term, "fragrance."

In addition to fragrance, baby toiletries contain an amazing list of chemicals that are known to be irritating to sensitive skin. Sodium lauryl sulfate is a common chemical used to make shampoos and bubble bath foams. Yet is one of the main culprits that cause shampoos to sting the eyes. It is a surprise to many parents that products marketed to babies are not necessarily more chemical-free or milder than products for adults.

Most babies don't need a lot of sweet-smelling soaps and lotions. A warm-water wash with a mild, plant-based soap will do just fine. Steer clear of soaps labeled as being "antibacterial." The more we use antibacterial chemicals, the more opportunities bacteria have to evolve defenses against these chemicals. Later, when we really need them, they won't work. Besides, antibacterials do nothing to protect against the cause of the common cold, viruses. If someone in the house is sick, wash your hands frequently with warm water and soap before touching the baby.

Before buying skin care products for your baby, check out the Internet consumer database Skin Deep, *www.cosmeticsdatabase.com,* a project of the Environmental Working Group. You can enter the name of a product you are contemplating buying and see its safety profile.

ECO-TIP: CHEMICALS TO AVOID IN BABY CARE PRODUCTS

× **Boric Acid and Sodium Borate (diaper cream): These chemicals can irritate infant skin.**

× **2-Bromo-2-Nitropropane-1,3-Diol or Bronopol (baby wipes): This chemical is a skin, eye, and lung irritant and can break down into formaldehyde and nitrosamines, both of which are probable carcinogens, according to the EPA.**

× **Ceteareth and PEG compounds (baby wipes, shampoos, body wash, sunscreen): Chemicals that may contain impurities such as cancer-causing ethylene oxide and the suspected carcinogen 1,4-dioxane.**

× **DMDM Hydantoin (baby wipes, shampoos, body wash): An allergen and irritant that can break down to form formaldehyde.**

× Oxybenzone or Benzophenone-3 (sunscreen): Can cause allergic reactions and form other chemicals called free radicals that can harm cells. It also may have hormone-like effects.

× Parabens (baby wipes, shampoos, body wash, sunscreen, lotions): Hormone-like chemicals suspected of causing reproductive and developmental harm as well as cancer.

× Phthalates (shampoo, body wash, and many other products): Often labeled simply as fragrance, these chemicals have hormonelike activity and may damage the kidneys, liver, lungs, and developing testes.

× Triclosan and Triclocarban (antibacterials in liquid soap, toothpaste): Contribute to bacteria resistance, are toxic to aquatic life, may be toxic to the liver, and have hormone-like effects.

× Triethanolamine or TEA (sunscreen, lotions): Causes skin irritation and allergic reactions, and can form nitrosamines, which the EPA says are probable human carcinogens.

SOURCE: Environmental Working Group's Skin Deep Cosmetic Safety Database: Safety Guide to Children's Personal Care Products. www.cosmeticsdatabase.com/special/parentsguide

Fun in the Sun

Sunburns are no fun, but neither should a baby completely avoid the sun.

But how much is too much? Parents may have a tough time judging whether

baby has had too much sun, so some doctors recommend that babies under

six months should avoid sun exposure entirely. Like most things, the answer

is a little more complicated.

SUN PROS AND CONS The sun has a crucial role in helping the body make vitamin D, which is actually a hormone rather than a vitamin and is necessary for the absorption of calcium and bone growth. Vitamin D deficiency results in a condition called rickets, which causes an abnormally large head, curved bones, and poor muscle development. New studies show that vitamin D also protects against diseases such as cancer and cardiovascular disease.

The current AAP recommendation is that babies be given vitamin D supplements until they begin drinking vitamin D fortified milk. Yet many researchers think the amount recommended, 200 international units per day, is too low. Consult with your pediatrician before deciding on giving more than the AAP recommends, since high levels of vitamin D can be toxic.

Some parents take issue with replacing sunlight with a daily vitamin—especially in light of the fact that many vitamins are produced using environmentally unfriendly processes and an increasing number of them are coming from overseas factories primarily in China, where lax oversight has permitted a number of recent food-related poisonings.

Experts find that just a few minutes a day of sunlight is enough to produce all the vitamin D a baby needs, so some physicians have started saying it is OK to let babies enjoy some sun exposure starting at just a few days after birth. Exposure should be strictly limited to a few minutes, especially if the sun is strong. Exposure should not occur during the hours of 10 a.m. and 2 p.m., when sun is the strongest. Do not use sunscreen on baby, both because it blocks vitamin D production and because of the chemicals in sunscreen.

If you live in a northern latitude where sunlight is in short supply during the winter, however, you may want to consider supplements. Studies indicate that the low angle of the sun in winter may not provide enough of the right wavelengths of light for vitamin D to be produced in the skin. Also, during the winter you probably shouldn't be stripping your child down to his skivvies in freezing weather just to build up his vitamin D. Sunning your baby near the window is not a replacement for direct sun exposure, because glass windows can block the type of light needed for vitamin D manufacture.

SUITING UP FOR THE SUN The sun may help make vitamin D, but it can damage sensitive infant skin. The best way to protect your newborn from the sun is by covering him up entirely, in long pants, long sleeves, hat, and socks. Sunscreen should not be used before the age of six months, because of the chemicals it contains, according to the Environmental Working Group. Parents may also apply it inconsistently.

Clothing is a wonderful alternative to chemical sunscreen lotions and sprays. Look for items that are rated for their ability to block the sun. The ultraviolet protection factor (UPF) is a clothing rating system that is analogous to the SPF (sun protection factor) system used for sunscreens. (Note that UPF ratings are not federally regulated the way SPF ratings are.) Several retailers sell baby and child swimsuits and shirts (sometimes called "rash guards," because they were originally invented for surfers) that cover most of the body with UPF-rated protection.

UPF 50 clothing keeps out 98 percent of harmful UVA and UVB radiation. Both types of radiation contribute to the risk of developing skin cancer. Of course, most types of cloth will block some rays, but if you are planning a day at the beach, it is best to use UPF-rated clothing. Keep your baby under a sun umbrella or tent (these come with UPF ratings as well) as much as possible.

SUNSCREENS EXPOSED As your baby becomes more active, it will become impossible to cover him at every moment. For babies six months and up, one option is a sunscreen rated SPF 30 or higher.

Sunscreens work by blocking the sun either physically or chemically. The physically blocking sunscreens contain titanium dioxide or zinc oxide, two white-colored chemicals that literally deflect the sun's rays. They are effective against both UVA and UVB radiation, the two types of sun radiation that cause skin cancer.

More commonly encountered in your neighborhood drug store are the chemical-based sunscreens. Instead of physically blocking solar radiation, the chemicals absorb it. Most chemical creams protect well against UVB but not UVA radiation; however, some newer formulations can protect against both.

Some of the common chemical sunscreen ingredients are octinoxate, homosalate, padimate-O, and benzophenone-3 (also called oxybenzone). All of these compounds have been found to have hormone-like effects in laboratory animal tests, according to the Environmental Working Group. They are also allergenic to many people.

Two safer chemicals are mexoryl SX and avobenzone (Parsol 1789). Mexoryl is active against both UVA and UVB, while avobenzone primarily blocks UVA and is used in combination with other chemicals that block UVB.

Which type is better, chemical or physical blockers? In term of both health effects and sun protection, the physical blockers are clearly better. The physical blockers do not have hormone-like effects. They are relatively inert and do not penetrate deeply into skin, whereas many of the chemical blockers can penetrate the skin. In fact, oxybenzone is found in the bodies of about 97 percent of Americans, according to a study conducted by the CDC. In terms of effectiveness, titanium dioxide and zinc oxide are effective at blocking both UVA and UVB radiation, whereas the chemical blockers mexoryl SX and avobenzone break down in sunlight and lose their effectiveness.

When it comes to protecting the environment, both physical and chemical sunscreens may be toxic to aquatic life. All types of sunscreens wash off when swimming. To reduce damage to the environment and to protect skin, UPF-rated swimsuits are better than relying on creams and sprays. Check online retailers to find full-body UPF-rated swimsuits for kids.

One disadvantage of the physical blockers is that they can be hard to spread. Today's formulations are easier to handle than ever, but be wary of ones that contain nanoparticles. Although several studies have shown these nanoparticles are incapable of penetrating deeply into the skin, it is advisable to avoid using nanoparticle formulations until more is known about them. Also, some studies suggest that nanoparticles harm aquatic life.

TIPS FOR USING SUNSCREEN:
- ✓ Use a sunscreen with an SPF higher than 30 that protects against both UVA and UVB radiation.
- ✓ Apply liberally and reapply every two to three hours or sooner, even if the label says waterproof.
- ✓ Sprays and aerosols are best avoided in babies and small children, who squirm a lot and may inhale the chemicals.
- ✓ Buy new sunscreens at the beginning of the season. The chemicals break down over time.

For a list of safer and more effective sunscreens, see the Environmental Working Group's sunscreen guide at *www.ewg.org/files/2009sunscreenguide.pdf.*

Baby Gear

If you have a gear geek in your family, chances are that person is going to love baby care. New lightweight materials and design innovations have transformed bulky strollers and car seats into durable, ergonomic products designed for modern lifestyles. One place not to skimp is on safety. Once safety is taken care of, your wallet and your environmental sensibilities are the limit.

CAR SEATS   A car seat is essential—you cannot get your new baby home from the hospital without one. Motor vehicles are the leading cause of death of children between the ages of 2 and 14, according to the National Highway Transportation Safety Administration (NHTSA).

Infant seats are designed for use by infants up to 22 or 32 pounds at most, depending on the style. It may be only a matter of six months before your baby is ready for a larger seat. Although they are only used for a few months, infant seats often come with a convenient handle so that the infant can be carried from car to living room. The carriers double as infant chairs and many parents find them extremely convenient. Some models can be popped into a stroller frame.

To reduce the amount of plastic, polyurethane foam padding, and other nonrenewable materials that you consume, consider buying a child restraint seat that spans multiple ages. Some chairs span the weight range from newborn (5 pounds) to first grader (55 pounds). If these chairs fit your other lifestyle needs, they can be a good option for reducing the amount of synthetic materials you consume. With every piece of gear, ask yourself, How many months or years will I use this? Will I use it on subsequent children? Can I pass it on easily to a charitable organization or a friend?

Every child must use a car seat or booster seat until age four in most states. However, the American Academy of Pediatrics recommends that children should continue to use booster seats until the child reaches about four feet nine inches in height and is between 8 and 12 years of age. Laws vary by state, so check your state's regulations. Don't forget to check the laws of the states you'll be traveling to on your summer vacation (see Chapter 10 for more information). Given the risk of automobile accidents, you may want to follow the AAP's guidelines even if your state has laxer regulations.

A car seat must meet federal safety standards and strict crash performance standards. When buying a new car seat, check to make sure it has been certified by the NHTSA. While all NHTSA-rated seats are safe, some are better than others in terms of ease of use. The easier a car seat is to use, the more likely the parents will be to properly install it. Most localities have organizations that will install the seat for you or help you through the process. Check your local police department, hospital, even car dealerships. You can search for the one nearest you at the Child Safety Seat Inspection Station Locator on the NHTSA website *www.nhtsa.gov/cps/cpsfitting/index.cfm.*

THE FACTS

The typical middle-income American family spends on average $13,590 on their baby by the time the child turns one year old, according to *Consumer Reports.*

GREEN ON A SHOESTRING

"Reuse" is one of the main tenets of the green movement, but the car seat is one item that you should consider carefully before buying used. Many charities no longer accept used car seats for donation

and many thrift stores refuse to sell them. Restraint belts can fray and important safety parts and instructions can get lost. That doesn't mean that you cannot pass car **seats** down to younger siblings or friends as long as you know that the seat is in good shape and has never been in a major accident.

If you are considering accepting a used seat from a friend, or buying one, ask the following:

✓ How old is the car seat? Older car seats may not be compatible with the LATCH restraint system, which began to be required in 2002. In fact, car seats come with an "expiration date," required by law. The date is usually six years after the date of manufacture.

✓ Does the seat have any visible cracks? Plastic can become weakened over time, a process hastened by exposure to temperature fluctuations over years of use during hot summers and freezing winters.

✓ Does the seat have a label with the date of manufacture and model number?

✓ Does the seat have the instructions? You may be able to get them online if you have the model number.

✓ Are the safety belts frayed or worn?

✓ Do you have all the parts? You may not know if an important safety belt is missing. Check the diagram in the instruction manual.

✓ Has the item been recalled? You can check for recalls and sign up for recall notifications from the federal government by visiting the website of the NHTSA's Office of Defects Investigation at *www.safercar.gov.*

Consumer Reports recommends not buying used play yards and cribs. Make sure any used baby product you're considering hasn't been recalled. For the latest recall information, visit *www.recalls.gov.* When buying new, send in the registration card so you'll be alerted to any recalls automatically.

STROLLERS AND OTHER FASHION STATEMENTS Once upon a time, baby gear was understated, not a fashion statement. Products were as unobtrusive as possible in neutral grays and beiges, perhaps so as not to clash with Mom's paisley dresses and platform shoes. Today's products are often more bold: Bright red strollers come to mind. Unless safety is your aim (a bright red stroller is probably most likely to be seen by a motorist), think twice before paying extra for a color scheme that you may tire of later, or a color such as pink that may be inappropriate for future siblings.

Many of us know people who have three strollers: One for everyday walking, one for jogging, and an umbrella stroller that rolls up small for trips on subways, buses, and airplanes. Before buying all these items, ask yourself, Do I really need the sturdiness of a jogging stroller for my morning exercise routine, or will a regular stroller with sturdy wheels do the trick? Can the jogger double as your stroller for shopping and regular use?

When it comes to nursery furniture, think dual use. Look for a changing table that can convert to a dresser, a crib that can convert to a toddler bed. Or find ways to go without. If you change your baby on a clean blanket placed on the floor, you won't have to worry about falls and spills. About 2,000 to 3,000 injuries each year are caused by accidents involving changing tables, according to *Consumer Reports.*

Whenever possible, try to choose mattresses and other cushiony furniture made from natural fibers instead of synthetic ones. This doesn't mean you have to go out and splurge on an entire new bedroom set for baby. A well-washed 100 percent cotton crib sheet that has been around a few years probably has a lesser impact on the environment than a brand-new organic cotton crib set.

WHEN BUYING FOR BABY Try to reuse and repurpose existing furniture whenever possible. But if you simply *must* buy baby furniture, keep these tips in mind:

× Avoid wood products containing particleboard, which offgases volatile organic compounds (VOCs), including cancer-causing formaldehyde. Pick solid wood furniture certified by the Forest Stewardship Council (FSC) or buy used furniture.

× Instead of a mattress made from polyurethane foam, choose a natural mattress made from wool, cotton, or natural latex rubber. These are naturally fire-resistant and don't need to be treated with flame-retardant chemicals.

× Steer clear of vinyl products such as waterproof mattress covers. Vinyl, or polyvinyl chloride (PVC), is made using toxic processes, yields

GREEN DICTIONARY

POLYURETHANE FOAM
Found in car seat pads, mattresses, furniture, and practically anywhere you need a soft seat, polyurethane foam is made from nonrenewable petroleum sources. Since it is flammable, polyurethane foam is often treated with chemical flame retardants, which can be toxic. For a more natural cushion, look for wool, cotton, or natural latex mattresses.

cancer-causing dioxins as manufacturing by-products, and is often softened using hormone-disrupting phthalates. Vinyl also generates fumes in your baby's room that can irritate airways. Instead, look for mattress covers made from wool or rubberized cotton. Even polyurethane laminate is a better choice than vinyl.

✗ Don't go for stain-resistant coatings, which are made with toxic chemicals that can persist in the environment indefinitely. (See Chapter 2 for a description of these chemicals in the section on nonstick cookware.) Skip items treated with stain-resistant chemicals in favor of naturally stain-resistant wool.

For more information go to *www.watoxics.org/safer-products/chosing-safer-products-mattresses-and-changing-pads.*

Greening the Womb

Life may begin at conception, but "green living" begins *before* conception. Doctors call it "preconception health care." The goal of preconception health care is to remove or decrease risks to unborn babies from maternal smoking, alcohol use, exposures to chemicals at work and home, obesity, and nutritional deficits.

GREEN YOUR LIFESTYLE Even if you are a nonsmoker who exercises, take a few minutes to ask yourself if you are living as healthily as possible. Do you use chemicals around the house or at work? Do you eat foods that are high in pesticides and other toxic substances? Certain pesticides and industrial chemicals, such as PCBs, can build up over years in the body and later are released during pregnancy and nursing. If a family member smokes, try to convince him or her to quit before you get pregnant.

EAT HEALTHFULLY Another question to ask yourself is whether you are eating as healthily as possible. You want to have optimal nutrition in place *before* you get pregnant. Folate and other nutrients are essential in the first few days and weeks of pregnancy when the essential systems of the body are forming. Make sure your diet is high in fruits and vegetables and whole grains. Choose lean meats over fatty ones and try to get some low-mercury fish into your diet on a regular basis. Take a multivitamin that has folate (folic acid) to reduce the risk of birth defects.

GET DAILY EXERCISE AND DRINK LOTS OF WATER You are not only eating for two, you are drinking for two. Consume filtered tap water in your own reusable bottle. If you are overweight, try to get down to a normal weight before conception. Children who are born to mothers who were obese early in pregnancy are more likely to be overweight as preschoolers, according to a 2004 study in the journal *Pediatrics*.[21] A 2009 study in the *Journal of the American Medical Association* found that maternal obesity nearly doubles the risk of giving birth to a child with a neural tube defect.[22]

EAT SAFER SEAFOODS A diet rich in seafood is great brain food for babies because many kinds of fish are rich in omega-3 fatty acids, which are important for neurological development. (For more about omega-3s, see Chapter 2; for seafood, see Chapter 3.) However, fish can also be rich in brain-damaging mercury which can be passed in utero to baby. A good middle ground is Alaska salmon, which is wild-caught and is naturally low in mercury. Steer clear of sushi-grade tuna such as maguro (bluefin tuna) and ahi (yellowfin tuna). A study conducted by scientists for the *New York Times* in 2008 found that mercury levels in sushi purchased at five Manhattan restaurants exceeded the FDA's action limit of one part per million, the level at which the FDA can legally remove the fish from sale.[23] For help choosing safe sushi, see the list on the Natural Resources Defense Council's website at *www.nrdc.org/health/effects/mercury.*

GO ORGANIC When choosing fruits and vegetables, choose organic or locally grown produce from a farmer who you know avoids pesticides. Most pesticides have been tested individually, not as the medleys of chemicals that are used in modern agriculture. A nonorganic diet exposes you to combinations of chemicals. Yet few studies have looked at the health risks of pesticide combinations. If you must buy conventional produce, steer clear of imports, which may use pesticides not licensed in the U.S.

Typical American cattle are raised on corn-based feed supplemented with hormones. (See Chapter 3 for more information on modern cattle production.) Some researchers suspect that hormones in beef can have effects on fetuses in the womb. A study published in a 2007 issue of the journal *Human Reproduction* found that men whose mothers consumed a lot of beef had lower sperm counts and more fertility problems than men whose mothers ate less beef.[24]

BEWARE OF FOOD-RELATED ILLNESSES Steer clear of foods that carry the risk of infections. Raw and unpasteurized milk, soft cheeses, raw eggs, and cookie dough should be avoided because they can carry harmful bacteria. Cook all meats and eggs thoroughly. After preparing meat, wash all cutting boards and utensils thoroughly with hot, soapy water.

AVOID ENDOCRINE DISRUPTERS Most canned food linings contain bisphenol A, a chemical that has hormone-like effects. Studies show that bisphenol A can leach from the can lining into foods. The Environmental Working Group in 2007 tested several brands of canned foods for bisphenol A content. They found BPA levels in chicken soup and canned ravioli at concentrations that were just five times lower than the doses shown to cause permanent damage to developing male reproductive organs in studies using rats and mice.[25]

STEER CLEAR OF SOLVENTS Switch to greener household cleaners. Avoid starting renovation projects that will expose you to fumes from paints, glues, and solvents. If you must renovate, test for lead paint before any sanding is done. Stay clear of gas stations if you can help it. Have your spouse or friend fill your tank, or go to a full service station and keep the windows closed. Find an environmentally friendly dry cleaner that doesn't use perchloroethylene (PCE) or other toxic chemicals.

AVOID WINE AND OTHER ALCOHOL Start your new abstemious lifestyle several weeks before you try to get pregnant. There is no safe amount of alcohol for your unborn baby. Researchers now realize that alcohol causes a spectrum of disorders of varying severity. Fetal alcohol syndrome disorders include lifelong physical, mental, behavioral, and learning disabilities.

Take Action

▸ Do your best to limit your consumption of natural resources and generation of waste by choosing a type of diaper that fits your lifestyle and green values.

▸ Ask a friend to host a "green" baby shower for you so that your loved ones bring eco-friendly gifts you can use.

▸ Whenever possible, choose clothing made of organic, natural fibers without chemical dyes.

▸ Save money by shopping for gently used clothing and baby gear.

▸ Select sleepwear that is snug-fitting rather than treated with chemical flame retardants.

▸ Wash baby clothes and bedding in mild detergents that don't contain artificial fragrances or chemicals.

▸ Consider air-drying your laundry to save energy and money.

▸ Provide the highest quality milk to your new baby by breast-feeding as much as possible during the first year of life.

▸ When using formula, choose a reputable brand based on cow's milk. Consult with your pediatrician on formulas for children with cow's milk allergies.

▸ Limit your baby's intake of soy, which contains plant estrogens.

▸ Reconstitute powdered formula with filtered tap water. Have your water tested if you suspect contaminants, live in an older home where lead in pipes may be an issue, or use well water.

▸ Avoid fluoridated water when mixing powered baby formula.

▸ Choose baby bottles that do not contain bisphenol A.

▸ Shop for organic baby food or make your own.

▸ Choose safer soaps and lotions for your baby by visiting the Environmental Working Group's Skin Deep Cosmetic Safety Database at *www .cosmeticsdatabase.com.*

▸ Cover up baby with UPF-rated clothing to prevent sunburn. For safer sunscreens, see the Environmental Working Group's sunscreen guide at *www.ewg.org/ files/2009sunscreenguide.pdf.*

▸ Go easy on the baby gear by considering whether you really need what you are about to buy.

▸ Put safety first by checking ratings and installing car seats correctly.

THE SCIENCE BEHIND IT

Bisphenol A

Bisphenol A (BPA) is a chemical that looks to our bodies like the female hormone estrogen. Many scientists believe that it alters the function of the hormonal system, which controls a complicated system of messages that direct puberty, reproductive cycles, development, and growth.

When even small amounts of bisphenol A are given in laboratory animal studies, the results include feminization of the male reproductive organs, infertility, precancerous cell changes in the breast and prostate, early puberty, and behavior problems. Bisphenol A has also been linked to obesity and diabetes.

Bisphenol A is a major component of polycarbonate plastics, which have been used for baby bottles because they are durable and relatively shatterproof. The chemical is also used in dental sealants and composites. BPA is now being removed from baby bottles, but it is still present in the linings of canned food, including baby formula.

BPA is also present in the bodies of 92 percent of a nationally representative sample of Americans, according to a CDC survey.[26] Children had higher levels of BPA than adolescents, who in turn had higher levels than adults.

In terms of BPA's effect on human health, a comprehensive look at BPA by the U.S. National Toxicology Program (NTP), published in 2008, found some cause for concern in infants and young children, but little concern about BPA's effects on adults. The NTP expressed concern over BPA's potentially harmful effects on the brain, behavior, and prostate gland in fetuses, infants, and children at levels to which they are now being exposed.

The NTP found only minimal reason for concern that BPA may be driving down the age of puberty in females and did not find evidence to support the concern that BPA exposure in pregnant women could cause birth defects or reduced birth weight.[27]

In 2008, Canada took steps to ban the sale of polycarbonate baby bottles containing bisphenol A. Similar efforts are being considered in the United States.

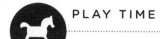

PLAY TIME

Toys and Activities for a Healthy Child and Planet

PLAY IS A YOUNG CHILD'S PRIMARY OCCUPATION. THROUGH PLAY, children develop their imagination, their understanding of the world around them, and their critical thinking skills. Through play, children also have the opportunity to learn about their environment, and how important it is to protect it.

Yet so many toys today are designed to entertain, rather than to encourage creative play. Many toys tie into TV shows and movies instead of allowing children to unleash their imagination. Most video games can improve a child's hand-eye coordination but do little to stimulate creativity. Few of the toys and games in stores today help children learn about nature, let alone get outside and explore it.

Creative play is so important to a child's development that the American Academy of Pediatrics (AAP) recommends that doctors bring the subject up with parents at well-baby visits. The AAP advises that "all children are afforded ample, unscheduled, independent, nonscreen time to be creative, to reflect, and to decompress."

In choosing toys that enhance creativity, parents also have to choose toys that are safe for their children and the environment. Toy trains coated in lead paint and rubber ducks made with hormone-disrupting phthalates are just two of the toxic toy scares that parents have navigated recently. The environmental damage done by producing petroleum-based plastics is significant, yet we so easily forget about it because most toys are made in overseas factories.

While indoor play is important, outdoor play is also essential for a child's development. Outdoor play offers children a sense of freedom, a sense of being an explorer, and an opportunity to exercise the mind and body. Many children spend very little if any time in nature today, leading to what author Richard Louv calls "nature deficit-disorder" in his book, *Last Child in the Woods* (Algonquin Books, 2005).

Kids spend less time outdoors than kids did in previous generations. This is partly because the nation has become increasingly suburbanized, but also because parents have less time to take children to natural environments where they can explore. Many children are "overscheduled" in extracurricular activities. Other kids, whose parents can't afford pricey classes, live in neighborhoods that lack opportunities for safe outdoor play and exploration. They spend time indoors watching TV or playing video games while their parents are at work.

In this section, we'll explore how to pick the right toys for your child's development, what materials in toys can be toxic to health and the environment, and how to navigate a culture where kids are expected to stare at screens. We'll also cover healthy outdoor activities like gardening, playing on the playground, and caring for a pet.

Toys for the Ages

Providing stimulating and enjoyable toys is perhaps one of the more pleasurable jobs of parenthood. Through websites and catalogs, parents can order a variety of toys to suit every green tendency, foster imagination, and offer years of play.

ZERO TO NINE MONTHS Children need few toys at this age, but try telling that to newly minted grandmothers, aunts, and other well-wishers. In lieu of toys, you might ask your friends and family to give money for diapers or a college fund. If that fails, read on for some suggestions.

During the first year, babies are developing basic motor skills as well as fine motor skills such as grasping items. Toys that hang over a bouncy seat or crib can give babies something to grab or bat. These toys can produce rewards such as squeaky noises or rattling sounds that can help teach baby cause and effect. Remember everything will go in the mouth so look for toys made of the safer materials described later in this chapter.

GOOD TOYS FOR BABIES:

✓ Rattles made from Forest Stewardship Council (FSC)-certified wood

✓ Stuffed animals made from organic cloth that baby can grasp and use for teething

✓ Crib toys that babies can bat at and grab

✓ Lots of parent and caregiver interactions that don't cost a thing

THE TODDLER YEARS Once a baby starts crawling and learning to walk, toys that encourage movement and exploration are excellent choices. Young toddlers will enjoy rolling a ball down a ramp and chasing after it. They love to push objects like toy lawn mowers and strollers.

Look for simple unadorned toys that give the imagination a workout. A plain doll without hair and elaborate facial features gives the child the opportunity to decide: Who is this person? What is he or she like? Stuffed animals are wonderful because children can create their own characters starting with a few physical characteristics.

THE FACTS

First graders get an average of 70 new toys a year, or roughly one every five days, according to the Campaign for a Commercial-Free Childhood, an advocacy organization.

GOOD TOYS FOR TODDLERS:

✓ Balls

✓ Things with hinges, such as boxes, cupboard doors

✓ Dolls that have few adornments

✓ Any object that the child can pull on a string

✓ Water toys for bath time

✓ Unbreakable mirror

✓ Cardboard box that your child can put things in and dump them out of

✓ Sand box (See the Eco-Tip on silica-free sand.)

✓ Push toys like doll strollers and lawn mowers

✓ Ride-on-top toys that child pushes with feet

✓ Stuffed animals

✓ Puppets

PRESCHOOLERS Children continue developing their imagination as they enter preschool age. Help inspire your children by reading to them, telling them stories, and listening while they come up with their own stories.

GOOD TOYS FOR PRESCHOOLERS:

✓ Bikes: A "running bike" or "balance bike" that lacks pedals will help your child develop his or her motor skills.

✓ Balance beam: Set up a two-by-four in your apartment or backyard.

✓ Dress up: Clothes and hats or pieces of fabric make great dress-up items.

✓ Indoor slide or child's gym for when the weather is bad.

✓ Sand box (See the Eco-Tip on silica-free sand.)

✓ Wading pool

✓ Swing that goes in all directions, not just back and forth

GREEN ON A SHOESTRING

Invest in the following toys when your child is young, and he or she will play with them for years. What is more they are durable so they can be passed on to younger children or even the next generation.

✓ **BLOCK SETS** Large wooden block sets of 60 pieces or more offer large graspable pieces that toddlers can use to develop fine motor skills. Children of eight years or even older will enjoy building bridges and houses.

✓ **PLASTIC SNAP-TOGETHER BUILDING BLOCKS** Small plastic blocks (such as Lego products) offer hours of creative play.

✓ **DOLLHOUSES** A quality dollhouse can last a child from two years old to ten years old, depending on your child. If the child complains that she is bored with the house, help her "redecorate" by adding new furniture, hanging homemade curtains, and painting the walls.

✓ **TRAIN SETS** Wooden train sets with lots of pieces provide endless combinations of track. But beware, you could invest quite a lot of money buying this type of toy for your child. Try to buy used when possible.

✓ **STUFFED ANIMALS** They aren't just for looking nice in the corner or sleeping with at night. To lots of children, they have lives of their own and offer hours of creative play.

✓ **DRESS-UP CLOTHES** Children love playing dress-up. As they get older, they can use the clothes as costumes in plays they write, direct, and act in.

KITCHEN TABLE TALK

Little Helpers

In developing countries, women usually have no choice but to include young children in their work. Many women spend entire days on survival tasks like hauling water, growing crops, cooking meals, and washing clothes at a riverbank. And their children accompany them. These young children help their mothers in whatever ways they can.

In our industrialized lifestyle, we forget that kids can make excellent helpers. Parents are often focused on getting the job done as quickly as possible so that they can relax with their kids. Another approach is to involve kids in the job itself. Get your child to help you around the house with sweeping, watering the plants, folding clothes, stirring pancake batter in the kitchen, or sorting out recyclable plastics using the numbers on the bottom. (See Chapter 2 to see what those numbers mean.) Make your child feel included in the household rhythm.

What Little Toys Are Made Of

So you know what sorts of toys will expand your child's horizons, but what should they be made of? We'll go over the materials found in kids' toys and let you know what items are safe and less harmful to the environment. You can choose toys made from organic cotton, unvarnished wood, and fabrics dyed with natural herbal dyes.

PLASTIC Plastic is made from a nonrenewable resource, and it has notorious waste-disposal problems. It isn't all bad, though. Plastic's longevity is not a bad quality in a toy. If possible, seek quality plastics and toys that will last. Children today are still playing with plastic dolls purchased in the 1970s.

That said, some plastics are worse than others. A lot of our most treasured toys are made with polyvinyl chloride (PVC), usually just called vinyl. Rubber duckies for the bath, baby's teethers, and many dolls are examples of toys that have been made of this chemical. PVC is also found in shower curtains, bath mats, kids' backpacks, and many waterproof household items. The manufacture of PVC is harmful because it results in release of hazardous dioxin. It has a characteristic "chemical" smell that can irritate the eyes and cause headaches in some individuals.

Whether you suffer from headaches or not, it is best to steer clear of PVC for another reason: PVC usually contains phthalates, which are chemicals that make the plastic soft enough to work with. Phthalates are potentially hazardous hormone-bending chemicals that should not be used in products for young children. A U.S. ban on certain phthalates went into effect in February 2009. The law permanently banned three phthalates: DEHP, DBP, and BBP in concentrations of more than 0.1 percent in "children's toys" or "child care articles." The phthalates DINP, DIDP, and DnOP were also provisionally banned in some items. However, some of the replacements have not been fully tested, so it is a good idea to look for nonplastic toys for children during the "mouthing" years.

Many vinyl (PVC) toys and lunch boxes also have been found to contain lead, a neurotoxic metal.

The U.S. Consumer Product Safety Commission defines a child's toy as "a product intended for a child 12 years of age or younger for use when playing." These include bath toys and books, dolls, balls, and pool toys. Child care articles covered by the ban include products used by children, ages three and under, for sucking, feeding, teething, or sleeping. These products include bottles, utensils, placemats, bibs, teethers, pacifiers, booster seats, and cribs. Playground equipment, musical instruments, bikes, and sporting goods are not affected by the ban on phthalates.

AVOIDING HARMFUL TOYS:

× Until your child stops mouthing objects, usually around age three, you should expect that any new toy is going to end up in your child's mouth. Shop accordingly.

× Don't buy toys at discount stores unless you are familiar with the manufacturer and the product is labeled.

× Call companies to ask what chemicals are in their toys.

× If you are using soft plastic toys purchased before February 2009, consider replacing them with phthalate-free versions.

WOOD Wooden toys are extremely durable and may be passed down through generations. The wooden train set you purchase for your toddler could someday become your great-grandchild's favorite toy.

ECO-TIP:
RECYCLE THOSE PEANUTS

When you order items through the Internet, they often come with a lot of packaging. Foam packaging peanuts made from expanded polystyrene (EPS) can be dropped off for recycling at several sites across the nation. There is also a "mail-back" program where you can return used EPS packaging materials. See *www.epspackaging.org*.

GREEN DICTIONARY

GREEN "MEME"

A "meme" is a unit of information that is transmissible from person to person. Spread green memes wherever possible. Help your children spread the word about recycling, walking instead of taking the car, and other planet-friendly practices.

In addition to trains, some of the wonderful toys made from wood include cars, baby rattles and teethers, and even entire kitchen sets. Most of these toys can be found in catalogs and on the Internet rather than in chain retailers. Order in advance for birthdays and holidays.

When shopping for wooden toys, look for ones made of solid wood rather than plywood or pressed board wood. The glues used to hold wood parts together usually contain formaldehyde, which is irritating to the eyes and skin in many people and may contribute to cancer risk. If you are unsure if an item is made of solid wood, turn it on its side and look for strips of wood or particles pressed together.

Many wooden toys are coated with a lacquer or varnish. Look for unvarnished toys or toys with natural coatings such as beeswax.

Wooden toys are made from a renewable resource, but they are not always eco-friendly. Deforestation of rain forests worldwide is taking place at a rapid clip. Look for products certified by the Forest Stewardship Council (FSC) as being from a certified well-managed forest. Or purchase toys from small domestic toymakers that obtain their wood from sustainably harvested forests.

COTTON Cotton is a wonderful natural fabric but conventional growing consumes large quantities of water, pesticides, and synthetic fertilizers. Cotton is usually bleached and then dyed with azo-based dyes that can cause allergic reactions in some people and have been linked to cancer in laboratory animals. New clothing and toys can contain dye residues that can irritate the skin.

Washing new cotton toys before you hand them over to your child can help remove dye residues. Or better yet, look for organically grown cotton stuffed animals and dolls. Many of these are dyed with plant-based dyes that are nontoxic and vibrant.

METAL Toys with metal parts may contain lead or other toxic metals. Unfortunately consumers have little information to go on when choosing metal toys. Look for labels that expressly say that the product was tested for lead. Choose reputable brands. You may want to call the manufacturer to ask about the safety of the product.

If you have a young child in the house, avoid toys that contain small magnetic balls or blocks that may be swallowed by a small child. If more than one magnet is swallowed, the magnets can stick to each other in the digestive system and cause life-threatening conditions.

Children's jewelry, clothing, and shoes may come adorned with charms that may contain lead. If these charms are swallowed your child could ingest a high dose of this toxic metal. Avoid these especially if you have young children in the house.

A 2009 federal law, the Consumer Product Safety Improvement Act (CPSIA) requires that manufacturers and importers test for lead products marketed to children under the age of 12. This law will give some peace of mind to parents who are concerned about lead.

When confronted with the possibility that your child's belongings, from toys to vinyl lunch boxes, may contain lead, you may be tempted to pick up a lead-testing kit from the paint store. But according to the Consumer Product Safety Commission (CPSC), these test kits are not reliable. The CPSC tested four commercially available kits and found that more than half of the test results were erroneous. Most of these were false negatives, meaning that the kit failed to detect lead when it was in fact in the product. None of the kits could reliably detect lead if the product had been covered with a nonlead coating.

ECO-TIP: SILICA-FREE SAND

When filling up the sand box, look for sand marked "play grade" and "silica-free." This will ensure that the sand has less of the crystalline silica dust that is linked to silicosis and lung cancer if one breathes the stuff for many years. Most of the sand available for purchase in the United States is made of silica (silicon dioxide, or SiO_2) but the play-grade brands contain less of the very fine, inhalable silica. Some sand may also contain tremolite, a form of the human carcinogen asbestos, so avoid all-purpose sand from hardware stores.

FACE PAINT, MAKEUP, AND TATTOOS Face-painting is a crowd-pleaser for the kids. You'll find face-painting booths at carnivals, amusement parks, and even museums. Professional painters use high-quality paints because they know there will be customer complaints if children develop rashes or other reactions.

When shopping for face paint for home use, choose the highest quality paint you can find. Some brands sold at party stores have been found to contain unsafe levels of microbes and have been subject to U.S. Food and Drug Administration (FDA) recalls. The Campaign for Safe Cosmetics found lead in kids' face paint kits, according to an October 2009 report.

The FDA regulates the ingredients in cosmetics, including children's face paint and theatrical paint. The agency approves the use of certain pigments, and states whether they may be used on the skin, around the eyes, and on the lips. Check the label to make sure the manufacturer uses FDA-approved ingredients.

TIPS FOR SAFE FACE PAINT:

✓ Check www.recalls.gov for product recalls.

✓ Follow the directions on the package.

✓ Check the package label to make sure that the pigment used is FDA-approved. You can view a list of FDA-approved pigments at www.fda.gov/ForIndustry/ColorAdditives.

✗ Do not apply face paint to the eyes or mouth unless the product is FDA-approved for that use.

✓ If your child is prone to allergies, test the paint by putting a small dab on his or her arm and waiting a few days before applying it to the face.

✓ Remove face paint before putting your child to bed.

✓ Consider making your own face paint using cold cream, cornstarch, and natural dyes. (See Chapter 9 for more on food-based dyes.)

MAKEUP AND NAIL POLISH Some children enjoy dressing up with makeup and nail polish. Or perhaps your child is performing in a play or dance recital and wants to wear some makeup. Before you doll up your child, read labels carefully and choose high-quality products. Not all FDA-approved additives are safe for children.

NAIL POLISH Adult nail polish may contain dibutyl phthalate, toluene, and formaldehyde, three toxic chemicals that children should not inhale. Dibutyl phthalate is a hormone-disrupting chemical that is toxic to the human immune system and is potentially harmful to wildlife if released into the environment. It is banned for use in nail polish in Europe but is still permitted in the United States. Toluene is neurotoxic and is listed as one of the U.S. Environmental Protection Agency's (EPA) priority pollutants under the Clean Water Act. Formaldehyde is linked to cancer, according to the International Agency for Research on Cancer (IARC) and the EPA.

If your child must have nail polish, check out some of the "greener" cosmetic lines that now produce peel-off nail polishes. These have less toxic ingredients.

PERFUME Fragrances often contain phthalates because these chemicals help carry the scent into the air. However many phthalates are hormone disrupters, and some are potentially toxic to the immune system, reproduction, and fetal development, according to the U.S. National Research Council. Look for products containing plant-based fragrances.

LIPSTICK Several brands of red lipstick contain lead, so it is a good idea to avoid using the bright red colors and to stick to safer pinks and other colors. Check the safety profile of your favorite brands at the Environmental Working Group's Skin Deep Cosmetics Safety Database at *www.cosmeticsdatabase.com*.

TEMPORARY TATTOOS Like makeup, temporary tattoos (also called skin decals) are required to utilize only FDA-approved colorants. The agency has, however, received many complaints from parents whose children developed rashes or other allergic reactions.

One type of skin decal to be wary of is the black henna temporary tattoo. These tattoos may contain a highly allergenic chemical called paraphenylenediamine (PPD), according to the FDA. PPD is a coal-tar product that is not FDA-approved for use on the skin. It can cause serious allergic reactions that result in rashes, blisters, and scarring.

Natural henna is brown, red-brown, or orange-brown. Note however that henna is FDA-approved only for coloring hair, not skin.

Getting Crafty

One of the joys of having kids is being able to release your own inner child.

Parenting is a great excuse to roll up your sleeves and play with clay, finger paint, and all those creative and messy arts and crafts that are staple activities for kids. Crayons, chalk, paint, colored pencils, and modeling clay can provide hours of fun and creativity. Check here on how to buy safe and environmentally friendly products.

ART SUPPLIES THAT ARE SAFE FOR KIDS AND THE PLANET The act of creating art unleashes a child's inventive spirit and puts him or her in control of her environment. Encourage your young children to experiment with colors and materials. As they get older, you can teach them techniques or enroll them in art classes. It is amazing what kids can create given gentle instruction.

When dabbling in the arts, all parents and instructors need to be on the lookout for toxic materials that could prove hazardous to kids and the environment. Washing hazardous chemicals down the drain spreads these harmful chemicals into water supplies, where they are toxic to wildlife. Paints, markers, and glues can contain solvents that can harm the nervous system, including the brain. Some ingredients may be flammable or irritating to the skin. Others have been found to increase the risk of cancer in animal studies or human studies.

Children are more susceptible to toxic chemicals than adults because per body weight they inhale more air. Children's brains, lungs, nervous systems, and other organs are still developing and are differently susceptible to toxic substances as compared to adults. Children often spend hours bent over an art project, inhaling fumes. They usually work without gloves so chemicals in paint and glue may seep through the skin. Young children may take a curious sip from a paint bottle or lick their paint-coated fingers.

Unfortunately both children and their parents often fail to read labels or follow instructions. No eager child wants to postpone an art project to track down that lost pair of protective goggles or take a trip to the store to pick up gloves. Parents are often the worst offenders, and by their own negligence pass on the disregard of safety to their children. Instead, parents should model good safety behavior by reading labels and putting on the goggles, gloves, or other required precautions.

The CPSC requires the labeling of art materials known to cause long-term adverse health effects. The Federal Hazardous Substances Act (FHSA) bans the use of ingredients in children's art supplies that cause long-term or short-term toxicity or are flammable. However, it provides exceptions for products that are properly labeled and are meant for children who are mature enough to read and understand the warnings.

Using safer art supplies is the responsible thing to do, both for your children and for the environment. Creating these chemicals in the first place can cause environmental pollution if the chemical plant does not follow procedures carefully. Workers in these plants may be exposed to toxic chemicals. Whenever possible, choose nontoxic materials.

STEPS FOR SAFE USE OF ART SUPPLIES:

✓ Always supervise.

✓ Purchase only products bearing the statement "Conforms to ASTM D-4236," a safety standard for art materials.

✓ Look for products certified by the Art & Creative Materials Institute (ACMI), a membership association of more than 200 art and craft material manufacturers.

✗ Do not purchase supplies that contain cautionary warnings on the label, especially if your children are under the age of 12.

✓ Use only products that are labeled as intended for children.

✓ Wear gloves and eye protection when needed.

✓ Work in well-ventilated areas where clean air flows toward the artist's workspace and contaminated air flows out a window or ventilation duct. A fan that blows air around a closed room could send contaminants toward children.

✓ Teach children to read labels and follow safety instructions.

✓ Keep food and drinks away from the art area.

✓ Store supplies safely out of reach of children.

✓ Dispose of old supplies that are not labeled with safety information.

✓ Dole out small quantities of supplies in order to minimize spillage and chemical exposure.

✗ Avoid materials that contain lead, cadmium, or other heavy metals, which are commonly used as pigments in adult art supplies.

✓ Cover cuts and sores with bandages before beginning projects to minimize entry of chemicals through cut skin.

✓ Wash hands thoroughly after the project is completed. Never use toluene, turpentine, kerosene, or other solvents to clean the skin.

✗ Avoid products that generate fine dusts that can be inhaled.

✓ Choose water-based products over solvent-based ones.

✓ Keep sharp tools in good working order and store them in areas where children cannot reach them.

✗ Never use food containers for storage of hazardous art materials.

✓ Take hazardous materials to your local collection facility—don't put them in the garbage.

✗ Do not substitute prescription eyeglasses for safety goggles. Put goggles over eyeglasses.

MATERIALS AND THEIR HAZARDS All of the materials below are enjoyable to kids and come in safer versions. Check labels before purchasing.

CERAMIC GLAZE Glaze may contain metals that give glazes their luster. These metals may include arsenic, uranium, lead, chromium VI, lithium, beryllium, cobalt, antimony, cadmium, nickel, barium, vanadium, soda ash, potassium carbonate, feldspars, and fluorspar. Some glazes may contain solvents (see below). Look for lead-free brands and follow the manufacturer's instructions.

CLAYS Clays can contain hydrated aluminum silicates, which in turn contain crystalline silica dust. Long-term exposure to crystalline silica dust can cause a severe lung injury called silicosis, as well as lung cancer. Clay may also contain asbestos, which is linked to a type of lung cancer called mesothelioma. Avoid breathing clay dust. Polymer clays, which are squishy at room temperature but can be hardened in a kitchen oven, usually contain polyvinyl chloride (PVC). Safer choices include 100 percent beeswax with natural dyes and earth clay, available at online retailers. Or make your own by mixing flour, salt, and water using this recipe:

HOMEMADE PLAY CLAY
1 cup flour
1/4 cup salt
2 tablespoons cream of tartar
1 cup water
1 tablespoon vegetable oil
natural coloring (see Chapter 9 for suggestions)

DRAWING SUPPLIES Drawing requires little more than a pencil and paper. When selecting pencils choose ones without cautionary or warning labels. Select nondusty chalk. Soy crayons are a renewable alternative to petroleum-based crayons. Choose charcoal that is nondusty and use a wet mop to clean up dust afterward. Choose recycled paper or reuse computer paper that has been printed on one side only.

GLUES Choose glues labeled for use by children. Read labels and choose the least toxic product available. Glues, especially rubber cement, can contain formaldehyde, solvents such as n-hexane, and toxic adhesives. Avoid instant glues because they are extremely strong and can bind skin and eyelids.

INKS Solvent-based inks contain chemicals that cause fatigue, dizziness, and short-lived feelings of euphoria. The fumes may be inhaled or the ink absorbed by the skin. Choose water-based and water-soluble inks. If permanent markers must be used, make sure the room is ventilated, or use them outdoors.

KNITTING AND CROCHETING When choosing yarn, look for natural animal fibers such as angora or other types of wool. Choose prewashed fibers to avoid contamination with molds or animal diseases. Organic versions are available. Plant-based natural fibers include cotton, flax, and sisal. Synthetic fibers made of acetate, acrylics, nylon, polyester, or rayon are also available. However these are made from nonrenewable resources with toxic chemical ingredients, creating worker exposures and potential environmental hazards if not disposed of properly.

PAINTS Some paints may contain toxic metals, give off hazardous odors, or both. Avoid any pigments made with chromate or other toxic metals. Choose water-based paints that are intended for use by children.

PAPERMAKING This is a fun activity but may involve using potentially irritating chemicals, such as chlorine bleach, washing soda (sodium carbonate), ammonia, lye, and hydrogen peroxide. Any of these can be extremely toxic if accidentally swallowed, so this activity should not be done with young children. Wear gloves and goggles and follow manufacturer safety recommendations when working with these chemicals.

SPRAY FIXATIVES These may contain hazardous solvents. Avoid using around children. (Spray paints marketed as safe for kids may be free of solvents but are an inhalation hazard.) If you must use spray fixatives, do it outdoors.

WOOD WORKING This activity can be fun for older children. When choosing projects consider the source of the wood. Find FSC-certified wood or scavenge pieces from your own yard or furniture that is slated for disposal. Both you and your child should wear a dust mask when sawing, and you should ventilate dust to the outdoors.

Beware of plywood and particleboards because these usually contain glues that offgas irritating and potentially cancer-causing formaldehyde. Many people also have allergic reactions in the form of skin rashes, itchy eyes, nausea, and vomiting. Sawing and sanding plywood and particleboard could release formaldehyde and vapors of carbon monoxide, hydrogen cyanide, and phenol, which are all toxic. Avoid working with pressure-treated lumber, which has been treated with potentially harmful chemicals under pressure to protect it from rotting. (See the section on playground equipment for a discussion of the chemicals used.)

GREEN ON A SHOESTRING

Here are some suggestions for making your own toys:

✓ **FINGER PUPPETS** Sew finger puppets out of old clothes. Have your child glue on bits of cloth for eyes and decorate the puppets with markers.

✓ **NESTING BOWLS** Use a nested set of mixing bowls from your kitchen. Or, check the thrift stores or garage sales for bowls.

✓ **MUSICAL INSTRUMENTS** An upside down bowl or box makes a great drum. Use wooden spoons for drumsticks. Make a maraca by placing dried beans inside a folded paper plate and stapling it shut. Make a guitar out of a tissue box with a paper towel roll as the neck of the guitar. Tape a few strings across the open part of the tissue box.

✓ **DOLL** Make a doll from a bandanna and some pillow stuffing. Tie a string where the neck should be and use string to section off arms and legs.

✓ **DRESS UP** Check the bargain bins at fabric stores or buy dresses from thrift stores. Add plenty of ribbon and let your child make her own fashion designs.

✓ **WHAT-IS-IT BOX** Tape a shoe box shut, decorate it, and cut a hole in one end big enough for your child's hand to fit through. Put inside items such as pinecones, smooth stones, rough stones, and sticks. Have your child identify things by their feel.

✓ **FUN WITHOUT TOYS** Some playtime activities cost no money, use no natural resources, and produce no greenhouse gases. They include tickling, playing hide-and-seek, making a pillow fort, and playing peekaboo, patty-cake, or other finger games.

CHEMICALS TO AVOID IN CHILDREN'S ART SUPPLIES Art supply manufacturers are not required to list ingredients on the label, so it is best to stick with products marketed expressly for children. The following ingredients are frequently found in art supplies sold to adults or older children, according to the CPSC. Always use precautions when doing crafts with your older children. Do not use these with younger children.

× **ACETONE (SOLVENT, AEROSOLIZED PAINTS)** Irritates the airways, can cause dizziness.

× **BENZENE (SOLVENTS, GLUES)** Flammable. Known human carcinogen, can cause dizziness, fatigue, and confusion, and is toxic to the liver.

× **FORMALDEHYDE (ADHESIVES AND GLUES)** Irritates the eyes, nose, skin and throat, causes headaches and dizziness, and is considered by the EPA to be a probable human carcinogen.

× **D-LIMONENE (PAINT THINNER, ALSO CALLED CITRUS OIL)** Highly flammable. Irritates the airways, eyes, nose, and is a stomach irritant if swallowed, causing nausea and vomiting.

× **ACIDS (USED IN DYEING FABRICS AND PAPERMAKING)** Can burn skin and irritate the eyes.

× **BLEACH (USED WITH FABRICS AND PAPERMAKING)** Can cause skin damage, eye damage, and headaches.

× **GLYCOL ETHERS (CLEANING SUPPLIES)** Cause birth defects and reproductive harm in animals; can cause dizziness and fatigue as well as anemia and kidney toxicity.

× **N-HEXANE (GLUES)** Highly flammable. Toxic to the nervous system and irritating to the skin, eyes, and nose.

× **MINERAL SPIRITS (OIL PAINTS, VARNISHES)** Highly flammable and can cause severe lung damage if accidentally inhaled.

× **TOLUENE (MODEL AIRPLANE GLUE, PAINT REMOVER)** Highly flammable. May cause reproductive toxicity and damage to the central nervous system, liver, and kidney. Inhaling large amounts can cause giddiness, euphoria, and interfere with heart rhythm.

× **TURPENTINE (PAINT THINNER, VARNISHES)** Flammable solvent that can cause lung damage if fumes are inhaled. Can also cause dizziness, headaches, and seizures.

× **XYLENE (ACRYLIC PAINTS)** Flammable solvent that can irritate the lungs, skin, eyes, and mouth. Can also impair thinking and movement.

× **METALS (POWDERED PAINTS, GLAZES, ENAMELS)** Lead and manganese are neurotoxicants; chromium VI (found in potassium dichromates and other dichromates) and cadmium are known human carcinogens.

× **DUST (PLASTER, CHALK, WOOD)** Can lodge deep in lungs and provide chronic irritation.

Outdoor Play

Fresh air and physical activity are two vital ingredients for raising a healthy child. We'll take a look at how to create a safe and Earth-friendly outdoor play area for your entire family to enjoy.

CHEMICAL-FREE YARD To create a safe place for kids to play while protecting streams, rivers, and the plants and animals of the planet, you should think twice before reaching for the biannual bottle of "weed and feed." Ninety million pounds of weed-killing herbicides are applied to lawns and gardens each year, according to the EPA.

Pesticides and herbicides kill not only the harmful insects or weeds you want to kill, but also can be toxic to beneficial insects, amphibians, and plants. Of 30 commonly used yard pesticides, 24 are toxic to fish and aquatic organisms, 16 are toxic to birds, and 11 are deadly to bees, according to the advocacy group Beyond Pesticides.

All of these species are worth preserving and many provide benefits around the yard and garden. For example, amphibians such as frogs and toads eat flies, aphids, mosquitoes, and other pests. Some species are pollinators, helping plants reproduce. The endangered Karner blue butterfly is one such insect. The butterfly population has dropped due to habitat loss and poisoning by insecticides. To protect the Karner blue butterfly the EPA has prohibited the use of the insecticide methoxyfenozide on cranberry bushes in several counties in Wisconsin.

Another important pollinator affected by pesticides is the honeybee. In the last several years honeybee populations have declined rapidly, leaving farmers and researchers scrambling to explain why. Researchers are converging on a theory behind the cause of what is now termed colony collapse disorder (CCD), according to a 2009 article in the magazine *Scientific American*.[1] These experts suspect that pesticides are sickening or weakening bees and making it difficult for them to find and return to their hives. These bees are made weaker still because the loss of biodiversity in farm fields means the bees are not getting adequate nutrition. These two factors—pesticides and poor nutrition—make honeybees more susceptible to viruses. The fungicide chlorothalonil and the pesticide class known as neonicotinoids have both been linked to CCD in studies.

To protect pollinators and other living creatures, including our children, it is a good idea to reduce or eliminate the use of toxic pesticides and herbicides. Many schools are moving to reduce the use of these chemicals around children. Yet ironically parents continue to purchase toxic products. Frequently people do not follow directions, applying chemicals without wearing proper protection and then tracking toxic chemicals into the home on the bottoms of their shoes.

Pesticides are designed to kill insects, but most of them target the same biological systems that humans have. For example several pesticides target the nervous system. The human and insect nervous systems work on similar principles. Pesticides that target the nervous system include the organophosphates, the carbamates, the pyrethroids, the ethylenebisdithiocarbamates, and the chlorophenoxy herbicides. According to the advocacy group Beyond Pesticides, 15 of the most commonly used lawn and garden pesticides and herbicides cause neurotoxicity, and 19 are linked to increased risk of cancer.

TIPS FOR AVOIDING PESTICIDES AND HERBICIDES IN LAWN CARE:

✓ If you need to kill off an area of grass, put a large piece of old carpet over it to starve the plants of light and oxygen. After a few weeks your grass will be dead. To find old carpet, keep your eyes open on your neighborhood garbage day, or check websites such as *freecycle.org*.

✓ If you are planning to replace grass with a garden or flower bed, remove

---

ECO-TIP: DON'T LET CHILDREN DRINK FROM GARDEN HOSES

Many brands of hoses contain lead, a neurotoxicant that can cause cognitive disabilities in young children. There is no safe level of lead exposure. Also, depending on how they are used, hoses may contain residues of gardening chemicals such as pesticides or fertilizers. Finally, hoses often sit in the sun where bacteria grow that could make children sick.

the grass with the roots intact so that the resulting grass sod can be transplanted into another location. You may be able to give the grass sod to a neighbor who wants to plant grass in his yard. Or try advertising the sod on a website like *craigslist.org* or *freecycle.org*.

✓ Remove weeds with a garden hoe, or better yet, have your kids dig them out with a small (child-safe) trowel.

✓ Herbicidal soap is a nontoxic alternative to conventional weed-killing chemicals.

✓ Organic lawn care is not regulated under the USDA organic regulations, something to keep in mind if you are hiring a lawn care company that advertises organic care.

PLAYGROUND EQUIPMENT Backyard play equipment can offer hours of enjoyment. If you are in the market for playground equipment, check into ones made of recycled plastic or FSC-certified wood.

RECYCLED PLASTIC PLAYGROUND SETS Recycled plastic playground equipment is an increasingly popular alternative to wood. It is durable and relatively inexpensive. Everyday items such as plastic food and beverage containers, shipping containers and wraps, and plastic bags are melted down and refashioned into recycled plastic decks, ladders, forts, sandboxes, and slides.

One type of playground plastic is recycled structural plastic (RSP) created from #2 HDPE (high-density polyethylene) containers, including milk jugs. According to one manufacturer, their average play set is made of more than 25,000 recycled milk jugs. The same company operates a take-back program to collect their playground equipment if a user decides they don't want it anymore. These products are incredibly durable, with some companies offering 100-year warranties.

When evaluating play sets, look for eco-friendly third-party certifications such as

✓ GREENGUARD, *www.greenguard.org*: A nonprofit, industry-independent agency that certifies that products have chemical and particle emissions that meet acceptable air-quality standards.

✓ Green Seal, *greenseal.org*: An independent nonprofit organization that establishes standards and certifies products such as personal care products, construction materials, household cleaning products, paints, and more.

✓ EcoLogo, *www.ecologo.org*: An environmental consulting firm that creates standards and certifies a variety of consumer and industry products.

✓ ISO, *www.iso.org:* The International Standards Organization is a non-governmental organization that is the world's largest setter of standards, including environmental standards.

✓ Scientific Certification Systems, *www.scscertified.com:* Independently certifies products using standards based on environmental impact, sustainability, and food quality.

WOOD PLAYGROUND SETS Wood is another popular option. Before you buy, check to see if the wood has been treated with any pesticides. In 2003, the EPA banned the use of chromated copper arsenate (CCA), an insecticide that contains 22 percent arsenic, in lumber for residential uses. Play sets built before then are likely to contain CCA.

Safer preservatives are now available for use in pressure-treated lumber. However, these preservatives are not risk-free. The EPA recommends that gloves be worn when working with pressure-treated lumber. The lumber should not be used for eating surfaces (such as picnic tables), and should not be burned because it generates toxic smoke and ash.

If you choose a wood playground set, ensure that the wood came from well-managed forests. Look for the Forest Stewardship Council (FSC) certification *(www.fsc.org).*

Some companies provide do-it-yourself kits that allow you to build your own playground. For some kits, you may need to buy the lumber yourself and do your own cutting, drilling, and assembly. This can be an advantage if you live near a supplier that offers FSC-certified lumber or you can find wood that you are confident came from well-managed sources.

Any play set should have a thick layer of mulch, wood chips, or sand beneath it. Nearly 60 percent of all injuries on playground sets are caused by falls to the ground, according to the CPSC, which publishes safety standards for home playground equipment at *www.cpsc.gov/CPSCPUB/ PUBS/323.HTML.* Steer clear of recycled tire rubber mulch, however. See The Science Behind It at the end of this chapter.

GREEN DICTIONARY

PRESSURE-TREATED LUMBER

Lumber that is subjected to pressure to allow pesticidal chemicals to penetrate the wood.

HAVE BIKE, WILL TRAVEL Bicycles are terrific for exercise, and kids are thrilled when they finally are able to ride without training wheels. Bikes are an eco-friendly method of transportation to and from school or a friend's house. The next time you have to drive your child to a friend's house for a playdate, consider biking with him there instead. You'll both get some exercise and fresh air, and keep a little bit of planet-warming carbon dioxide out of the air.

Most bicycles in toy stores today are made with aluminum frames stamped "made in China," making it hard for consumers to judge the environmental and labor conditions associated with their manufacture. But you can find an eco-friendly alternative: bamboo bikes. Several boutique bicycle manufacturers make bicycles with bamboo frames. You can also find do-it-yourself kits online.

BIKE TRAILERS, TRAIL-A-BIKES, AND BIKE SEATS When your child is too young to ride his or her own bike, consider purchasing a bike trailer, bike seat, or trail-a-bike. A bike trailer is towed behind the bike, a bike seat fits behind the adult seat over the rear wheel, and a trail-a-bike is a one-wheeled bike that attaches to the adult's bike, turning it into a bicycle built for two. With your child firmly ensconced on one of these devices, you can use your bike for errands or just to get a little exercise.

Safety experts recommend that babies be at least one year of age before being placed in a bike trailer or bike seat. Before that age babies do not have the muscles to maintain sitting up for long periods. Babies should not spend long amounts of time in a slouched position in a trailer. Also, the bumps on the road subject babies to continuous jiggling. Think how uncomfortable it is to ride on a dirt road in a car, and you'll get the picture.

When cycling with your small child in tow, think carefully about how best to avoid accidents. It may be best to stay on a bicycle-only path rather than sharing the road with automobiles. Although the risk of collision may seem low, the consequences of an accident could be disastrous.

Helmets are essential for the safety of a child in a bike trailer or bike seat, and are mandated by law in many states. No helmets are rated for children under one year of age, which makes sense because children under that age should not be in bike trailers or carriers.

HARD HEADS Most bike helmets are made of polystyrene foam surrounded by a polycarbonate plastic shell. They also contain nylon or polyethylene straps and a plastic buckle. All of these materials originated from petroleum deposits deep underground that were recovered from the earth, depleting its natural resources. However, safety experts have found that these are some of the most lightweight and safest (for the rider) materials available.

Helmets may also be made of ABS plastic. The manufacture of ABS involves the mixing of three probable human carcinogens, acrylonitrile, butadiene, and styrene. ABS is considered a safer plastic because the end user is not exposed to any hazardous chemicals. However, the manufacture of ABS involves several toxic chemicals, and these could be harmful to factory workers and the environment if safeguards are not in place.

Bicycle helmets must meet strict safety standards set by the CPSC. When choosing a helmet for your child, consider safety first. You can get more information on how to select a safe helmet at the Bicycle Helmet Safety Institute's website, *bhsi.org*.

HOW DOES YOUR GARDEN GROW? It is as simple as putting a seed in dirt and watering it. It can be done in a pot on a windowsill or patio. Or you can go all out and dig up part of the lawn and replace it with a vegetable garden capable of feeding the whole family.

Gardens are a great delight to many children. Where else can you chase butterflies and capture beetles? Vegetable gardens are just one of the many options. Here are some other types of gardens:

CHILD'S FLOWER GARDEN What child wouldn't like to have his or her own place to retreat and enjoy nature in a space that he or she created? Give your child a plot of land and help her remove the grass (see tip above on saving grass sod) and build a small fence (if necessary, to keep deer or other animals from eating the flowers). If you live in an apartment, create a refuge on a patio or put some potted plants by a sunny windowsill. Help your child decide what seeds to plant, and take her to a gardening center to buy them.

BUTTERFLY GARDEN Certain flower species attract butterflies. Several retailers sell premixed seed packets to create your butterfly garden. Or pick and choose your own. Consult your local agricultural extension office or websites to find out which types of flowers grow best in your area. Some butterfly favorites include common milkweed, marigold, and butterfly bush. Look for flower varieties that are native to your area.

RAIN GARDEN One of the problems with many suburban and urban developments is that rain runs from streets and driveways directly into storm drains, where it is whisked away rather than being allowed to seep back into the ground to replenish the underground aquifer. Return rainwater to the ground where it fell by constructing a rain garden. Build the garden in a depression where rain can collect after it runs off your patio, cement walkway, or driveway. Plant native plants in the rain garden so that the plants thrive with existing rainfall and do not need additional watering.

BOOK GARDEN Create a haven for your young reader by placing a child-size bench in the garden. Add stepping-stones, a birdbath, and a sundial. Complete your child's book sanctuary by erecting a trellis with a climbing flowering plant and a sun umbrella that can be opened up when it is hot.

BERRY GARDEN Nothing is more nutritious and at the same time delicious as a sun-warmed blueberry or raspberry. Children can spend hours picking berries—as long as they can pop them in their mouth right away. As they do they'll be getting more than their day's share of vitamins and antioxidants.

VERTICAL GARDEN If you don't have space for a garden, consider building or purchasing a tiered wall planter. These vertical planters allow you to place several small potted plants on a series of shelves. When you water the top plants the water drips down into the lower pots, making watering easy and efficient.

GREEN ON A SHOESTRING

A rain barrel is a no-brainer. Why not collect rainwater for free instead of paying your utility company for the water you use in your garden or flower bed. You'll save money and reduce your environmental impact because you'll draw less chlorine-treated water from the system.

Rain barrels are now popular items in gardening catalogs and high-end gardening stores. A closer look reveals that many are not all that different from a giant plastic garbage can, except that they are a little sturdier and have a spout near the bottom for drawing water.

You can easily create your own rain barrel out of any number of items you already have around the house. Your rain barrel can be as simple as placing a bucket under your downspout before a storm. Some food manufacturers use barrels and sell them cheaply. If you buy a used barrel, make sure it was not used for toxic chemicals. You can also check environmental groups or your local municipality to see if they sell discounted rain barrels.

If you make your own, be sure to cover the top with a screen to keep mosquitoes from breeding in the barrel. If you have young children in the neighborhood, you'll want to firmly attach a lid to prevent accidents. Finally, many homemade and store-bought rain barrels alike are rather ugly, so you might consider placing potted plants around it or growing a vine over it.

One final note: Until recently, rain barrels were illegal in the state of Colorado. Such bans were enacted to keep rainwater flowing to underground aquifers and rivers in places where water rights are precious. Check with your state to see if any laws prohibit use of rain barrels. If so, petition your government representatives to repeal the law.

TAKING A DIP Swimming pools are a great relief during a hot summer. Kids love them, and parents love anything that keeps kids occupied for hours. But pools are not environmentally harmless. They consume water, energy, and require treatment with hazardous chemicals. If you are considering installing a pool or already have one, consider how you can make it safer for swimmers and reduce its drain on environmental resources.

TIPS FOR SWIMMING WITH LESS IMPACT ON THE ENVIRONMENT:
✓ Join a community pool instead of installing your own.
✓ Choose an energy-efficient pool pump and use a timer to control its use. Pool pumps are one of the biggest energy users in the home.
✓ Install a solar-powered pump and skimmer. These only run during the daytime, but that is usually no problem during the long days of the swimming season.
✓ Install a rooftop solar pool-heating system. Water is heated in flat solar panels on the roof and then returned to the pool.
✓ Use a pool cover. It keeps heat from escaping and water from evaporating, especially in hot climates. The average uncovered swimming pool loses four to six feet of water each year to evaporation in the Phoenix area, according to the Arizona Department of Water Resources.
✓ Monitor your water chemistry carefully and add only the appropriate amounts of chlorine and acid.
✓ Choose environmentally friendly pool chemicals—several are now on

the market. Or look into installing a system that injects ozone gas into the water to kill microorganisms. These can reduce chlorine use by up to 90 percent.

✓ Consider installing a saline pool, which uses sodium chloride (salt) to keep algae away. Or go for a "natural pool" instead of a chlorine-treated pool. These pools clean the water by circulating it through aquatic plants.

Screen Time

Most children today spend long periods of time in front of a screen whether it be watching commercial TV, viewing videos, or playing video games. This section will help you limit screen time to promote a child's outdoor exploits, as well as give tips on how to select "greener" electronics.

VIDEOS AND YOUNG CHILDREN Despite bearing the names of famous scientists on their labels, videos for babies have never been shown to promote intelligence. In fact, most studies show that TV for babies does little for them and could potentially be harmful. Babies are geared to learn speech from human lips and have a difficult time picking it up from videos. Children are attuned to understand the rhythm of their caregivers' and family members' voices, not the voices they hear on TV. Their visual systems are immature, and they have no cultural frame of reference to understand the images they see. If TV or videos are used as substitutes for parent-child interactions or physical exploration, then TV is definitely harmful.

For all these reasons, the American Academy of Pediatrics (AAP) recommends that children under the age of two not watch any television or videos. This can be hard to do in some households, especially ones where older children may resent having their video habits interrupted by a new addition to the family. If possible, have your older children watch TV when their younger sibling is napping. Or move the TV to the parental bedroom for a few years and let your older children watch their favorite shows out of sight. Babies and young toddlers are unlikely to be interested in the shows anyway. They want to be like the older kids and be around their family members. In other words, they want the social aspect, which is exactly what is lacking when everyone's concentration is aimed at TV.

Around age two, children are more able to process the variety of voices on TV. They are more aware of the world and can more easily understand what they are watching. Around this age they may benefit from educational shows that are designed for young children. The actors speak slowly and clearly. The sets are simple and colorful, the characters cuddly. One study published in a 2005 issue of *American Behavioral Scientist* found that children who watch these shows knew on average about ten more words at age two and a half than nonviewers.[2]

After age two, parents should continue to limit their children's screen time, according to the American Academy of Pediatrics. One study of more than 4,000 adolescents found that the more hours of television they watched, the higher the odds that they became depressed during the seven-year follow-up period, according to the report in the 2009 issue of *The Archives of General Psychiatry*.[3] A study in the 2009 issue of the journal *Pediatrics* found that children's stress levels correlated to how much time they spent in front of screens (TV, movie player, and video games).[4]

Parental TV habits often feed directly into children's habits. Try not to have TV on as background noise. In households with background TV, adults talk less to their children, and this can have a negative impact on language acquisition and cognitive development, according to a 2009 article in the *Archives of Pediatrics and Adolescent Medicine*.[5]

Television and other screen-based diversions are potentially harmful not just for the content they provide but also for what they do not provide: opportunities for exercise, reading, playing stimulating games and doing puzzles, and interacting with other human beings.

HEALTHY TIPS FOR WATCHING:

✓ Develop your child's play skills instead of using TV as a babysitter. Try instead to encourage your child to play or read by himself.

✓ Give your child a "screen allowance." Decide on an appropriate amount of screen time, such as half an hour a day, or only on weekends, or whatever works for your family. Help your child decide what shows he wants to watch.

✓ Before letting your child watch a movie, check on its violence, language, drug references, and overall content. Several websites offer movie synopses geared toward parents. Two are *CommonSenseMedia.org* and *ParentsChoice.org*.

✓ Watch movies and TV shows with your child. Are any parts scary? Disturbing? Talk with your child about the movie, and ask how it made him feel. Watch for moodiness or other behavior changes over the next few days.

✓ Keep the TV and computer in the family area instead of in the child's room. A child who has a TV in his or her room is more likely to suffer from sleep problems and do poorly on tests at school, according to studies.

✓ Before purchasing a video game, check out sites that review games, such as *WhatTheyPlay.com*.

NOW THIS MESSAGE As green parents we want to help our children realize that acquiring lots of "stuff" is not good for the planet. The first "R" of reduce, reuse, and recycle means that we need to just say no to buying things that we don't need. The fewer new toys and clothes our children get, the less the drain on nonrenewable resources and the building of mountains of garbage in landfills.

Advertisers know that children have great powers over the buying habits of parents. Teens and children influence the shopping habits of parents to the tune of an estimated $200 billion per year, according to studies cited in a policy statement by the American Academy of Pediatrics. According to these sources, teens directly spend an additional $155 billion, and children younger than 12 years spend about $25 billion annually.

Many children are too young to understand the purpose of advertising, according to the AAP policy report, which goes on to say that children under eight years of age are "cognitively and psychologically defenseless against advertising." In the 1970s the U.S. Federal Trade Commission (FTC) found that it was unfair and deceptive to advertise to children under age six. The Children's Television Act of 1990 placed a limit on the amount of time that commercials could be shown during children's programming: 10.5 minutes per hour on weekends and 12 minutes per hour on weekdays.

Other countries have gone much farther and enacted complete bans against showing ads that promote products for children. The country of Greece bans toy ads during the hours that children typically watch TV. Sweden and Norway have banned all advertising aimed at children under the age of 12.

Marketing to children not only instills desires for certain products and toys, it has a deeper message: that consumption is essential to personal identity. The message goes beyond simply that buying stuff makes a person happy—it is that buying a *particular* item or brand makes *you who you are*. The "cool" children are the ones that have the latest electronic gadget or wear the hip brand of clothing. While there have always been "cool" kids, "nerdy" kids, and

THE FACTS

The U.S. has 5 percent of the world's population yet uses 25 percent of the world's resources.

everything in between, marketers now consciously try to create fads and trends through tie-ins to popular TV characters and movies.

This problem will not go away any time soon, so parents need to create strategies to counteract the marketing messages. Help your child build a strong identity around his or her unique likes and dislikes. Does your child have a favorite sport? Is he interested in music or languages? Could she help start a nature club to protect local resources or share nature with children younger than her? Cultivating hobbies can keep kids away from the television and give them activities to enjoy other than shopping.

TIPS FOR CONFRONTING ADVERTISING:

✓ Teach your children to critically evaluate commercials. What is this commercial trying to sell me and why? Is it something that I really need? Remind your children that the kids in the commercial are paid actors.

✓ Use technology to skip commercials. You can prerecord shows using a digital video recorder or watch the show using the on-demand feature offered by many cable companies. Or simply press "mute" on the remote control.

✓ Teach your child to enjoy and respect nature. This can help bolster your message that consuming wisely is essential for conservation.

GREEN SCREENS Although we try to promote outdoor play and family board games, the allure of the TV or computer screen is hard for any kid (and many adults) to resist. By the age of four or five, kids are already discussing the latest video games with their peers. Here are some tips on picking environmentally friendly screens.

When shopping for electronics, consider energy usage. Some of the large plasma TVs consume more energy than a typical household refrigerator. The two biggest factors in energy consumption are the technology and the size. For their size, liquid crystal displays (LCDs) consume fewer watts per square inch than do plasma screens.

To reduce your energy consumption, choose an ENERGY STAR-certified model with a power-saving mode. Look for the latest ENERGY STAR ratings since these are generally stricter than previous versions. ENERGY STAR's Version 3.0 for TVs mandates power consumption standards for TVs while turned on, whereas the previous standard applied only to energy usage of TVs when turned off (standby mode).

TVs do draw power while turned off so that they'll come on quickly when you press the "on" button. The Version 3.0 ENERGY STAR rating requires that standby mode use no more than 1 watt in standby mode. New standards will go into effect in May 2010 that require ENERGY STAR TVs to be 40 percent more energy efficient than conventional TVs.

COMPUTERS At some point in your child's academic career, he or she will need a computer. The "greenest" option is to have your children share a family computer, but if fights are breaking out regularly over computer usage, or the ten-year-old family computer crashes on a regular basis, it might be time to buy a new computer.

Before purchasing a new computer, give careful thought to what the computer will be used for and what features your child will need. Will you need a high-quality graphics card for video games and movies or will a basic one suffice? How much memory will you need? What about processing speed? Today's computers are more energy efficient than ever. Look for ENERGY STAR-certified models.

Along with power consumption another thing to consider is the amount of toxic metals and flame retardants used in your new box. You can find information about the amount of environmentally damaging metals and chemicals in computers through the Electronic Product Environmental Assessment Tool (EPEAT). Products can be certified as Bronze, Silver, or Gold-rated depending on how well they meet the standards. These standards restrict cadmium, mercury, lead, hexavalent chromium, and some brominated flame retardants. The standards also require the use of reusable or recyclable components as well as safer packaging and a computer take-back program. See *www.epeat.net* to find brands of desktops, laptops, and monitors.

Before you buy, find out if the manufacturer has a take-back program for disposing of computers. You may also donate your computer to a charity that provides computers for schools. According to the EPA, most people are storing their old computers in their closets and garages. Most of us simply don't know how to dispose of these items. If you have an old computer or two in your garage, don't put it out in the regular trash. Contact your local municipality to find out if they have an electronic waste initiative. If not, look on the Internet for programs.

Unfortunately much of the electronic waste generated in the industrialized world is being shipped to developing countries in Africa and Asia. In some places, children strip the computers of valuable metals and parts without wearing proper protection, according to Greenpeace International. Take-back programs can keep old computers from becoming toxic junk. You can encourage companies to be socially responsible by purchasing from companies that use fewer toxic materials and offer take-back programs.

When powering up your handheld devices, don't forget the rechargeable batteries. Today's rechargeable batteries are quite comparable in performance to their waste-generating cousins. They can also save you money. All batteries contain toxic metals but rechargeable ones can be used over and over until you are finally ready to dispose of them. When you do, consult your local government or the Internet for battery disposal and recycling options in your area. Some consumer electronic stores also accept batteries for recycling.

Books

Books offer children access to a wonderful world of imagination. Reading is a basic skill that, once learned, offers hours of entertainment. Children can choose from a range of topics from fairy tales to detective stories. Research shows that children whose parents read to them have better verbal skills.

CHOOSING ECO-FRIENDLY CHILDREN'S BOOKS Finding books printed on recycled paper is harder than it probably should be. Only one-third of the paper consumed in the United States is recycled paper. About one-fourth of the volume of trees logged each year is converted into paper, according to the Forest Stewardship Council (FSC). Every two seconds an area of ancient forest the size of a soccer field is destroyed, according to Greenpeace International.

Using recycled paper can make a dramatic improvement to the environment. Each ton of recycled fiber that replaces a ton of virgin fiber saves 17 to 24 mature trees and up to 7.5 tons of carbon dioxide–equivalent emissions, according to the Green Press Initiative, which works with publishers and paper manufacturers to find ways to use more recycled paper.

Children's books often contain glossy pages adorned with handsome illustrations, and recycled paper does not lend itself as well to the production qualities that publishing houses seek. As demand grows for recycled products, however, a number of large picture books are now appearing on recycled paper. The Dr. Seuss environmental classic, *The Lorax* (Random House), was reissued in 2008 on recycled paper.

Novels are more likely to be printed on recycled paper than are art-filled picture books. Several publishing houses have committed to increasing their use of recycled paper over the next several years. Consumer demand can help. The Canadian publisher of the popular Harry Potter books published one million copies of *Harry Potter*

GREEN ON A SHOESTRING

Libraries are the frugal green parent's friend. Not only can you check out books for free, libraries regularly hold book sales that often have wonderful children's books available. Libraries often hold children's programs that help get kids interested in reading.

and the Order of the Phoenix on 100 percent recycled paper, saving more than 39,000 trees, according to Greenpeace International. The U.S. publisher then issued the subsequent books on recycled paper.

Until more publishers start using recycled paper, one option is to buy used books whenever possible. This has become easier than ever using the Internet. When purchasing new books, look for ones that address environmental themes *and* are printed on 100 percent recycled paper.

Animal Companions

Pets are great companions for most kids. Most are fun to play with and all can teach responsibility. But pets come with their own environmental price tag. In this section we'll learn about some eco-friendly pet practices.

DECIDING ON A PET Animal companions come in all shapes and sizes. If your children are lobbying for a pet, you have plenty of options. Before succumbing to your child's pleading, consider how the new addition will fit into your family's lifestyle. If your child wants a dog, ask whether someone will be home during the day to keep the pet company or will it spend long hours alone? Who will walk the dog? Will the dog get the exercise and companionship he needs?

When considering a cat, consider who will do the less pleasant job of cleaning the litter box. Who will be responsible for feeding the animal? Although cats do not need to be walked, they need to be treated gently so that they learn not to bite or scratch. Are your children mature enough to avoid teasing or scaring their feline friend?

Lots of other furry friends are available in the cages of pet stores: rabbits, guinea pigs, and other small mammals. For children with allergies and asthma, a dander-free fish might be the ideal pet. Consider the cost of setting up a tank, as well as who will keep the water clean.

While some breeds of dogs are less allergenic than others, there is no such thing as a 100 percent hypoallergenic dog, according to the American Association of Allergy Asthma & Immunology.

FEEDING FIDO In the spring of 2007 a major pet food manufacturer announced it was recalling about 60 million cans and bags of cat and dog food due to

THE FACTS

The average household spends $1,843 per year to take care of a large dog and $1,035 to care for a cat, according to the American Society for the Prevention of Cruelty to Animals.

contamination with melamine, a toxic chemical. Melamine causes potentially fatal kidney disease and the contamination resulted in the deaths of hundreds of animals in the United States and other countries. As the investigation into the contamination unfolded, it became clear that this toxic chemical had been intentionally added to a pet food ingredient to boost protein levels.

The experience with melamine-laced pet food suggests a bigger problem with our food supply. Globalization means that food products pass through complex supply chains before ending up in final products. In addition to concerns about melamine, pet foods have been recalled over contamination with bacteria, fungal toxins, and excess vitamin D.

Another concern many people have about pet food is the presence of animal by-products. All commercial pet foods are required to meet certain nutritional standards. However, some brands contain more real meat and fewer by-products. Some are made from organic ingredients; others are made without chemical preservatives and colors. Be sure to read labels carefully rather than going with the claims on the front of the package.

In response to pet food scares, many consumers have started taking pet food production into their own hands. Up until the early 1900s, people fed their pets table scraps and home-cooked meals rather than buying pet food. The practice is becoming popular again as pet owners question the safety of global pet food production.

A number of books and websites now offer advice on making your own pet food. Choose a reputable book written by an animal nutritionist and consult your veterinarian. Cats have vastly different nutritional needs than dogs. Cats require meat in their diets whereas dogs can tolerate a greater variety of foods.

Take care to avoid human foods that make animals sick. Chocolate contains a chemical called theobromine, which is toxic to both cats and dogs. Both cats and dogs lack the enzymes required for digesting milk. Although animals evolved to eat raw meat, today's industrially produced meats and eggs may contain harmful bacteria such as *Salmonella* and *E. coli*, so cooking is advised.

For more information on human foods to avoid, see the American Society for the Prevention of Cruelty to Animals' website People Foods to Avoid Feeding Your Pet at *www.aspca.org/site/PageServer?pagename=pets_peoplefoodtoavoid*.

FLEA AND TICK CONTROL Fleas and ticks can make pets miserable. Americans spend more than one million dollars a year protecting their pets from these pesky insects. Yet some of the chemicals found in flea collars, baths, and sprays are far from healthy for pets or their owners. Many of the chemicals are toxic to the nervous system, reproductive system, organs, or are suspected or known to cause cancer. A recent study by the Natural Resources Defense Council (NRDC) found that flea collars leave potentially harmful levels of two toxic pesticides, tetrachlorvinphos and propoxur, on pet fur for up to a week.

Children are especially vulnerable to the toxic effects of pesticides because they inhale and ingest more chemical per body weight than do adults. Plus, children often spend more time curled up with pets, hugging pets, hanging on to pets, and coming in contact with pet fur on carpets than do adults.

If you have a pet and a child, try to avoid using flea and tick collars, baths, and sprays unless absolutely necessary. Here are some tips on flea and tick prevention without pesticides:

- ✓ Comb your animal daily with a flea comb.
- ✓ Give your dog a weekly bath.
- ✓ Wash your dog's or cat's bedding (or your bedding if your animal sleeps with you) every week.
- ✓ Vacuum rugs and carpets often.
- ✓ Maintain your yard so that you reduce long grass that can harbor ticks and overgrown shrubs that provide habitat for fleas.
- ✓ Herbal oils should be used with caution. Some can cause allergic reactions in humans and toxicity in animals. Oils to avoid are cinnamon, clove, d-limonene, tea tree, citrus, lavender, geranium, linalool, bay, rue, and eucalyptus. Pennyroyal oil is often recommended for flea control but can cause seizures, coma, and death in animals. Pennyroyal is also an abortive herb and should be avoided by pregnant women. Safer oils are cedarwood, lemongrass, peppermint, rosemary and thyme, according to the NRDC. Note that herbal remedies are not effective against ticks.

If these methods fail, you may need to opt for a pesticide treatment. Some flea and tick treatments are less toxic than others. The NRDC has compiled a list of less toxic flea and tick products as well as their active ingredients and relative toxicity. The list of products can be viewed at *www.greenpaws.org*.

The NRDC recommends avoiding products that list tetrachlorvinphos or propoxur as active ingredients. Propoxur is a probable human carcinogen according to the EPA. Tetrachlorvinphos is toxic to the nervous system and classified by the EPA as likely to cause cancer in humans. Permethrin products are toxic to cats and should be avoided.

PET WASTE DISPOSAL Your waste disposal duty will hinge on whether you have a dog or a cat, and if it is a cat, whether you keep it indoors or out.

Of course, all pets from goldfish to gerbils make waste, but we'll just cover the larger mammalian pets here.

CATS

If your pet of choice is a cat, you'll need to decide whether you are going to keep your furry friend indoors at all times or let him or her out into the yard for exercise and fresh air. Keeping cats indoors has many benefits for the environment, while allowing cats out has many benefits for the cats. Benefits of keeping cats indoors:

✓ No need to remove ticks and fleas using pesticides or by combing and bathing (if indeed it is even possible to bathe a cat).

✓ Animals are less likely to be killed by automobiles, predators, or disease.

✓ You'll be protecting birds and other wildlife. Felines are agile hunters that kill millions of birds each year, according to the National Audubon Society.

Benefits to cats that are allowed some time outdoors:

✓ Your cat may be happier being outdoors where there are so many insects and small mammals to chase.

✓ Our feline friends bury their own waste so you won't have to maintain a litter box.

✓ Your animal will get more exercise and is less likely to become overweight.

If you decide on an indoor-only cat, you will want to give some thought to the type of cat litter you put in the box. Conventional cat litter is made of clay, which contains crystalline silica dust. Continuous exposure to crystalline silica dust over years could lead to silicosis, a noncancerous but potentially fatal lung disease, or lung cancer. (See earlier in this chapter for information on crystalline silica in playground sand.) Every time you scoop your cat litter you expose yourself and potentially your family to silica dust. You also expose your cat.

In addition to dust, conventional cat litters exude chemical fragrances that are aimed at making the litter box acceptable to humans, not cats. Take a whiff of a conventional cat litter and ask yourself if such a strong perfume has ever existed in nature. These perfumes come from potentially toxic chemicals. Avoid chemically treated litters because cats spend much of their time licking and grooming, and they may ingest the chemicals in litter.

Instead, try a chemical-free cat litter made of pine, wheat, corn, or recycled newspaper. Some of these come in scoopable versions. Many are just as good at controlling odor. Some cat litter can even be composted, although experts recommend not composting cat feces because *Toxoplasma gondii*, a parasite that can damage the developing brain, can survive the composting process and last up to a year. These parasites cause birth defects in babies born to mothers who were exposed to *T. gondii* during pregnancy. They can also harm sea otters and other water-dwelling creatures.

DOG DUTY

Most dogs spend part of their day outdoors in a fenced yard or have a human who takes them for long walks. These humans are usually seen carrying a plastic bag with which to scoop up the poop. What is the best way to dispose of that poop? Many dog owners simply toss the doggie business into the garbage where it ends up in a landfill. The fact that it is encased in a plastic bag prevents harmful bacteria from leaching from the landfill into water systems. However, the plastic-encased poop will take years to biodegrade. Biodegradable plastic bags made from corn-based plastics are now available to conscientious dog-owners.

Another option for disposing of doggie poop is to flush it down the toilet. It is clean and efficient and accepted by many municipal water treatment systems. The water treatment plants strip the fecal matter of harmful bacteria. Check with your municipality to see if flushing is allowed. (Do not flush cat poop because *Toxoplasma gondii* can survive the water treatment plant and go on to contaminate surface waters.)

Take Action

▸ Cut down on your use of natural resources by buying fewer toys and instead give your young children safe household items like pots and spoons to play with.

▸ Look for simple toys that allow children to use their imagination rather than character-based toys that tie into movies and TV shows.

▸ Choose natural materials such as whole wood (not plywood) and cloth.

▸ Check for toy recalls at *www.recalls.gov* before purchasing new or used toys.

▸ Toys painted bright red, yellow, or orange may contain lead paint. Call the manufacturer to see if the product has been tested.

▸ Select face paint and cosmetics that are labeled as safe for children, or make your own face paint.

▸ Choose nontoxic art supplies that are labeled as safe for use by children. Look for products bearing the statement "Conforms to ASTM D-4236," a safety standard for art materials.

▸ Create a safe lawn and yard for your child to play in by using natural lawn care methods instead of synthetic chemical pesticides and fertilizers.

▸ Look for eco-friendly backyard play equipment made from recycled plastic or FSC-certified wood, or forgo installing backyard equipment and play instead at public parks.

▸ Skip the recycled rubber mulch in favor of wood chips or mulch.

▸ Convert part of your lawn to a wildflower or vegetable garden to increase the biodiversity of your area and cut down on energy-intensive lawn care. Try a reel mower to replace your gas- or electric-powered mower.

▸ Provide alternatives to TV watching, such as games and crafts, and encourage children to develop the ability to play creatively on their own.

▸ To avoid being pestered to buy things for your children, limit your young child's exposure to advertising and teach older children to be media-savvy consumers.

▸ Look for energy-efficient computers and television screens.

▸ When possible, choose books printed on recycled paper and books that encourage respect for nature and the environment.

▸ Choose pet food that is healthy and pet litter that is eco-friendly. Choose safer pesticides to tackle ticks and fleas.

THE SCIENCE BEHIND IT

Recycled Rubber Playground Mulch

In playgrounds across America, the sweet smell of mulch is slowly being replaced by another smell: recycled tires. A number of municipalities and schools are swapping natural materials like wood mulch for a crumbly black mix made from pulverized tire rubber. City governments point to the savings: Mulch and wood chips degrade and sand gets blown away or trekked home on the bottom of shoes, but tire rubber is forever.

Tire rubber does take quite a long time to break down, which is why the nation has nearly 200 million discarded tires sitting in landfills or illegal dumping sites. These tire piles have occasionally caught fire, and if they do, they can send toxic polycyclic aromatic hydrocarbons (PAHs), styrene, phenols, butadiene, and benzene into the air along with lead and arsenic from belted tires. Tire fires are extremely hard to extinguish: One fire in Virginia in 1983 burned for nine months.

Cities and states with tire dumps would naturally like to get rid of these black rubberized mounds. Some people view turning discarded tires into children's playground mulch as an ideal example of recycling unwanted garbage into needed products. But any parent who has spent any time standing on the cushiony peanut-shaped tire curds can point to a few drawbacks. One is the smell that emanates from recycled tire mulch. Another is that any child under the age of two sitting in the mulch is highly likely to put a piece of it in his mouth.

The smell of recycled tire mulch comes from the mix of 49 chemicals that are released into the air from automobile tires. Tires are made of synthetic rubber mixed with plasticizers, antioxidants, and metals like cadmium, arsenic, nickel and lead. To convert the rubber into mulch, manufacturers wash the tires and grind them into tiny pellets, using magnets to remove metals. They mix the pellets with polyurethane or another binding agent to create a smooth material that can be extruded into peanut-shaped mulch pieces. They can coat the black rubber mulch to make it bright blue, red, or another kid-friendly color.

Surprisingly few studies have evaluated the risk of rubber tire mulch to children. One study conducted by the California Office of Environmental Health Hazard Assessment (OEHHA) found that a child who plays on a playground surface made from recycled tires from age 1 to age 12 had an only slightly elevated cancer risk due to the presence of the carcinogenic chemical known as chrysene.[6] The OEHHA also found that if a small child swallows a piece of the mulch, the cancer risk would be insignificant.

The study is reassuring, but it looked at only a narrow range of exposure scenarios. For example, what happens if a child eats more than one piece of mulch? More research needs to be done to explore the health risks of tire rubber, including the potential for the latex to sensitize children to latex allergies.

Human health is not the only consideration. Environmentalists are concerned about the toxic chemicals in rainwater runoff from the playgrounds. The toxic chemicals found in tire rubber are hazardous not only to people but to wildlife.

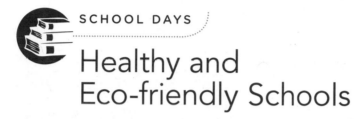

SCHOOL DAYS

Healthy and Eco-friendly Schools

TODAY'S KIDS SEEM TO GROW UP FASTER THAN THEY USED TO. TWO generations ago parents sent their children off to school at age five. Today school often begins at age three or four in the form of preschool or prekindergarten, and by age five the once momentous transition to kindergarten is just a blip in the minds of our worldly wunderkinds.

Of course, there are some big differences between preschool and elementary school. There are new buildings to navigate, big bathrooms that the youngest ones share with older kids, and new teachers to meet. While children are learning new skills, we parents and caregivers are learning how to let go of our little ones and let them develop and grow.

As our children learn the three R's of the academic world, however, we want them to continue to learn and practice the three R's of environmentally conscious living, that is, reduce, reuse, and recycle. Many schools now include environmentalism in their lesson plans, especially in the early grades when children study the natural sciences. Our young students receive many lessons on the environment, especially in the spring around Earth Day.

But school policies do not always match the classroom lessons on how to protect and preserve Earth. Many schools do not recycle paper, juice boxes, or water bottles. School lunchrooms often use disposable tableware made of polystyrene and other plastics. Many lunchrooms purchase premade foods in bulk from faraway suppliers and serve predominantly foods high in fat, sugar, and salt. Many school facilities are actually making children and staff sick due to a variety of harmful chemical exposures.

In this chapter we'll take a look at how you can help your child's school adopt more environmentally conscious and health-protective practices. We'll start with child care facilities and move into public schools.

Early Beginnings

Finding the best child care for infants and young children is the top priority for most families. Read on for suggestions on how to find a facility that cares for your child and the planet.

STARTING OUT RIGHT Numerous child care opportunities abound for babies and young children. You may choose a child care center run by a private individual or your employer, a not-for-profit day care run by a foundation or church, or an in-home program run by a neighborhood mom. When visiting child care facilities, health and safety should always be at the top of your list. Is the facility childproofed? Is the staff-to-child ratio adequate? Is the area clean and well maintained? Are practices in place to protect children from preventable exposure to harmful chemicals? Are the child care workers caring and nurturing, and do they have training in early child development?

Once you've found a child care facility that meets the most important needs for the care and safety of your child, you can sort facilities by their commitment to the environment. Many child care facilities have adopted an environment-friendly policy. However, many such facilities must weigh care for the environment against convenience and cost. Disposable items—such as diapers, plates, cups, napkins, and even toys—are viewed by most people as more hygienic and more convenient than reusable items. With the proper training of child care staff and supportive systems in place, however, reusable items can be just as safe as disposable ones.

ECO-TIP: **ECO-FRIENDLY CHILD CARE FACILITY CHECKLIST**

Does your child's child care facility:

✓ **allow cloth diapers?**

✓ **allow glass baby bottles?**

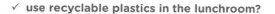

✓ use recyclable plastics in the lunchroom?

✓ serve nutritious snacks and lunches?

✗ avoid individually packaged, nutrient-poor snacks that generate a lot of garbage?

✓ allow children ample time for outdoor play?

✓ use nontoxic methods for killing pests and weeds in areas where children play?

✓ use eco-friendly cleaning products?

✗ avoid heating food in plastic containers?

✓ follow a preventive maintenance plan to address moisture control and promote healthy indoor air?

✓ test for radon every two to three years?

✓ test for lead paint (if built before 1978)?

✓ use eco-friendly art supplies?

✓ train their staff on environmental health practices and considerations?

The Children's Environmental Health Network (CEHN) organizes one of the only national programs dedicated to effective training for child care professionals in environmental health protection. For more information visit *www.cehn.org/cehn/education/childcare.htm*.

Another helpful program is the Eco-Healthy Child Care program, organized by the Oregon Environmental Council (OEC). See *www.oeconline.org/our-work/kidshealth/ehcc*.

K-12

Although you can choose a child care facility on health and safety principles,

the choice of kindergarten and beyond is usually determined by where you live. Many parents decide on a neighborhood or town based largely on the school system's academic reputation, not on its commitment to health and the environment. Help your school realize its educational potential by getting involved in bringing health protective and eco-friendly policies into action.

GET INVOLVED While academic quality is clearly the most important aspect of a school, you don't have to be content with a school that does not make the health and safety of your children a top priority. Join the parent-teacher organization. Find like-minded parents and start a green team, a recycling committee, or an initiative to reduce pesticide use in the school. Work with the principal and school board to develop alternatives to the current practices.

Today's children are being asked not only to get stellar grades, but also to show commitment to the community through participation in food drives, collecting school supplies for children with few resources, and activities in scouting and churches. Your child may want to start a program to promote recycling at the school or plant an organic community garden. Ask your child what issues he or she would like to work on, and help your child organize his or her friends and teachers to help. See Chapter 5 for more suggestions on how to get children involved in helping the environment and promoting healthy practices in their schools.

STOCKING UP ON SAFER SCHOOL SUPPLIES One of the facts of life in today's cash-strapped schools is that parents are being asked to send in a variety of school supplies at the beginning of the school year. Whether shopping for notebooks or pencil cases, eco-friendly school supplies are becoming easier than ever to find.

PAPER Look for products bearing totally chlorine-free (TCF) and processed chlorine-free (PCF) certification (See Green Dictionary). Although chlorine bleaching is much more environmentally benign than it used to be, chlorine-free processes are even better at keeping toxic waste out of rivers and streams.

In addition to looking for chlorine-free paper, choose paper with the highest percentage of postconsumer waste (PCW), which means paper that has passed through the hands of people like you who toss paper into recycling bins. Preconsumer recycled content consists of leftovers from the paper manufacturing process. While these leftovers

TOTALLY CHLORINE-FREE (TCF) AND PROCESSED CHLORINE-FREE (PCF)

PCF-certified paper contains at least 30 percent recycled content. The TCF label is given to virgin fiber paper products that have been certified by the Chlorine Free Products Association (CFPA) as not having been bleached with chlorine-containing compounds.

should be used, the purchase of PCW paper will signal to manufacturers the demand for paper that has been used by a consumer and tossed. America recycles about 40 percent of the newsprint, magazines, and office paper it uses, but this percentage could and should be much higher.

PENS Recycled plastic pens are available from green online retailers.

PENCILS A handful of pencilmakers now make pencils from Forest Stewardship Council (FSC)-certified wood or from postconsumer waste.

CRAYONS These childhood standbys are made from petroleum, a nonrenewable resource. Soy-based crayons are biodegradable and made from a renewable resource.

BINDERS AND NOTEBOOKS You can find one- and three-ring binders containing 30 to 40 percent postconsumer waste.

BACKPACKS AND BOOK BAGS Several manufacturers now make backpacks from recycled materials. One brand makes them from recycled plastic bottles. Others may be made of natural fabrics such as organic cotton or hemp. Avoid backpacks made with polyvinyl chloride (PVC), since these are made using toxic chemicals including hormone-disrupting phthalates. They also offgas irritating fumes.

WHERE TO BUY Check online retailers that specialize in green or recycled office supplies. Some large office supply stores are now stocking green pens, pencils, and other supplies in addition to 100 percent recycled paper.

SEEING THE FOREST, NOT THE TREES Trees are a renewable resource, but forests are not. Trees can be replanted, but forests are complex ecosystems that contain mixtures of tree species of differing ages and a variety of ground-covering plants. They are also home to numerous animals with complex predator-prey relationships.

Clear-cutting of forests deprives animals of their homes and disrupts the natural relationships between species. For example, some animals may survive clear-cutting and relocate to new habitats, while other species will be unable to successfully find new territory and will die off, altering the web of dependencies in the ecosystem.

When a natural forest is clear-cut, the trees that sprout up in the cleared space are often fewer in variety than in the original forest. They take decades to grow to maturity before they can provide the biodiversity that the land once afforded.

Tree farms are not a replacement for forests. They are usually managed with chemical treatments of fertilizers, pesticides, and herbicides. What is more, they are usually monocultures, containing a single species of tree, and they may lack the undergrowth that provides habitat for insects, birds, amphibians, and small mammals.

Americans recycle about 40 percent of all paper, but due to the availability of photocopiers and computer printers, the amount of paper we use has risen along with the recycling rate. Reducing our use of paper can help prevent clear-cutting of forests.

Do your part to reduce the demand for paper by reusing fliers sent home from school and encouraging your kids to draw and color on the back of your used computer paper. Encourage your school to transition its paper fliers to paperless e-mails. This could take a couple years, since parents who are accustomed to checking their child's backpack will have to become accustomed to checking their e-mail instead. Eventually most parents appreciate the ease and speed of online communication.

School Lunches

Parents rely on school cafeterias to provide nutritious snacks and lunches. However, cafeterias are under pressure to serve a lot of children fast, so they tend to fall back on kid-friendly favorites like pizza or nachos served in a disposable polystyrene dish. Read on for ways to encourage healthy eating and help change school lunchroom habits into ones that protect the planet and don't generate a lot of garbage.

THE DISPOSABLE LUNCHROOM Cafeterias need to get kids fed—and fast. In today's economy it is cheaper for a school to buy disposable plates, spoons, and napkins than it is to pay workers to scrape plates and run dishwashers. It is also potentially safer, because disposable tableware is sanitary and nonbreakable.

While plastics have their advantages, most are made from nonrenewable petroleum sources that are tapped in foreign countries. The manufacture of plastic can result in the generation of hazardous wastes that can contaminate the earth if not disposed of properly. Plastics never biodegrade but rather disintegrate into tiny pieces in a process that takes hundreds of years in landfills. Many plastics never make it to landfills and instead end up choking seabirds and sea mammals in far-off oceans.

Despite all the problems with plastic, there are no easy solutions. Schools have to weigh the negative effects of plastic against the consumption of water that dishwashers use, plus the added cost (often passed on to parents in taxes) to hire additional lunch staff. With the help of other parents, however, you may be able to convince your school's lunchroom staff to switch to more environmentally friendly practices, such as using plant-based, compostable plastics.

Greening the lunchroom can become an excellent learning experience for your school-age child. Your child may want to assemble a "green committee" with his or her classmates to raise awareness of the issue. The committee could develop a petition to circulate among parents asking them to support the transition of the lunchroom into a healthier and more eco-friendly environment. You can help by assisting your child in calculating the costs of switching to recycled paper napkins, for example. If the lunchroom manager can be convinced that eco-sound practices are viable, the manager might just go for it.

ECO-TIP: WHAT SCHOOLS CAN DO

✓ **Switch to reusable plates and cutlery if at all feasible.**

✓ **Use recycled paper products.**

✓ **Use plant-based biodegradable plastics.**

✓ **Purchase recyclable plastics (labeled #1 and #2) instead of polystyrene (#6), which is not widely recycled.**

✓ **Ensure that the lunchroom recycles as many items as possible. Water bottles (#1) and juice boxes can be recycled in many municipalities.**

CAFETERIA FOOD FIGHTS Over the last few decades, schools began offering sodas, cookies, and chips in vending machines, even in elementary schools. Fast-food restaurants began appearing in school lunchrooms, replacing the much bemoaned "cafeteria food" that students usually detest.

More recently, in response to parent complaints and concern over the rising rate of obesity among children, junk food has made a slow but steady retreat from schools. Soda companies have voluntarily agreed to restrict their offerings to 100 percent juice drinks and water in elementary and middle schools. And many school districts and state governments have committed to serving healthier foods.

That said, a glance at the average school lunch menu in the United States today finds that it is usually a repetitive offering of nachos, pizza, and chicken nuggets. These foods are high in fats and carbohydrates, but they can be made in healthier versions by incorporating whole wheat buns and crusts, low-fat cheeses, and healthy meats. If you see these kid-friendly favorites on your child's lunch menu, ask your lunchroom for details on the ingredients and nutritional content of the food.

Good nutrition is essential for academic success. Healthy foods promote increased attention and decreased fatigue. Proper nutrition is linked positively to higher grades and better performance on standardized tests. Well-nourished children are less likely to suffer from anxiety, depression, and hyperactivity.

Unfortunately defining good nutrition has become muddled in the minds of many parents, thanks in part to the food industry, which is always trying to improve the marketability of its products through labeling with health claims. Ironically, the healthiest foods don't come in packages. Fresh or frozen berries are both sweet and packed with vitamins; crunchy vegetables such as snap peas, carrots, and celery are kid palate-pleasers. Apples are packed with filling carbohydrates yet don't make kids sleepy the way a high-carbohydrate bagel or pretzel might.

Changing your school's lunchroom habits may seem like an insurmountable task. The administration or lunchroom manager may tell you that kids won't eat the healthier alternatives. It is true that many kids today have forgotten what simple fresh food tastes like. Their palates expect very salty and very sweet foods. Yet several case studies conducted by the Center for Food and Justice at Occidental College and the Community Food Security Coalition found that children not only accepted healthier options, in many cases they preferred dishes such as whole wheat veggie and chicken wraps with sides of seasonal fruits to less healthy fare.[1]

KITCHEN TABLE TALK

Lunchroom Envy

Chances are your brown-bagging child will at some point develop a severe case of lunchroom envy, somewhere around the middle of first grade. She'll gaze into her lunch box filled with whole wheat sandwich bread and chopped apples and carrots, then gaze wistfully at her classmates who are wolfing down chicken nuggets or nachos. She'll ask herself, "Why was I born into a family of healthy eaters in a world of tasty but unhealthy treats?"

While we want to feed our children healthy foods, we have to remember the old adage "anything in moderation." When parents strictly forbid items, they become objects of intense desire. Forbidding your child from eating school lunches usually has the unintended consequence of making those lunches seem even more appealing.

If your child craves cafeteria food, talk with her about the importance of getting a balanced diet containing lots of fruits and vegetables and limiting salt and fat. Feed her tidbits of information about the foods, such as that a container of chocolate milk has 28 grams of sugar, about as much as a candy bar. Depending on what you feel comfortable with, you might let your child eat cafeteria food once a week, or once a month.

Allowing your child to eat unhealthy meals now and again is fine for the active child who eats healthily most of the time and gets regular exercise. Unfortunately in America nearly a third of all children are overweight and must struggle daily to choose the healthy apple sitting right next to the tempting French fries. Healthy lunch advocates say the reason they are working so hard to overturn the pizza-nacho-nugget mentality is that all children should be able to eat healthily at school without being tempted by caloric, nutrient-poor choices.

Beth Feehan is one mom who is working to improve school lunches by bringing farms together with schools to provide fresh produce in New Jersey through that state's Farm to School Network. She is an advocate of school gardens where children can learn lessons in natural science while producing food that they can eat in the lunchroom. When children plant and tend their own garden, says Feehan, they build a sense of ownership and community. "I have come to believe that a school garden is the way to change students' taste buds and help them become open to trying things that grow in the ground," says Feehan.

Although the pace of change has been slow, Feehan's persistence is paying off as more schools become interested in finding ways to include local agricultural products in their lunch offerings. "I've come to understand that systemic change in this arena takes time," says Feehan, "but I've also learned not to go away."

Another reason cafeterias resist changing menus is the concern that healthy alternatives will drive up the price of lunch. Pizzas and nuggets are easy to freeze and store, whereas fresh fruits and vegetables go bad if not consumed within a few days. Small lunch staffs are not equipped to peel carrots or shuck corn. Cost barriers can be overcome but will depend on the availability of local produce, the growing season, the willingness of the school or district to make changes, and many other factors. Lots of schools have made the change to healthier foods. For more information on what you can do to make your school's lunches healthier, see www.betterschoolfood.org.

TIPS FOR HEALTHY LUNCHROOM EATING:

✓ Visit your child's lunchroom during the lunch hour. Does the cafeteria provide fresh fruits and vegetables? If so, are the kids eating them?

✓ Does the school primarily serve nachos, pizza, and deep fried foods? If so, are these modified to lower the fat and sodium content? Request that the school provide nutrition facts.

✓ Study the school lunch menu with your child. Point out the low-fat and healthier options like nonfat milk instead of chocolate milk and whole wheat hamburger buns instead of white-bread buns.

✓ If you are concerned about the nutritional quality of the food at your child's school, bring the issue up at a parent-teacher association (PTA) meeting or directly to the school principal. Or form a small committee of parents to identify problems and propose solutions. Enlisting like-minded parents will help your school's administrator understand that this is a concern of many parents today.

THE FACTS

Roughly 30 million children eat a cafeteria-prepared lunch at school every day of the week throughout the entire school year, according to the National Farm to School Network, an organization that advocates for bringing local produce to school cafeterias.

ECO-TIP: HEALTHIER SCHOOL PARTIES

Celebrating birthdays is a sacred ritual in many schools. This means that on average your child will have two to three birthday parties a month where sugary cupcakes, cookies, or another treat will be served. If this sugar overload is of concern, suggest to the teacher a monthly celebration that honors all the kids born that month. On that day, the birthday parents could send in one sugary treat, a kid-friendly fruit, and a crunchy snack such as crackers. This will cut down on the number of cupcakes the kids get and the number of days that the teacher has to handle sugar-hyped kids.

BROWN-BAGGING IT One of the best ways you can minimize your child's ecological impact and provide the nutrition your child needs is by using the good old lunch pail method. Bringing lunch from home cuts the amount of garbage flowing to landfills because you can pack food in reusable containers. You can send in recycled-paper napkins, or cloth ones if you prefer. You can send stainless steel spoons (although metal forks and knives may be prohibited due to safety reasons).

WHEN PACKING, CONSIDER THE FOLLOWING:

✓ Be on the lookout for lead in lunch boxes. Vinyl (PVC) lunch boxes have been found to be contaminated with lead dust. Many lunch boxes now advertise that they are lead-free.

✓ Purchase stainless steel food containers that can safely store hot foods so that you can send pasta, macaroni and cheese, soups and other foods that taste best when warm.

✓ Pack sandwiches in reusable sandwich boxes made of safer plastics (labeled #1, #2, or #5), or use freezer-quality plastic sandwich bags and have your child bring them home so that you can wash and reuse them. (Reuse them for nonfood uses if you are concerned about your ability to get them clean.)

✓ If you must send a disposable lunch (for a field trip, for example), wrap sandwiches in wax paper instead of plastic bags.

✓ Purchase a reusable beverage bottle made of stainless steel or a plastic that is labeled "bisphenol-A-free."

✓ See Chapter 2 for suggestions for healthy fruit and vegetable snacks.

LOCALS ONLY Children in the United States are notorious for not liking vegetables. This is no surprise when we consider that in most restaurants and homes, vegetables are an afterthought, pulled out of a freezer bag or a can and microwaved far too long before being spooned out onto the margins of the plate.

Fresh vegetables, however, are a delight to eat. A fresh raw baby carrot is bursting with sweet flavor. A deep red steamed beet is nature's candy and tastes nothing like the sour vinegar-seeped beet slices served with iceberg lettuce at the burger joint. Fresh veggies properly prepared are delightful to children—especially those who haven't been misled by oft-repeated clichés about how children hate vegetables.

Few institutions have committed as many sins against the vegetable as the school lunchroom. School lunchrooms are well known for destroying the flavor of any cuisine they get their hands on—they can even ruin pizza. But they are especially ruthless to vegetables: Mushy green beans that little resemble the springy sweet mouthfuls they were when first picked. Overcooked carrots. Oversalted corn. The list is endless.

One solution to this veggie abuse is to bring in local farmers. If you live in an area with local growers, chances are these family farmers are having trouble surviving in an economy dominated by global food production and transport. One way to help them out while improving school nutrition and pleasing childish palates is for schools to buy produce from local farms.

Farm-to-school programs help both farmers and children. Students can learn how food is grown, and how delicious fresh fruits and vegetables can taste. Children can take field trips to the farm to see firsthand how a working farm operates. The farm personnel can help with planting school gardens and holding cooking demonstrations. Schools can use the farm as an outdoor laboratory where kids can learn about soil, plant life, insects, and other topics.

Children can begin to understand why it is important to preserve farmland so that it survives as a lasting resource of locally grown produce for years to come. They can learn how their food choices affect not only their health but also the health of their environment.

Convincing your school to go local can take a major effort on the part of parents and community leaders. School districts are like massive ocean liners that can turn only very slowly, but turning can be accomplished with enough will from the community and the support of local leaders. Some state governments and foundations provide support for programs that connect farmers and schools. For more information, check out the website of the National Farm to School Network, *www.farmtoschool.org*.

School Gardens

A school garden is a wonderful way to combine the joy of watching seeds germinate and grow into plants with lessons in ecology and sustainability. Gardening can improve the science curriculum, teach lessons in nutrition, help children understand the importance of taking care of Earth, and impart lasting skills that could blossom into a lifetime hobby.

GROWING UP GREEN Growing a garden can be part of a science curriculum for young children learning about the biology of living things. Children can study plants, earthworms, beetles, and other crawly critters in a hands-on environment rather than a sterile classroom. A study in a Texas school found that children who combined science education with hands-on experience in the garden scored significantly better on a science achievement test than the children who did the classroom education only.[2] Some states, such as California, provide resources on how to link garden work with the state's educational curriculum.

School gardens can also provide valuable lessons in healthy eating. Many urban and suburban children have never tasted just-picked vegetables. They've sat through lesson after lesson on how they should be eating fruits and vegetables daily but they rarely encounter much more than the deep fried potato. When children plant and harvest their own food, they will be much more interested in tasting it.

In addition to providing garden-fresh foods, a school garden can help children gain a sense of responsibility about taking care of the planet. Children can discover that plants need a certain mix of nutrients, including nitrogen, potassium, and phosphate. Plants live in dependent relationships with other plants, with soil bacteria, and with other inhabitants of the soil. Maintaining biodiversity will help all species survive.

Finally, a school garden can be the start of a lasting hobby that will get your child to spend more time outdoors appreciating nature and learning to be a steward of nature. A school garden can inspire students to become more adventurous in their eating, and with parental help they may even be able to plant small vegetable plots in their backyards. If your child is inspired, he may set up a small business selling his tomatoes to neighbors.

THE FACTS

Nearly 9,000 U.S. schools participate in farm-to-school programs in 42 states, according to the National Farm to School Network.

GREAT IDEAS FOR SCHOOL GARDENS:

✓ Grow food for the school cafeteria. Work with the lunchroom staff to decide what to plant and when to harvest.

✓ Form a summer club to maintain the garden when school is not in session.

✓ If vegetables are too much of a commitment, plant a butterfly garden consisting of flowers that attract pollinating insects.

✓ Grow a rain garden consisting of plants that serve as a place for water to accumulate and sink into the soil, replenishing groundwater supplies.

Recess—Where Has It Gone?

Recess refreshes kids by giving them a much needed break during the school day. But many schools are cutting recess to use that time to cram more lessons into the day. Read on to find out what you can do to restore physical activity to your child's day.

RECESS REDUCTION Schools are under pressure to get academic results, and with good reason. About 15 percent of American high school students drop out before getting their diplomas, according to the U.S. Census Bureau. To squeeze extra hours of instruction into the day, schools are cutting extras such as art, music, and yes, recess. In a recent study published in January 2009 in the journal *Pediatrics*, nearly one-third of the 11,000 children studied had less than 15 minutes of recess or no recess each day.[3]

Recess reduction is now starting as early as kindergarten. Half-day kindergarten classes often do not have recess at all, because teachers are pouring more academics into the two or three hours per day than before. Schools are relying on parents to provide physical activities and trips to the playground before or after school.

Academic aspirations, however, are not the only reason for the retrenchment of recess. Changing cultural habits are another. These days many kids are driven to school and show up without appropriate cold-weather clothes. Teachers cannot send children out in freezing weather without hats and coats for health reasons. Ice on playground equipment is also a hazard. In warmer climates, air pollution can keep kids indoors.

Some teachers use recess as a reward for good behavior. Teachers may punish students for poor classroom conduct by taking away their recess for the day. Ironically it is often the kids who act out that benefit most from a bout of fresh air and exercise.

Removal of recess time could have the counterproductive effect of making it even harder for students to learn. Recess gives kids a chance to work off pent-up energy, oxygenate their brains, and return to class ready to pay attention. Several studies have found a positive relationship between time spent at recess and classroom behavior. The *Pediatrics* study mentioned above found that children who had at least 15 minutes of recess daily behaved better in class than children with no recess. Other studies have found that exercise has a beneficial effect on the school performance of children with dyslexia.[4]

The loss of recess may also be contributing to obesity rates among children. In some schools, a snack period has replaced the 15-minute mid-morning recess. Rather than offering healthy snacks, parents or teachers may provide cookies, chips, or another calorie-rich, nutrient-poor food. These foods may also be available in vending machines on school grounds. The brief head-clearing recess, therefore, has been replaced by a sugary snack that fuels hyperactivity in some children and makes others feel like taking a nap.

If recess is becoming rare at your child's school, try speaking to other parents, the teacher, and the principal about your concern. It may be that the educators and parents are feeling the same way you do. Also talk to the children. If enough of them voice their need for recess to their teachers, their pleas could result in changes. In the meantime, try building exercise into your child's day. Walking or riding a bike to school invigorates the brain far more than sitting in a diesel-powered bus. Take your child to the playground after school.

Getting There

Today's kids use a variety of modes of transportation to get to school. Your child may walk, ride a bike, take the school bus, ride public transportation, or ride along with you in the car on your way to work. We'll look at how to choose a transportation method that is good for the planet and your child's health.

HOOFING IT Walking to school is now viewed as something that was done in the good old days, like sending a message by telegraph. It is something we did back when streets were safe and life was unhurried. Today's parents tend to think of walking as a pleasant diversion that fits nowhere into a reality where both parents are rushing to the office, and homes are sited far from schools.

There are many reasons why kids don't walk to school. In new housing developments, schools are typically built at the edge of communities along major roads instead of embedded in neighborhoods. More kids grow up in households where both parents work outside the home, or in single-parent households where Mom or Dad must work long hours to keep the family afloat. Many kids live a mile or more from school and would have to cross major boulevards to reach the school. For many families, walking to school *is* completely out of the question.

Yet a growing number of families are rediscovering this lost pleasure. Parents are realizing that their young children not only *can* walk, they love to walk. Children love to smell fresh air, pick dandelions off lawns, and talk to friends or siblings along the way. Walking can be a special time to spend with Mom or Dad, when time slows and children can revel in not having to feel rushed.

Of course, walking is also great exercise. With so many children at risk of becoming overweight or obese, walking is a good way to keep in shape or to work off that after-dinner dessert. For parents who have trouble finding time to squeeze a workout into their busy day, walking may be just what the doctor ordered.

Walking for exercise takes some practice if you are not used to it. Start slow. If the school is far away, you may want to start building up your child's endurance by walking around the neighborhood. With a little practice, most first graders can easily walk a mile to school in around 20 minutes.

WALKING SCHOOL BUS Not every parent can take the time to walk their child to school because there are younger siblings to care for or for many other reasons. If you cannot walk yourself, you might look into setting up a "walking school bus" with neighbors. In a walking school bus, parents who are walking with their kids pick up kids from neighborhood houses along the way. Instead of each parent walking every day, parents can take turns chaperoning kids to school.

If you are interested in starting a walking school bus, talk to your friends and neighbors. Offer to chaperone the walk. When other parents see how easy it is, they may be tempted to join you.

GREEN ON A SHOESTRING

Cut your carbon footprint and your car's gas bill by walking to school regularly.

GREEN DICTIONARY

**WALKING
SCHOOL BUS**

A group of children that walks to school with one or more adults, who "pick up" children from the houses along the way.

SAFETY IN NUMBERS Safety is a prime concern, especially if you will be supervising several children. Points to consider when organizing a walking school bus:

✓ Are there sidewalks?

✓ Do intersections have the appropriate pedestrian traffic signs?

✓ Are drivers conscientious of the need to slow down for pedestrians?

✓ Do the children have enough supervision? To ensure safety on the walk, the Centers for Disease Control and Prevention (CDC) recommend one adult for every six children. For children under six, one adult per three children is advised.

✓ Is criminal activity a concern?

If your neighborhood isn't safe for walking, work with other parents in your community to make it safe. Form a pedestrian-advocacy organization. Such organizations may be able to help your town obtain state or local government funds to improve safe-walking conditions. Contact school officials and enlist their support. The school may be able to provide a crossing guard for dangerous intersections. Your local police department may be able to post signs or send the occasional police officer to remind drivers to be on the lookout for pedestrians.

FOR MORE INFORMATION ON ORGANIZING A WALKING SCHOOL BUS:

• Walking School Bus, *www.walkingschoolbus.org:* Learn how to organize a walking school bus and how to escort your children to school safely.

• International Walk to School Day, *www.walktoschool.org:* The international walk to school day is a great time to raise awareness about walking to school. It is usually held in October.

• Safe Routes to School, *www.saferoutesinfo.org:* This federally sponsored organization provides resources to encourage and enable more children to walk or bike to school safely.

BUSING BLUES School buses are a wonderful convenience. However, most buses in today's fleet run on diesel fuel, which generates exhaust that contains cancer-causing chemicals and small particles that can damage lungs. According to the Natural Resources Defense Council (NRDC), tailpipe emissions can find their way into buses, exposing children to toxic fumes. In a study published in January 2001, the NRDC found that for every million children who ride in school buses for an hour or two every day, 23 to 46 of them eventually may develop lung cancer related to exposure to diesel fumes.[5] The small particles in diesel

THE FACTS

Of the roughly 450,000 public school buses in the U.S., 390,000 are powered by diesel fuel, according to the EPA.

exhaust can increase the risk of lung diseases like bronchitis and may trigger or worsen asthma attacks.

The U.S. Environmental Protection Agency (EPA) is promoting the replacement of older, more polluting diesel buses with ones that generate fewer emissions. Over the last decade the agency has increased the pollution standards to force manufacturers to produce cleaner buses. The agency has also produced a number of recommendations to help reduce the exposure of children to bus fumes. These include recommending that buses do not idle in front of schools and encouraging bus retrofitting or replacement of older, polluting buses.

If your child rides the bus, ask your school district what efforts they have made to protect children from diesel fumes. Does the school have a "no idling" policy for buses waiting outside the school? Could the buses be retrofitted with pollution control mechanisms? When it is time to replace buses, help steer your district toward the least polluting options. Encourage practices that lower diesel fumes inside buses. For example, opening windows when weather permits drastically reduces the accumulation of fumes inside the bus. Children who have the longest rides will be exposed to fumes for the longest period of time, so those children should sit in the front where fumes are least.

School buses that run on propane gas or compressed natural gas (CNG) are available in some areas. Consider gathering parents into a committee to lobby for the school district to adopt these alternative fuel buses when they replace their fleet.

RUSH HOUR For many parents, driving their kids to school is necessary. Their school may not provide a bus due to cost-cutting measures. Parents may need to leave for work before the bus picks up in the morning. Many children attend before-school programs as well as after-school programs that don't include busing, and driving becomes inevitable.

Yet driving can be a headache as well. With so many parents doing it, drivers become ensnared in traffic jams and sit in long lines of cars waiting to drop off their kids at the front door of the school.

If your school's traffic pattern is a nightmare, chances are other parents are feeling the same way. Try to coordinate a carpooling effort among your neighbors. You'll reduce your greenhouse gas emissions and keep traffic down at the same time. Another option that might work for you is to park a few blocks from the school, well outside the traffic zone, and walk with your child to the school. Try to find a place to park that cuts down on the amount of driving you'll have to do to get to your commuting route. Although it may take a little bit of extra time, you and your child may appreciate the exercise.

Back-to-school Clothes

Shopping for back-to-school clothes is an annual ritual for many families.

By purchasing only the items we need and choosing natural fibers and

organically grown cotton, we can cut down on the impact on our planet.

FASHION FOUL-UPS Among the pre-18 set, nothing says more about you than what you wear. Let's face it, kids can be unmerciful to peers who don't keep up appearances. No parent wants to be responsible for ruining a child's positive self-image. But there has to be a middle ground between making sure our kids are suitably clothed in today's society and not running the family fortune into the ground—nor ruining the planet in the process.

Start by talking with your child from a young age about the difference between needs and wants. We want new toys, but we have plenty of them already. We want ice cream, but we need to eat our nutritious dinner first. We don't always get everything we want. Often we later realize that we didn't really want what we thought we did.

As your child matures you can help her or him understand where fabrics such as cotton and rayon originate, and who makes them into clothing. Children (and many adults) never question the path that a consumer good travels from its origins in the earth or in a field, through a factory and across an ocean, and finally into the shop where we purchase it. Help your child understand that consumer goods have a life cycle that involves natural resources. We don't want to squander natural resources.

Finally, your child will be curious about the world, and this is an opportune time to bring up the fact that many of our world's inhabitants are unable to afford as many material possessions as we have. Many are unable to purchase essential items like shoes or medicines. Many more don't even have decent housing or clean water to drink. Your child may be surprised to know that nearly one-fifth of the world's population doesn't have access to any type of toilet or outhouse—they simply "go" out in a field, according to the World Health Organization.

These are depressing statistics, but they may foster in your child the desire to improve the world and make sure that resources reach the people who need them, and that fewer resources go to waste among people who already have all the shirts, pants, and designer handbags they need.

ON THE TRAIL OF DONATED CLOTHES When you pack up your child's used clothes to donate them, they may not be headed to the places you think they are. Numerous charities collect used clothing. What they do with it afterward varies quite a bit.

A few charities pass clothing directly to needy individuals. Homeless shelters, for example, might collect coats that can be handed out to shelter residents immediately. Many charities, however, sell the clothes and use the money to fund their work. These charities may maintain their own thrift stores or sell the clothes to other stores, including for-profit thrift stores or companies that ship clothes overseas.

Clothes shipped overseas are often sold rather than donated to needy individuals. Some countries have banned the importation of used clothing because it undercuts sales of locally produced items. Clothing resellers defend the practice on the grounds that in many parts of the world there are few options to purchase low-cost clothing.

Clothing that is too worn or torn to be resold can be sold to clothing recyclers that convert it into stuffing for furniture or into insulation. For example, one type of housing insulation is made from recycled denim jeans.

WHAT TO DO WITH OUTGROWN CLOTHES:
- ✓ If you want your clothes to go to the truly needy, instead of being resold, do your homework on the charity before donating.
- ✓ When your child's clothes wear out, convert them into household cleaning rags.
- ✓ If you are into crafts, save scraps of fabric to make a quilt or doll clothing.
- ✓ Repair rips in clothing yourself instead of replacing clothing.

TOXIC TOGS Clothes may contain dyes that can cause allergic reactions. If your child has an itchy rash, consider that the source could be his or her clothing. Some people with chronic foot dermatitis found out it was caused by a dye in the socks they wore.

Clothing can contain chemicals left over from its manufacture. Some clothes have been found to contain formaldehyde, which is irritating to the skin and eyes. Lead has been found in screen prints on T-shirts as well as on snaps and buttons that adorn children's clothing. Lead has also been found in shoes, flip-flops, and sunglasses. Check the U.S. Consumer Product Safety Commission (CPSC)'s recall website at *www.recalls.gov*.

Numerous products made for children are listed on the CPSC's recall list. The sheer number of products should decline in the next few years as a new law

---

GREEN ON A SHOESTRING

At back-to-school time, set reasonable expectations with your children about how many items they'll be getting new. Explain that they are helping the environment by accepting hand-me-downs from older cousins or siblings.

called the Consumer Product Safety Improvement Act (CPSIA) kicks in. This law mandates that no item marketed to children under the age of 12 contain more than 600 parts per million lead. (This number will go down to 90 ppm lead in future years.) The law applies to everything from clothing to baby strollers.

GREENER GYM SHOES Gym is the typical kid's favorite school subject. To reduce the risk of injuries, many schools require that kids wear athletic shoes for gym class. At back-to-school time, one of your countless errands may be to take your child to the shoe store to get fitted for a quality pair of athletic shoes.

When it comes to choosing "greener" shoes, the options have improved over the years. The consumer outcry over shoes being made in overseas sweat-shops under inhumane working conditions has yielded tremendous benefits. Many of the major shoemakers have switched to safer materials that don't endanger worker health or have instituted commitments to reasonable hours and wages as well as worker benefits.

Several shoemakers have product lines that feature recycled materials. Others have committed to reducing waste and using renewable energy, such as wind power. It is sometimes hard though to verify claims because only one major athletic shoe producer is still making shoes in U.S. factories rather than exclusively overseas.

That said, some shoe companies now work with several third-party certifiers to ensure safe and environmentally conscientious conditions in factories. Companies have reduced the amount of toxic chemicals that workers handle. One manufacturer has dramatically reduced the amount of harmful volatile organic compounds (VOCs) produced during shoe production. Another replaced the toxic metal chromium with a less toxic leather-tanning procedure. See Tips for Choosing Eco-friendlier Shoes below.

ECO-TIP: AVOID POLYVINYL CHLORIDE (PVC)

PVC plastic contains toxic phthalates and other chemicals that endanger the health of workers who manufacture and work with PVC plastics. The production of PVC results in generation of the cancer-causing chemical dioxin. Less toxic plastics that are now being used as substitutes for PVC include ethylene vinyl acetate (EVA) and thermoplastic polyurethane (TPU).

TIPS FOR CHOOSING ECO-FRIENDLIER SHOES:

✓ Look for brands that offer information about environmental impact.

✓ Choose brands that have phased out PVC. See the report "Cleaning Up Our Chemical Homes," issued by Greenpeace in 2007, *www.green peace.org* for a list of athletic shoe companies that have phased out the use of toxic chemicals in their products.

✓ When your child outgrows shoes, pass them on to a friend or neighbor, or donate them to an organization such as the nonprofit Soles for Souls, *www.soles4souls.org*, that passes shoes on to needy children.

✓ Some shoe stores collect used athletic shoes that are then broken up into parts. The rubber and foam are recycled.

For other school footwear, check the many online green retailers that have sprouted up over the last several years. Shoe designers have taken up the green shoe challenge, and you can now find sandals made of FSC-wood and flip-flops made from recycled tire rubber. Some online shopping sites rate shoes for their use of sustainable materials, organic fabrics, recycled rubber, and fair worker conditions.

GREEN ON A SHOESTRING

Buy quality brands of footwear so that the shoes don't start falling apart before your children outgrow them.

Environmentally Safe Schools

Our children spend roughly six hours per day at school and we expect school facilities to be safe. But not all schools use practices that are healthy for our children or the planet. Schools may be situated on or near contaminated sites, may have problems such as mold or radon, or may routinely use toxic cleaning and pesticide products. The good news is that more schools are identifying and remediating these problems. Parents can help by notifying school officials when they suspect a problem.

UNCOVERING A SCHOOL'S MURKY PAST A child care facility in New Jersey opened on the site of a former thermometer factory. The fact was revealed only when several children tested positive for mercury. A new high school in Los Angeles was built on a former oil field and opened only after millions of dollars were spent on systems to vent potentially explosive methane gas and toxic hydrogen sulfide.

Several notorious cases of schools being built on top of contaminated land have emerged over the last 50 years. In some cases, toxic building materials were used in school foundations. Depending on the type of contamination, toxic fumes can seep up from the soil or foundation and into the school or child care facility. Often these toxic substances cause learning disabilities that are not noticed until the child is older.

Avoiding toxic schools is essential, but how is a parent to know what secrets a school is hiding? Many times the school district officials or child care facility's owners are also completely in the dark, so you will have to do your own investigation. Take a look around the area. Is it in an industrial area, or a former factory area? Ask the school staff or owner how long the school has been there, and what the building or site was used for prior to its becoming a school. You can also check newspaper archives and talk to longtime area residents. Check with your state's department of environmental protection or the website *scorecard.org* to see if the area has been identified as an area in need of cleanup.

BREATHING EASY ABOUT YOUR SCHOOL'S AIR Toxic waste is not the only contaminant that may threaten schools. Roughly half of the 115,000 schools in the U.S. have indoor air quality problems, according to the EPA. Some of the most common toxic substances in schools are radon and mold. Radon is a natural radioactive gas found in the ground and is the second leading cause of lung cancer after smoking. It is tasteless, odorless, and colorless. Radon levels can fluctuate over time, so monitoring needs to be done every few years. A radon-remediation system can be installed to reduce radon levels.

Mold can grow due to leaky roofs and plumbing problems, poor building design that allows the accumulation of moisture in the air, or improperly maintained ventilation systems. Mold can trigger asthma attacks and lead to chronic lung irritation. Mold can usually but not always be removed from schools.

Asthma is responsible for 14 million lost school days annually in the U.S., according to the EPA. It is found in 1 of every 13 school-age children and is rapidly rising in the population, especially among preschool-age children.

If your child is complaining of headaches or has respiratory problems that seem to clear up during the summer or winter school holidays, suspect that the problem could be the school's air. Bring up the problem to other parents, and see if anyone else is having similar issues. Talk to the school principal to find out if any of the staff has complained. If your suspicion is strong, request that the school district test the indoor air.

Also, find out if any renovations are planned during the summer and ask what ventilation measures will be taken to clear the air before the children return to school in the fall. If the school is undergoing renovations, children may be exposed to paints, solvents, flooring materials, and other building materials that offgas VOCs. Insist that your child's school provides ways to shield children from exposure to VOCs during renovations.

Lung irritation and asthma attacks can also be triggered by pest problems. Mice, rats, cockroaches, and dust mites produce droppings that can cause asthma attacks and allergies. If your child's school has pests, encourage the school to first try nonchemical methods of removing pests as part of an integrated pest management (IPM) approach.

With IPM, school groundskeepers first try to eliminate the conditions for pests and use nonchemical treatments, before resorting to chemicals. For example, school officials would first improve the cleanliness of the school by making sure that food crumbs are swept up daily, garbage cans are covered at all times, and pest shelters and pathways are found and removed. Weeds and standing water should be removed from around the perimeter of the facility to reduce the attraction of pests to the building. Chemical poisons should be used only as a last resort and for the most limited time possible, preferably during holidays when children and staff are absent from the school. Traps and baits should be tried before using pesticide sprays.

Other sources of indoor air pollution are chemicals in science labs and shop classes. Copying machines, computers, and other office equipment all give off VOCs. Your child's school may use especially strong cleaning supplies that leave irritating smells and residues behind.

SYMPTOMS ASSOCIATED WITH BAD INDOOR AIR:

× Headache	× Sinus congestion
× Fatigue	× Shortness of breath
× Nausea	× Sneezing
× Dizziness	× Nose irritation
× Cough	× Itchy or watery eyes
× Throat irritation	× Skin rash or irritation

See the Healthy Schools Network at *www.healthyschools.org* and the EPA's Healthy School Environments at *www.epa.gov/schools* for more information.

OUTSIDE SCHOOL WALLS Indoor air is not the only concern when it comes to schools. Sources of outdoor air pollution near the school can cause unhealthy conditions that affect children while they play on playgrounds or sports fields. Outdoor air problems can stem from close proximity to major highways and industrial refineries as well as from underground contamination. Highways can provide toxic components of gasoline combustion, such as benzene and polyaromatic hydrocarbons (PAHs). Industrial plants may give off lead, cadmium, nickel, or other toxic metals in the form of fine dust that settles on playing fields and playground equipment. Underground storage tanks may be leaching oil and its breakdown products into the soil, where they seep up into the air around the school.

Nor are all outdoor air threats from man-made sources. Pollen and fungal spores may irritate children on playgrounds and come in through windows and get trapped in the classroom, making allergy-sensitive kids miserable for some parts of the year. And dust is a major air contaminant in some parts of the country: In California's Central Valley, the combination of intensive agriculture and water diversion makes the air some of the most polluted in the country.

If you suspect your child's school has outdoor air quality issues, talk to the school district about ways to lessen the impact on children. Or contact your regional or state environmental department. The problem may be much bigger than anything the school can handle, but if enough parents complain, the county or state may be able to address the problem.

TEMPORARILY YOURS Portable classrooms are often used when the area's school-age population outgrows the school's facilities. Yet these portable classrooms sometimes become permanent fixtures. These classrooms may be trailers that traditionally are built using lightweight wood products such as plywood and pressed board. These wood products are held together by glues, which can contain the toxic chemical formaldehyde. Many people are sensitive to formaldehyde and develop skin rashes, itchy eyes, and headaches. Long-term exposure to formaldehyde may increase the risk of cancer and lung disease. Poor ventilation and moisture control in these classrooms can also lead to serious mold and mildew issues.

If your child is attending class in a trailer, be alert for symptoms of formaldehyde exposure such as itchy eyes, skin rashes, and headaches. Look for signs of breathing problems or worsened asthma due to mold or mildew. Check with other parents to see if their children are experiencing similar symptoms. It may be that the problem can be solved through better ventilation. If your child's school is purchasing trailers, talk to administrators to make sure they are selecting trailers built without formaldehyde-emitting materials.

THE GRASS IS NOT ALWAYS GREENER Many school districts are replacing grass-covered athletic fields with artificial turf because it requires no cutting, herbicides, or pesticides. High schools, colleges, and town recreation departments are increasingly interested in artificial turf. Artificial turf requires little or no watering, whereas the typical natural grass playing field consumes 50,000 gallons a week during the growing season, according to the Synthetic Turf Council, a trade group that represents artificial turf manufacturers.

Despite these benefits, artificial turf presents some serious concerns for the environment and children's health. Some artificial turf has been found to contain potentially dangerous levels of lead, a metal that is toxic to the brain and can cause lifelong cognitive problems in children, according to the EPA. If your child's school uses artificial turf, ask the principal or groundskeeper whether it has been tested for lead. Fields that are old and visibly worn are most likely to release lead in the form of dust. Not all types of artificial turf contain high levels of lead, so testing will need to be done.

Parents will want to keep their children off of lead-contaminated fields entirely. The CPSC recommends that all children playing on lead-contaminated turf wash thoroughly after playing, and wash clothing and shoes. The CPSC has called for voluntary industry standards to eliminate the use of lead in artificial turf.

Artificial turf also contains a cushioning layer of ground rubber from recycled automobile tires. Many parents are concerned about the toxic metals and chemicals in recycled tire rubber. See The Science Behind It at the end of this chapter for more information on artificial turf.

Homeschooling

Homeschooling is an increasingly popular choice for families. Teaching children at home means you can instill environmental values without having to make the compromises that many of us make when we send our children to schools.

Homeschooling is a logical choice for many families. Some families are seeking the option of teaching religious values. Others are military families who move every couple years. Others choose homeschooling because one or more of the children have a learning pattern that does not fit into the 25-students-per-class public school model. Still other parents think that public school stifles creativity and encourages consumerism.

Homeschooling provides an excellent opportunity to teach your children to live an environmentally conscious lifestyle. You can make the experience even more exciting by taking field trips to the recycling center, garbage dump, or science museum. Homeschooling families often get together to have group lessons. Consider teaching one on endangered species, the food chain, the need for biodiversity and habitat preservation, or another environment-related topic.

Teaching at home is also one of the most eco-friendly ways to educate your children. Since you don't have to transport children to school either in your car or on a diesel-powered bus, you cut your family's greenhouse gas emissions significantly. You can use paper scraps, old computer paper, and last year's school supplies; you don't have to buy new items each year. Your child has much less need for new clothes and backpacks so you'll cut down on your family's use of the planet's resources. Several homeschooling groups offer opportunities to swap books and other learning materials.

Take Action

▸ Choose a child care facility that provides a safe and nurturing environment for your child while reducing toxic exposures around the facility.

▸ Whenever possible, reuse school supplies from last year. When buying new, look for eco-friendly supplies, such as recycled paper and PVC-free backpacks.

▸ Work with your school district to find alternatives to disposable tableware in schools.

▸ Find out what is in the lunches at the school. Are the cafeteria offerings laden with fat, sugar, and salt? With like-minded parents, work on changing cafeteria offerings.

▸ Suggest that classroom birthday parties be celebrated on a single day each month so that parties take less time away from studies. Offer to bring kid-favorite fruits like grapes and strawberries.

▸ When sending lunch with your child, use reusable containers. Work with your child to understand the importance of eating a healthy lunch.

▸ Organize a "walking school bus" for your neighborhood.

▸ Work with the school district to bring farm-fresh produce into the cafeteria whenever possible.

▸ Help establish a school garden where the students can fulfill science curriculum goals in a real-life setting.

▸ Encourage your school to return recess to its proper place as a much needed opportunity to exercise the body and refresh the mind.

▸ Try to walk or ride a bike to school with your child at least a couple days a week.

▸ When it is time for your school district to replace buses, advocate for the purchase of cleaner-burning vehicles.

▸ When choosing back-to-school clothes, help your child understand how new clothes are made, and what toll they take on the environment. Choose gently used clothes and clothes that are not made in sweatshops.

▸ Donate used clothing to a needy family or a worthwhile charity.

▸ Check *www.recalls.gov* for recalled clothing items that contain lead or other toxic chemicals.

▸ Find out if your school has a history of contamination with toxic chemicals. If you suspect toxic contamination, contact your school administration to find out what they are doing to address the problem.

▸ Suggest that the school adopt an integrated pest management approach, where toxic chemicals are used as a last resort and only when children are not at the school.

▸ If your school is considering installing artificial turf, make sure the decision-makers are aware of the potential toxicity.

THE SCIENCE BEHIND IT

Artificial Turf

When inspectors from the New Jersey Department of Environmental Protection arrived at a Newark school football stadium in 2007, they were conducting routine tests for signs of contamination from a nearby metals scrap yard. They found that the school's artificial turf contained levels of lead that were nine times greater than the allowable level in soil. Yet, the scrap yard did not produce lead dust, so where did the lead come from?

Eventually inspectors pinpointed the source: The lead was coming from the artificial turf itself. The pigments that make the "grass" green contain lead because the metal improves colorfastness. The fake blades of grass are made from a nylon or nylon/polyethylene blend that contains significant levels of lead. Although a July 2008 report by the U.S. Consumer Product Safety Commission found that the levels of lead in artificial grass were too low to provide any real danger to children, many scientists believe there is no safe level of exposure for children. In New Jersey, entire playing fields were ripped up and replaced at a significant cost.

Lead is only one of the concerns about artificial turf and its impact on the environment. Artificial turf also contains black, gritty rubber granules that serve as padding at the base of the blades of artificial grass. These rubber granules are made from recycled automobile tires, a fact that worries some public health groups because the crumbs contain toxic chemicals including volatile organic compounds (VOCs) and heavy metals that can be toxic. Synthetic turf manufacturers convert 25 million used auto tires into rubber for artificial turf each year, according to the Synthetic Turf Council. These small black particles could be ingested or inhaled by small children, exposing them to toxic substances.

The rubber also contains latex and some studies indicate that latex exposure via artificial turf may increase the risk of developing a latex allergy. A further concern is the high incidence of "turf burns" that occur when kids skid along the artificial turf. These turf wounds could aid the spread of the antibiotic-resistant bacteria known as MRSA (methicillin-resistant *Staphylococcus aureus*).

Another reason to oppose artificial turf is that it is made from a nonrenewable resource. Petroleum is the starting material for nylon and polyester. The small black rubber granules can spread to nearby waterways where they may prove toxic to fish and other aquatic organisms. However, the environmental impact of synthetic turf is difficult to compare to the gallons of water, pesticides, and other chemicals applied to living grass.

Finally, artificial turf also gets quite hot in the summer. Surface temperatures can top 100°F. To cool it down, some schools and municipalities find that they have to water the artificial grass that they purchased because it didn't require watering.

EARTH-FRIENDLY FESTIVITIES

Parties, Holidays, and Celebrations

CHILDREN ARE EXCELLENT ANTIDOTES TO HOLIDAY FATIGUE. IF you've ever felt weary of the banal repetition of holiday songs, the annual trotting out of tired-looking tinsel and garish decorations, or the forced cheerfulness of parties, just look into a child's eyes, and you'll experience a revival of holiday magic.

Whereas adults mark time in months or years, children judge the passing of time by how many weeks it is until Christmas, or how long ago was Valentine's Day. The Fourth of July tells them what month it is, and Halloween tells them it is fall. Children who can easily answer a question about what they did before Thanksgiving may have trouble telling you what they did in November.

If you survey the average child about what he likes about holidays, gifts and sweets will probably top the list. Who could imagine Halloween without candy, Christmas without presents, or Thanksgiving without pumpkin pie? Yet most children also love the family time that holidays represent. Children get to play with their cousins. School is out and Mom and Dad are home from work. Schedules are relaxed. Holiday perks include sleeping late and having a nice, leisurely pancake breakfast instead of a rushed bowl of cereal.

Foods, decorations, gifts, and sweets have become the staples of holidays, but these material goods are merely symbols that convey deeper messages such as "I love you" and "I care about spending time with you." Yet these messages can get lost in the desire to throw the perfect holiday party or provide a memorable birthday experience for a child.

Sometimes we try to make an event or holiday so perfect that we end up running over budget and purchasing items willy-nilly without a thought of what impact our consumption is having on our planet. The United States already uses more natural resources than any country in the world, despite making up just 5 percent of the world's population, so you can imagine how holiday binges drain our planet's resources.

It helps to remind ourselves now and then that holidays are about spending time with family and friends, not buying stuff. One of the easiest green steps you can take is to *reduce* the amount of gifts, wrapping paper, candy, paper goods, plastic tableware, tinsel, ribbon, tape, and paper plates you bring into your home each holiday. Not only is this good for the planet, it saves you money.

Of course, *reuse* is another essential green holiday tradition. It is easy to reuse many holiday items from year to year. Many families have Christmas ornaments that are pulled out of storage each year, and some become family heirlooms. You can reuse decorations, tablecloths, cloth napkins, durable party plates, and even those ubiquitous plastic Easter eggs.

Recycling should also be on your holiday to-do list, but it comes in third after reduce and reuse. Recycling consumes resources, and is not available in all areas for all materials, so why not avoid buying the stuff in the first place? And when you do have to buy items, try to find products made from recycled materials whenever possible.

It can seem overwhelming to adopt "greener" practices around the holidays, especially the holidays that feature the theme of giving. But there are so many ways to give that don't involve purchases. One of the best gifts a parent can give to a child is time. And think about this: By reducing, reusing, and recycling, you are giving a priceless gift back to the planet.

When "greening" your holiday, it sometimes helps to set yourself a challenge, such as "I will give all presents wrapped in reusable materials instead of wrapping paper" or "I will serve organic vegetables at my holiday party." Get your kids and spouse on board, and put them to work finding creative ways to reduce your holiday impact. They may decide to make all the family Christmas cards out of used computer paper, or turn orphaned socks into puppets for their younger cousins.

Adding "be green" to an already lengthy holiday to-do list is not as hard as it sounds. It is surprisingly easy to make small changes that can add up to big differences in the amount of resources you consume and the amount of garbage you toss. This chapter will provide you with plenty of tips on how to integrate eco-friendly practices into the fine art of event planning.

THE FACTS

The U.S. consumes the greatest share of the world's supply of corn, coffee, copper, lead, zinc, tin, aluminum, rubber, oil seeds, oil, and natural gas. For meat and many other commodities the U.S. has the greatest per person consumption.

Birthday Parties

An eco-friendly birthday party does not mean a single candle atop a meager sugar-free crust of bread. You don't have to do away with the friends, the presents, the goofy party hats, or the favors. Instead choose the parts of the party that matter to your child and find substitutes for eco-unfriendly party items.

KEEP IT SIMPLE, SILLY Having an eco-friendly birthday party may seem daunting in today's consumer-driven culture. In days of yore, the birthday party consisted of rambunctious kids running around the Formica kitchen table. Today's parents are likely to outsource parties to bounce houses, video arcades, laser tag facilities, waterslide parks, bowling alleys—the list is endless. These activities are certainly crowd-pleasers, but before plunking down the plastic for a big birthday bash, make sure that you are doing something that is within your means and will be meaningful to your child.

A lot of children are perfectly content just having a few friends over to have cake. You can reduce your impact on the environment by keeping parties simple in the first few years of life. As your child enters elementary school and gains the inevitable painful awareness that his family doesn't do things the way "everyone else" does, you will want to talk with your child to set reasonable expectations about what types of parties fit your eco-conscious lifestyle and budget.

When it comes to parties, it helps to start managing expectations when your children are young. Children should learn that they live in a world of limited resources of the natural *and* financial kinds. Try to stay true both to your bank account and to your eco-friendly values. In parties as in most other aspects of life, going green is likely to save you a lot of green.

If you are ready to host an off-site party, several eco-friendly party settings are available. You may live near a nature reserve that offers birthday party activities led by professional wildlife experts. Or try the zoo or natural history museum. If you live near the beach, a visit to the shore could be exactly what your child desires. In each case you have the opportunity to blend education and tips on preserving the environment into your child's birthday experience.

ECO-FRIENDLY PARTY LOCATIONS

- Nature preserves
- Zoos

GREEN ON A SHOESTRING

Hosting large parties at eco-friendly venues may not be in your budget. There are lots of ways to save on parties. You may want to have a family tradition of having a large party every other year instead of every year. On the in-between years you could have your child invite a few friends over for cake, or just have a family celebration.

- Beaches
- Parks
- "Pick-your-own" farms
- Botanical gardens

ECO-FRIENDLY THEMES (WHICH CAN BE DONE AT HOME)

- Gardens galore: Provide seeds, pots, and dirt and let kids plant their own flowers.
- Backyard camping: Set up tents and have the kids come with sleeping bags to watch the stars and play flashlight tag.
- Scavenger hunt: Hide recyclable items at a nearby park. Provide teams of kids with lists of the items, which they can then exchange for prizes.
- Eco-art: Have the children bring items that were headed for the garbage and turn them into works of art.
- Dinosaurs: Make fossils from clay before the party and let the kids go on a fossil dig in a sandbox.

ECO-FRIENDLY DECORATIONS AND FAVORS An eco-friendly party starts with the invitations. One of the easiest green things you can do is send the invitations electronically instead of mailing them. You'll save on postage and the cost of buying the invitations. You'll also save the planet from the greenhouse gas emissions of the mail truck, the bleach used to whiten paper pulp, and the loss of trees that are cut and converted into pulp.

When shopping for party decorations and favors, a good question to ask is: "Do I need this, or will it just become junk five minutes after the party?" Step back and ask yourself which traditions can be modified to be less of a blow to the environment. Could you substitute silly hats from the dress up box for party hats? Can you buy sturdy decorations—such as windsocks or cloth spirals—that you'll be likely to save and reuse next year? Can you buy durable cotton table-cloths and decorate them with fabric markers? (This could be a good activity for the kids to do while waiting for all the guests to arrive.)

ECO-TIP: WHAT HAPPENS TO HELIUM BALLOONS WHEN THEY GO UP IN THE SKY?

When your child lets go of a helium-filled balloon, where does it go and what happens to it? The balloon rises about 5 miles into the atmosphere above Earth, until the icy temperature and low atmospheric pressure cause it to explode into small fragments. The fragments rain down onto Earth and have been found in the stomachs of numerous sea creatures from dolphins to leatherback turtles. The ribbons can entangle animals or choke them if swallowed.

Although balloons are made of latex, a natural product that is biodegradable in sunlight and air, they also contain pigments, preservatives, and plasticizers. And even latex doesn't biodegrade in a dark, oxygen-deprived landfill. Helium is a nonrenewable gas that has environmental impacts when it is mined, stored, and shipped to your nearby party store. Because of the potential to harm wildlife, most eco-friendly party hosts choose not to purchase balloons.

If you must have helium balloons, tie them securely around your child's wrist. If possible, avoid silver-colored Mylar balloons, which are not biodegradable. If you do buy Mylar balloons, you can save them and refill them with helium for another occasion. Or use them to wrap a gift.

PLANET-FRIENDLY ALTERNATIVES TO BALLOONS:

✓ **Use reusable windsocks posted on long poles.**

✓ **Put up hanging decorations or fly small flags. Party stores and discount stores frequently sell these with seasonal and holiday themes.**

The last step in hosting a party is sending a thank-you note. You can do this via e-mail as well. Another popular trend is to send the thank-you note home with the party guest as part of the "goodie bag." Choose recycled paper or do something creative like writing the thank-you note on a wooden toy (train whistles are popular).

GIFTS GONE OVERBOARD The tradition of giving gifts at birthdays is centuries old. Yet any parent of a child about to tackle a mountain of presents from 20 preschool classmates could be forgiven having misgivings about the custom. Could any child possibly enjoy playing with that many toys? Could the money spent on these toys be better spent providing food to the nearly 60 million children worldwide who don't have enough to eat? And what are the wrapping paper, packaging, and plastic doing to our environment?

If your child is having a small party of a few close friends who know his or her interests, then it is likely that the gifts will be appreciated. But if you've invited the entire class plus extended friends and relatives, your child may get far more toys than he or she can use.

So what is a parent to do? You can always write "no gifts" on the invitation, but this message is likely to be ignored by some guests and embraced by others, so that when party time comes, some kids will show up with elaborately wrapped gifts while others will be empty-handed, causing embarrassment to the party guest or, more likely, to his or her parent.

An increasingly popular custom is to suggest that in lieu of gifts, party guests make a small donation to a charitable cause chosen by the birthday child. For example, if your child is an animal-lover, he may be glad to know that his birthday party is helping to feed abandoned shelter dogs. If your child has a soft spot for endangered species, she may like to help out a charity that tries to prevent the cutting of rain forests. If you hold the party at the local firehouse, you could collect money for the volunteer firefighters fund.

Charities have caught on to the trend, and many will send your child a certificate, stuffed animal, or other small gift in return for donations. However, you may want to discourage your child from accepting thank-you gifts. You don't want your child to think he or she will get a new toy every time he or she does a good deed.

When the day of the party arrives, be prepared for some children to bring gifts while others bring a donation for the charity or a card showing that they donated online. (Some parents won't have read the invitation, or some may choose to bring a gift anyway.) However, the guests who don't have a gift in hand will have the satisfaction of knowing that they honored the birthday child in another and perhaps more meaningful way.

And do the birthday children miss the presents? They certainly might if they receive no presents whatsoever. Keep in mind that you may have to buy your child a few gifts (but then, you may have been planning on doing this anyway, and *you* know exactly what he or she wants).

Charitable birthday giving is a growing trend. At least one Internet-based company now offers to manage charitable gift giving for your child's birthday. The company offers to send e-mailed invitations that include a link to your child's chosen charity. Parents can log on to monitor the RSVPs and donations. However these tasks are easily done using your own e-mail program, too.

Before selecting a charity, investigate how much of the organization's budget goes to administrative overhead. A good investigative resource is Charity Navigator at *www.charitynavigator.org*.

You will be surprised how many parents are relieved to dig in their purse or pull out their checkbook rather than make a run to a toy store to pick up a gift for a child they don't know very well.

Other enterprising ideas for limiting conspicuous consumption:

- ✓ Encourage guests to bring a used toy. This works best during the first few years of life when children could care less who gets what toy.
- ✓ Ask each child to bring a copy of his or her favorite book to be given to a literacy program for underserved kids.
- ✓ Have children bring nonperishable food items for delivery to a food bank.

VOLUNTEER BIRTHDAYS Today's kids' parties are usually about entertaining the children with games, shows, or activities. But what if we could channel all the rambunctious energy that children bring to parties toward helping accomplish a goal that benefits the planet? That is the concept behind volunteer birthday parties.

At a volunteer party, the kids get involved in doing a project rather than just being entertained. They might clear trails in a nature preserve, plant seeds in a community garden, plant trees at a local park, or collect trash on the beach. A stint of time doing these activities (how long depends on the age of the children) could be followed by cake and more traditional party activities.

To find organizations in need of volunteers, go to *www.volunteermatch.org*.

GOOD THINGS COME IN LESS PACKAGING Good old-fashioned wrapping paper looks nice but has the unfortunate fate of being used for only an hour or so before being tossed into the garbage—or if you are in luck, tossed into the recycling bin. Instead of succumbing to the onetime use of wrapping paper or gift bags, choose reusable materials or recycled materials.

ECO-FRIENDLY WRAPPERS

- ✓ Buy a reusable cloth grocery bag and have your child paint a rainbow or balloons on it. Put the birthday child's name on it.
- ✓ Decorate a reusable tin or basket.
- ✓ Wrap the present in a hand-painted T-shirt or bandanna.
- ✓ Use old road maps, glossy magazine pages, or the comics section from the Sunday paper.
- ✓ Collect your computer paper that has been printed on one side only. Have your child decorate the unused side with stickers or drawings.
- ✓ Sew your own reusable fabric birthday bags or purchase them online.
- ✓ Several green retailers and toy stores now sell reusable birthday-themed gift bags.

ECO-TIP: **GIVING A GIFT THAT COUNTS**

Choosing a gift for one of your child's friends can be a daunting task for the eco-minded parent. You may feel that many of the toys on store shelves lack imagination. See Chapter 7 for examples of creative and ecologically friendly toys. A one-year subscription to a kid-themed nature magazine is a good choice. Books are nearly always welcome, too.

HEALTHIER BIRTHDAY FARE The staple fare of birthday parties is, of course, the birthday cake. Depending on your personal views, you may think it is OK to splurge on calorie-rich, nutrient-poor foods once a year. Or, you may be looking for ways to reduce the sugar load coursing through the veins of your party guests.

Whatever your inclination, party hosts can find plenty of healthy and tasty options to replace the traditional party foods. You may be surprised how many kids think grapes and blueberries are just as delicious as candy-coated chocolate pieces. Dried fruits such as pineapple bits or raisins are usually crowd-pleasers. Popcorn is a naturally low-fat treat that kids love. Fruit smoothies rank up there with ice cream sundaes on most kids' lists of favorite foods.

When it comes to the pièce de résistance, the cake, you have plenty of options. Health food cookbooks abound with recipes that use fruit juice concentrate or honey in the place of refined sugar. Note that the overall amount of sugar may not be less when using these sugar substitutes. These ingredients are after all still sugar, just in a more natural form. They still contribute to weight gain and tooth decay, but lack the processing that white granulated sugar undergoes. Steer clear of artificial sweeteners, dyes, and preservatives. Learn more about why you should avoid food additives in Chapter 2.

Regardless of the type of sugar you use, you can boost the nutritional content of the birthday cake by making a carrot cake or frosted blueberry muffins. Adding fruit or a sweet vegetable will raise the level of vitamins and minerals without sacrificing flavor. Just remember, you won't please every partygoer no matter what you do. A lot of kids don't like traditional cake—they find it too sweet.

One of the best beverages to accompany cake is milk. Milk provides the antidote to the biting sweetness of cake. Yet few people think to serve it at parties, perhaps because it has a reputation for being too healthy. Make milk available at your parties. A lot of kids will appreciate it. Serve plenty of water to keep kids hydrated during the party, especially if children are playing outdoors.

Making your own cake is the easiest way to steer clear of food dyes and other unwanted additives. Most people are surprised at how easy it is to make a cake. It takes only a few more ingredients than a cake mix does, and the baking steps are identical whether you start from scratch or use a mix. When you make your own cake, you know what is in it. An alternative to the do-it-yourself model is to find a trusted bakery that can provide you with an ingredient list.

Frosting is also easy to make although it does take practice to turn out a decorated cake to match the designs available in bakeries. Give yourself plenty of time to do the frosting the night before the party. You might want to invest in a frosting dispenser that makes it easy to make borders and flowers and to write your child's name.

When decorating, skip the food coloring, which contains artificial dyes. Instead mix frozen raspberries into the frosting to make pink. Use frozen blueberries to make bluish purple icing. (See more suggestions for food-based dyes in the Easter section of this chapter.) Or shop health food stores for food dyes and colored sugars made from all-natural ingredients.

SERVING ITEMS AND DECORATIONS Step into a party store and you'll see aisle after aisle of character-themed party supplies. If your child has a favorite TV character or superhero, you may be tempted to pick up a few items. The key is to pick up *only* a few items, such as a character-themed centerpiece, rather than buying the whole collection.

Instead of stocking up each year on character-themed plates and cups, consider a radical idea: Go reusable. Why is this a radical idea? We've become accustomed to thinking that all party supplies should be disposable. We are concerned about the spread of germs, and we don't want to be up late washing dishes after the party. But today it is possible to purchase colorful plastic or durable ceramic plates and cups that are dishwasher-safe and reusable. See Chapter 2 for a rundown on the best plastic choices. Purchase a set now and you can use them for many parties to come instead of having to scramble to buy disposable items each year.

Another Earth-friendly practice is to replace paper napkins with cloth ones. These are easy to purchase at houseware stores, but you can also make your own out of any leftover fabric you have lying around the house.

If reusable doesn't do it for you, consider buying biodegradable plates and tableware. You can now find plates and cups made of sugarcane or biodegradable and compostable corn-based or potato-based plastics. Again, these are a less eco-friendly option than going reusable, because manufacturing and transporting the biodegradable plates takes energy. If you cannot compost the plates, at least try to recycle the paper products. Note that most municipal recycling programs will not take paper items that have food stains on them.

EARTH-FAVORABLE FAVORS One of the treats of going to a party is coming home with a small gift or bag of loot, usually referred to as a "goodie bag." The traditional goodie bag has for the past several decades been filled with cheap plastic toys and a few pieces of candy. The plastic toys disappear into the innards of your house and occasionally surface from beneath a sofa cushion or bureau. But how often do they get played with?

When choosing party favors, instead of going for the small plastic snakes and noisemakers, consider giving a single substantial gift that your party guests will enjoy for some time to come. Small but fun and useful gifts include a flashlight, a book, a packet of markers or crayons, a sketchpad with pencil, or a beach pail-and-shovel set. Look for quality but low-priced items that offer creativity and fun.

Halloween

Halloween is a favorite among children and adults. Kids love dressing up, but it is usually the candy that they treasure most. With a little effort, however, you can provide a moderately healthy and entirely happy Halloween experience.

COSTUME CRAZINESS Coming up with a costume idea is a favorite activity for kids and their grownups. Parents might want to satirize a political or media figure, while kids want to dress up as their favorite superhero or TV star. Maximize creativity and tread lightly on the planet by steering clear of pricey store-bought costumes and emphasizing to your child the fun of making his or her own costume.

Easy to make homemade costumes:

- Fairy
- Princess
- Cat
- Nurse
- Doctor
- Witch
- Ghost
- Fireman

- Baseball player
- Frankenstein
- Dracula

If you are buying a costume here are some things to watch out for:

× **PVC MASKS** PVC releases volatile organic compounds (VOCs) that can irritate eyes and lungs. Some VOCs are linked to cancer in workers who breathe large amounts over long periods of time.

× **HALLOWEEN MAKEUP** Some brands have been recalled due to bacterial contamination. Choose a reputable brand of face paint or use adult makeup. See the Environmental Working Group's Skin Deep Cosmetics Safety Database at *www.cosmeticsdatabase.com* for suggestions. Don't let your child fall asleep in his makeup. Wash it off before bedtime. (Additional suggestions can be found in Chapter 7.)

GREEN ON A SHOESTRING

Your child may be craving a certain TV character or fairy-tale princess costume, but you don't want to spend a lot of money on an item that will be worn once and takes its toll on the planet in the manufacture of the polyester fabric, ribbons, and sequins. Here are some tips on satisfying costume wishes without compromising your values:

✓ Buy used costumes from online auction sites or classifieds—best to do this "off-season" before the Halloween demand ramps up.

✓ Organize a costume swap in your neighborhood or parent's club.

✓ Cruise garage sales.

✓ Shop the post-Halloween sales for items you know will get worn again.

✓ Check thrift stores—again, go off-season for best selection and prices.

✓ Make a costume out of clothes your child already has. Superman-themed pajamas can become a costume—just add a blanket as a cape.

✓ Make a princess costume out of a fancy dress from an older sibling.

SWEETS AND TREATS Halloween is the one night of the year when all our efforts to get our kids to eat healthily go flying out the window. But you don't have to give in to the madness: You can help your healthy eater avoid the sugar-coated craziness. Just remember that a little candy in moderation will probably do little harm if your child eats healthily most of the time. In fact, psychologists say that it can be damaging to forbid sweets altogether, because children crave what they are forbidden to have and these cravings can lead to eating disorders later in life.

But how do you convince your child to go easy on the candy (or forgo it altogether), when this is one of the central traditions of this holiday? Parents over the years have come up with lots of tricks for reducing (or eliminating) the treats. Some parents skip trick-or-treating altogether by taking their children to parties (see Tricks to Avoid Treats below). But if your child simply loves trick-or-treating, or you can't bear to deprive your child of a custom that you enjoyed so much as a child, there are ways to reduce the amount of candy your child eats after trick-or-treating. Read on:

AVOIDING CANDY OVERLOAD WHEN TRICK-OR-TREATING:

✓ Feed your child a full dinner before she goes trick-or-treating so that she won't snack along the way.

✓ Talk to your child about what is in candy and why she should limit how much she eats.

✓ Make sure your child brushes his or her teeth after eating candy—don't let the sugar sit on teeth for long periods of time.

✓ Have your child collect change for a worthy cause instead of collecting candy. For example, kids can collect for the United Nations Children's Fund (UNICEF) via door-to-door trick-or-treating. See *UnicefUsa.org* to get a bright orange-colored collection box.

AFTER YOUR CHILD COLLECTS THE TREATS, HERE ARE SOME TRICKS THAT PARENTS USE FOR LIMITING HOW MUCH GETS EATEN:

✓ Set a limit on the amount of candy he or she can eat each day.

✓ Have your child select his favorite candies and discard the rest.

✓ Offer to trade your child's bag of loot for a toy he has been craving.

✓ Start a tradition of a "Halloween Fairy" or "Magic Pumpkin" who comes to collect the candy that night and leaves a book or other meaningful gift in its place.

✓ Buy the candy from your child. If your child is saving up to buy a toy or pay for a trip, he or she may appreciate money more than candy.

Throwing out candy is a waste of packaging, ingredients, and resources. So what should you do with candy that you've collected from your child? Some municipal composting facilities will collect candy, or you can throw it in your backyard compost pile (take the wrappers off first).

You can also pass the candy out to trick-or-treaters that come later in the evening, or you can donate the candy to a children's home or nursing home. If you are thinking about these options, think also about the fact that you are distributing a nutrient-deficient food to some of society's most vulnerable people: the poor and the elderly. Many of these individuals, including those living in nursing homes, do not have adequate dental care. A third of our nation's children are expected to become obese adults. Do you want to contribute to this trend?

TRICKS TO AVOID TREATS If you are serious about cutting down on your environmental impact *and* promoting health, you'll probably want to avoid purchasing candy altogether (and not allow your child to collect it).

Below are some ways to replace the tradition of trick-or-treating with healthier activities that your children will love. If your child has health problems that prohibit eating the fats, sugar, dyes, and preservatives in candy, the suggestions in this section will be helpful.

- Take your child to a Halloween party instead of taking him or her trick-or-treating. Many communities offer such parties. If none are in your area, host one for your child's friends.
- Get together with other families on your block to organize a progressive Halloween party. The children gather in costume at the first house where they play a Halloween-themed party game. Every 20 minutes or so they move to the next house where they play a game or make a craft. They can win prizes and stuff themselves with healthy snacks at each house instead of collecting candy.
- For your older children, suggest that they stage a party at a nursing home, senior center, or home for people with disabilities. Your child will gain a greater understanding of how other people live and see the value of *giving* to the community rather than engaging in an annual ritual that is all about *taking*.
- When hosting a Halloween party, it is easy to incorporate healthy snacks into the offerings. Late summer vegetables, such as carrots, peppers, and sweet potatoes, come in shades of orange and yellow. For black, use raisins or olives. Be creative and arrange thinly cut veggie strips into the shape of a human skeleton.

FRIGHTENINGLY EASY DECORATIONS Go easy on the planet and your wallet by having your kids make the decorations instead of buying them. Craft books and websites are good places to look for ideas, or try these favorites:

- ✓ Make spooky spiders using black construction paper and black chenille stems (aka pipe cleaners). Use the chenille stems to make spider legs and attach them to a black paper circle cut out. Hang them from the ceiling.
- ✓ Paint faces on pumpkins using nontoxic paints. Check Chapter 7 for tips on choosing safer art supplies for use by children.
- ✓ Adapt your favorite sugar cookie recipe to make orange and black cutout cookies. Make orange coloring by adding grated orange peel to the recipe. Use powdered cocoa to make the black (actually brown) cookies. Cut the cookies using Halloween-themed cookie cutters.

If shopping for decorations, choose durable ones that can be used for Halloweens to come. Store all decorations in well-marked sturdy containers so you can find them next year. Look for decorations made of wood from well-managed forests and natural-dye cloth, preferably made by local craftspeople so that jobs and money stay in your area. In the past few years, Halloween decorations have been marketed like never before. Halloween spending has been steadily rising over the years, and the average person now spends about $65 on candy, decorations, and costumes, according to the National Retail Federation. It is now common to see people stringing electric lights and erecting giant inflatable skeletons on their lawns. When choosing decorations, remember the planet and go lightly on the lights.

Thanksgiving

We bemoan the effect of the Thanksgiving meal on our waistlines, but the traditional Thanksgiving meal is actually one of the healthiest dinners around. In addition to naturally low-fat turkey meat, fall vegetables like pumpkin and squash are rich sources of antioxidants and other nutrients. Stick with seasonal foods and you cannot go wrong.

ALL THE FIXINGS If you think about it, the first Thanksgiving dinner was the ultimate locally sourced, organically grown holiday meal. The Pilgrims and

KITCHEN TABLE TALK

Host a Healthier Halloween?

Is it even possible to make this candy-laden holiday the slightest bit healthier or better for the environment? Yes, it is not only possible, as Seattle mom Corey Colwell-Lipson discovered, but kids *love it.* She founded Green Halloween, a community movement that is now spreading across the nation.

The revelation that kids love Halloween even without cartloads of candy came as a surprise to Colwell-Lipson, when, in 2006, someone gave her young daughters bubbles instead of candy. The bubbles were an immediate hit with the group of pint-size trick-or-treaters, and Colwell-Lipson realized that kids are eager for alternatives to candy.

She soon found that other moms and dads are looking for alternatives, too. She discovered that a lot of her friends and neighbors wanted to provide healthier and more eco-friendly choices but were hesitant to alter the time-honored tradition of trick-or-treating. Her mother Lynn Colwell came on board to help spread the word about ways to cut down on consumption at Halloween through their website *GreenHalloween. org.* They've also partnered with nonprofit groups to bring the event to a national audience.

At *GreenHalloween.org* you can find creative ways to make your child's Halloween healthier while helping the environment by cutting down on the use of preservatives, food dyes, and candy wrappers. Halloween treats that are better for the environment include organically grown and fair-trade chocolate (see Easter later in this chapter for more information) and certified organic lollipops and fruit roll-ups that contain natural flavors and real fruit.

One aspect of Halloween trick-or-treating that is hard to get away from is the individually wrapped candy. All those wrappers take their toll on the environment, piling up in landfills and taking years to degrade. If you decide to give candy, Colwell-Lipton advises giving just one piece rather than a handful.

If your conscience won't let you give candy, you can give small change (pennies, dimes, nickels, and quarters), Halloween-themed pencils, rubber stamps, seed packets, homemade play dough, or small notepads. Or give an item sure to get some use in the near future: a toothbrush! Look for items made from recycled materials when possible, and resist the urge to buy cheap plastic toys.

But won't kids miss the candy? First of all, they'll probably get at least some candy from other houses. Second, kids are thrilled with unique and unexpected gifts. Use your creativity and come up with small gifts that you think children will enjoy. You may even want to make the gifts from items you have around the house.

Finally, remember to plan ahead to give yourself enough time to make gifts or buy items or organic sweets on the Internet, says Colwell-Lipton. "If you wait until the last minute," she says, "you could end up spending more than you want to, or grabbing that bag of store candy."

Native Americans had to grow, gather, and prepare every item they served. No synthetic pesticides or artificial fertilizers were used. Food miles (the distance a food travels from source to plate) were in the single digits.

Fall is a wonderful time to eat like a "locavore." Foods that are harvested in the fall include sweet potatoes, squash, yams, carrots, beets, potatoes, and leafy greens such as kale. A few days before the holidays, get out your sharpest knives and chop the vegetables in advance. The more prep work you can do, the easier it will be to cook most or all of the meal from scratch.

Fall vegetables are some of the healthiest foods around. Beets are high in folate, potassium, and manganese. Kale is off the charts when it comes to beta-carotene (vitamin A), and vitamins K and C. Winter squash is a good source of beta-carotene, vitamin C, and potassium. All of these vegetables contribute to dietary fiber.

When planning your holiday meal, go lighter on the carb- and fat-laden side dishes in favor of more squash, sweet potatoes, and leafy greens. If skipping the mashed potatoes would be an abomination in your household, try adjusting the recipe to use nonfat milk and less butter. Go easy on the gravy, too.

For your holiday baking, consider substituting some of the white flour with whole-grain flour. For example, you might try making your own bread rolls this year using whole wheat flour. Have the kids get involved with measuring the ingredients and kneading the bread, or use a breadmaker.

Fall-gathered apples will be at their crunchiest, perfect for pies. Try making pies yourself instead of buying store-bought ones. If you go with store-bought pies or shells, check the ingredients list and look for brands without preservatives and artificial colors or flavors. Pies labeled "no sugar added" sound great because they imply that they contain only the natural sweetness of fruit. But often "no sugar added" means that the product contains artificial sweeteners, which children should avoid. See Chapter 2 for more information about artificial sweeteners.

LET'S TALK TURKEY Today's commercial turkeys have been fattened on a diet rich in grains and fillers and given antibiotics to prevent diseases that are transmitted in large, crowded turkey houses. Slaughtered turkeys may be injected with water and flavor-giving chemicals to make them plump and juicy before they are frozen. This year, consider one of the following:

Organic turkeys are certified by U.S. Department of Agriculture (USDA) as having been raised without antibiotics and fed a diet of certified organic grains from pesticide-free fields. The turkeys must be given access to the outdoors (although the birds don't always seize the opportunity to leave the security of the turkey house). A 2006 study found that antibiotic resistance was far less common among organically raised turkeys and chickens than it is on conventional farms.[1]

Heritage turkeys are breeds that are no longer in commercial production. Several farmers and organizations are trying to bring back turkey varieties that have nearly disappeared from existence. These varieties have names like Beltsville Small White, Jersey Buff, Narragansett, Standard Bronze, White Holland, and White Midget. They are usually raised under conditions similar to organic turkeys but they may not be certified. You can learn more at *heritage foodsusa.com*.

Go fresh. If organic or heritage turkeys are too costly for your budget, try to find a locally raised turkey that has not been frozen. If you don't live near a farm, you may be able to find one that can be shipped to you. You will taste the difference. See *localharvest.org* to find a turkey farmer in your area.

These turkeys will be more expensive, especially since many supermarkets give free turkeys to loyal shoppers. Still, they are worth the extra money not only because the meat has not been doused with additives, and not only because the birds were probably raised in more humane conditions than conventional turkeys, but also because the meat simply tastes superb.

GREEN DICTIONARY

HERITAGE TURKEY
A heritage turkey belongs to a breed that is naturally mating; has a long, productive outdoor lifespan; and grows at a slow rate. (Conventional turkeys must be artificially inseminated, are slaughtered at maturity, and grow very quickly.)

Winter Holidays

Nothing chases away the winter blues like holiday decorations and lights.

Nothing brings back the blues like a high electricity bill for holiday lights.

Some of our most endearing holiday traditions are endangering the environment.

Whether you celebrate Christmas, Kwanzaa, or Hanukkah, we'll look at ways to cut down our carbon emissions and environmental impact without sacrificing holiday cheer.

HOLIDAY DECORATIONS Outdoor decorations have become very popular over the last decade. No longer is a simple string of lights around the roof considered adequate. Today many houses go all out with lights, inflatable snowmen, and even prerecorded music. Some households compete to see who can put up the most ostentatious display.

If you are serious about conserving natural resources, consider forgoing this trend. You'll save money on your utility bill but perhaps even more important, you'll reduce the amount of electricity you use. (See Eco-Tip: Where Does My Electricity Come From?)

Instead, rethink the standard decorations and create your own meaningful ornaments and wall hangings with the help of your children. Make wreaths from leftover branches from your Christmas tree. Make paper chains from strips of used computer paper. Hang holiday cards from years past on a string to liven up the room.

And speaking of cards, sending holiday cards is a wonderful tradition, but many people are finding they can transmit the same love and warmth by sending a card via e-mail instead of sending a paper version. When you send your season's greetings electronically, you can usually include a lot more pictures and text than you could fit in a paper envelope. If you must do paper cards, select ones made from recycled paper.

If you are determined to put up lights, look for LED (light-emitting diode) lights. These lights have a cheerful brightness and use one-tenth the electricity of conventional bulbs. They generate a lot less heat, so they are less of a fire hazard. Put your lights on a timer so that you don't have to constantly remember to turn them off when you go to bed.

Another option is to invest in solar-powered holiday lights, which come with a small photovoltaic panel and are ideal for outdoor use. These panels require just a few hours of sunlight to charge a battery. The lights come on automatically at dusk and burn brightly until dawn or until the charge runs out. They are ideal for decorating mailboxes, trees, shrubs, or outlining doors and windows.

ECO-TIP: WHERE DOES MY ELECTRICITY COME FROM?

If you live in the U.S., chances are your electricity comes from coal. Coal-fired power plants generate nearly half of all electricity used in the U.S. Coal is one of the most polluting fuels around, so it is no surprise that the generation of electricity is the largest contributor to greenhouse gases in the United States.

Natural gas, nuclear power, and oil combined make about 42 percent of our nation's electricity. Hydroelectric power contributes another 6 percent. Less than 3 percent of the electricity is made from nonhydroelectric renewable sources such as solar or wind power, according to the U.S. Energy Information Agency's 2007 data.

Consult your electric utility bill to find out how electricity is generated in your area, and try to reduce your electricity use by shutting off lights, turning off electrical appliances, and refraining from smothering your house with strings of electric lights.

CHOOSING A TREE The Christmas tree is more than just a holiday decoration—it becomes the focal point of the house. Yet not all trees are created equal. Consumers now have the choice of a cut living tree, a live in-a-pot tree, and, of course, an artificial tree.

CUT-YOUR-OWN OR PRECUT TREES Cut-your-own or precut trees have many benefits over their artificial cousins. One benefit is that trees provide a living carbon sink (during the tree's lifetime before it is harvested and installed in your living room) that sequesters carbon dioxide while giving off oxygen. When the holiday season is over, the trees can be composted or turned into mulch for use in parks and playgrounds. Christmas tree farms are often family owned and make enough of a profit that the land can stay in the hands of farmers instead of being sold to real estate developers. These trees provide habitats for animals and reduce erosion by keeping soil in place. The trees are a well-managed crop, with new seedlings being planted to replace cut trees.

Keep in mind, however, that most trees are grown using conventional agricultural practices. Many are treated with pesticides and weed killers. These chemicals are unlikely to still be on the tree when you purchase it because they are broken down in sunlight, but avoiding using these chemicals is good for wildlife and the environment. Look for growers with eco-friendly practices.

Your choice of tree will of course be influenced by your budget. Most farms charge more for trees than you would pay at the lot outside a big box store. If you go with a local farm, make sure you are getting your money's worth. Your local farm may truck trees to the farm to supplement the ones they grow locally. You may find that the precut tree you selected at your local farm was actually grown several states away.

Some farms advertise organically grown trees. If you are tempted to buy an organic tree, ask the seller about the growing conditions. Were synthetic pesticides or herbicides used? Were any provisions made to maintain soil quality on the tree farm? The USDA does not certify trees as organically grown, so you are going to have to take the seller's word on it.

At the end of the Christmas season, be sure to recycle your tree. Many communities offer curbside pickup while others offer a central drop-off location. Your tree will be shredded into mulch and used under swing sets and playground structures in nearby parks. Your children will get to enjoy the tree again, only this time under their feet.

Check websites like *localharvest.org* for information on local, sustainable, and organic tree farms.

LIVE IN-THE-POT TREES Potted trees are becoming a popular option. These may be balled and burlapped (B&B), container-grown, or grown in the ground until they are dug up and potted. Unfortunately, few consumers do their homework before purchasing them. When these consumers encounter trouble planting them or maintaining them, the trees often end up in landfills.

Before buying a live containerized tree, figure out which species to buy and what to do with it after the holiday. Check for native species that will grow in your yard with minimal care. If you live in a very cold climate, check with your local agricultural extension officer for region-specific advice.

Some species can be kept in the pot and used year after year, while others need to be planted in the yard to survive. If you are going to plant the tree in the yard after Christmas and you live in a region where the ground freezes, you'll have to dig the hole in late fall.

Trees that grow well in pots include cedars, spruces, and pines. These grow slowly enough that they won't outgrow the pot. Prune them periodically to maintain their shape.

Trees that need to be planted in the yard after the holidays are Douglas fir, grand fir, and noble fir. When planting the tree, choose a location with plenty of room for growth. A Douglas fir can grow 40 feet or more by the time your infant has become old enough to get her driver's license. Make sure you don't plant the tree too close to the house because the roots could impact the foundation.

Whichever tree you choose, keep it indoors for as little time as possible. Evergreens survive the winter by going into dormancy. When they encounter indoor, warm temperatures, they break out of their dormant state and begin growing. If you try to put them outdoors after they've lost their winter hardiness, the trees may die of cold damage. To prevent this from happening, potted trees should ideally be kept indoors for a week at most, according to tree experts at the Oregon State University Extension Service.

While the tree is indoors, make sure it gets plenty of water, and keep it away from direct heat sources like radiators and furnaces. Use LED lights, which stay cool, rather than using conventional lights, which get quite hot and can damage the tree.

When you are ready to plant the tree outdoors, don't transport the tree straight from a warm house to the freezing outdoors. Give the tree a chance to adjust to colder temperatures by placing it in a garage or unheated patio for several days. Once the tree is outside, plant it promptly so that the roots don't freeze in the pot.

ARTIFICIAL TREES Artificial trees take the headache out of transporting the tree and cleaning up all those pine needles that the kids track all over the living room. However, there are a number of good reasons to avoid artificial trees. They are often made of PVC, the manufacture of which releases harmful dioxins. Artificial trees often smell artificial, and that smell is made up of volatile organic compounds (VOCs) that can be irritating to the eyes and throat as well as trigger asthma attacks. The trees release toxic fumes if they are burned or incinerated. The trees are made overseas and shipped far distances, so our purchase of them contributes to the release of climate change gases. Lead, a toxic metal, is another concern because lead is sometimes used in green pigment.

If at all feasible, avoid buying an artificial tree. In addition to all the reasons listed above, children usually can't stand them. Many children live for the annual ritual of selecting a tree, even if it is just from the lot outside the grocery store. If the pine needles are driving you crazy, make a deal with your children and have them do the sweeping.

Holiday Gift Giving

Gift giving has become a tradition for many holidays. Finding the right gift, however, can be a challenge. So many of us already have too much stuff cluttering desktops, kitchen cabinets, and fireplace mantles. These items neither bring happiness nor do any good for the planet. Here are some tips on finding meaningful gifts for our loved ones and friends.

HOMEMADE GIFTS Think back to the last handmade gift you received during the holidays. Chances are you were touched by the idea that your friend or loved one sat down and took the time to make your gift. Most people will appreciate a handmade gift just for the very fact that it is handmade.

Children can make excellent helpers when it comes to making gifts. Depending on their age, they can paint and assemble presents. When choosing a craft to make for friends, try ones that allow your child to show off his or her creative side. Your child does not have to be an expert painter or have a flair for the arts. Most kids like getting their hands in paint and helping Mom or Dad with big jobs. Choose something uncomplicated and make the first one yourself so that your kids get a sense of what they need to build.

Some simple crafty gifts that kids can make:

HAND-PAINTED T-SHIRTS OR APRONS Use fabric paint and have your children make handprints on the item.

PINECONE CHRISTMAS TREES Roll a pinecone in glue and sprinkle glitter on it.

PICTURE FRAMES Kids can paint and decorate simple wooden frames.

HOMEMADE COOKIES Combine an activity kids love (baking cookies) with a craft of decorating gift tins. Buying tins can be expensive. Instead, collect glass, plastic, and metal food containers throughout the year and decorate them with holiday themes using glued-on paper and stickers.

HANDMADE HOLIDAY GREETING CARDS Use holiday-themed stamps and ink.

Whenever possible use materials from around the house that otherwise would have headed to the garbage. One family painted holiday messages on wood shingles left over after demolishing a small shed, then gave the painted signs to family and friends. Another family created festive tiles by gluing photos of their friends' children onto tiles left over from refurbishing a bathroom.

FAIR-TRADE GIFTS When you pick up a holiday gift stamped "Made in (insert far-off country here)," do you ever wonder who made it? Was it made by a young wife in a factory filled with dangerous fumes? Or an artisan who received just pennies for long hours of work? Or a child who goes to a "school" that doubles as a factory during lunchtime? Often we simply don't know.

The fair-trade movement tries to bring a human face and a humane approach to buying gifts made overseas. The goal of fair-trade is to provide realistic wages to the craftspeople and return profits to their communities rather than to exporters or retailers.

Fair-trade gifts come in many shapes and sizes and are not limited to coffee-table knickknacks. It is possible to buy fair-trade clothing, furniture, foods, home décor, housewares, jewelry, toys, personal accessories, and many other products. Often these items do not cost more than conventionally produced goods because fair-trade organizations work directly with producers, cutting out the "middlemen."

Entire communities benefit from the production and sale of fair-trade items. The money may go to pay children's school fees, purchase or grow more nutritious foods, or pay for health care costs. Women are empowered because their traditional roles as clothing makers and artisans become more valued in the community. Fair-trade organizations help craftspeople procure the starting materials for their work while mitigating environmental impacts.

You can double the impact of your holiday gift money by purchasing a craft item made by indigenous craftspeople in a developing country. Your dollars go toward improving the standard of living in that area, and your gift goes

FAIR-TRADE

Fair-trade gifts are made by craftspeople who earn fair wages, work under safe conditions, and produce products that do not exploit natural resources. The goals of fair-trade are to:

• Create economic opportunities for marginalized peoples.
• Develop transparent relationships between producers and sellers.
• Ensure prompt and fair payment for goods produced.
• Support safe working conditions.
• Provide opportunities for business expansion.
• Cultivate respect for the environment.
• Respect cultural identity.

THE FACTS

According to the World Bank, 2.7 billion people live on less than $2 per day.

to someone who will appreciate the uniqueness and fine craftsmanship of the gift. North American consumers spent $160 million buying Fair Trade Federation–member goods in 2007. Sales of these goods doubled from 2004 to 2006, according to the Fair Trade Federation.

Fair-trade merchandise can be found at boutiques, craft fairs, and online. Look for the Fair Trade Federation (FTF) logo, which indicates the retailer is a member of the Fair Trade Federation, *fairtradefederation.org*, a trade association that promotes North American organizations committed to fair-trade. Member retailers are listed on the FTF website, and may display the FTF logo or use the words "Member of the Fair Trade Federation" on their products. (Certifications for fair-trade foods and coffee are covered later in this chapter.)

To learn more about fair-trade products, see the World Fair Trade Organization at *www.wfto.com* and Fairtrade Labelling Organizations International at *www.fairtrade.net*.

GIFTS OF GOOD Not all gifts come in packages. An increasingly popular eco-friendly choice is to give a gift to a charity in the gift recipient's name. A donation is a terrific gift for the child who already "has it all."

For those children that don't already have it all, you may want to give clothes, shoes, gloves, hats, or jackets. You may want to ask the parents what the child needs. Or try to choose toys that are made of durable materials and will provide years rather than months of playtime. For more good ideas on children's toys, see Chapter 7.

GIFTS OF SERVICE A lot of us have too much stuff, or have too much stuff we don't need, use, or want. Holiday gift giving unfortunately can result in getting more unwanted stuff.

A growing tradition is to give the gift of services rather than stuff. A grandparent who is looking for a meaningful gift might give piano lessons or a ballet class. This way grandma spends her money on something the child likes rather than a toy or item of clothing, which may be quickly shoved to the back of the closet.

Or, give the gift of services that you (or your child) can perform. These sorts of gifts are great for kids who don't have a lot of their own money to spend. Younger kids might give "coupons" for tasks like emptying the dishwasher or putting away groceries. Older kids might give "coupons" for services like babysitting a younger sibling or washing the car. Kids of all ages can give coupons for hugs.

Other good "coupon" gifts include offering to:

- Shovel snow.
- Make dinner.
- Weed the garden.
- Take the dog for a walk.
- Mow the lawn.

One of the greatest gifts parents can give is time with your children. It doesn't cost any money and usually consumes little in the way of resources, but it can mean a lot. For example, if you have a young baby at home, you may want to give the gift of one-on-one time with each of your older children.

BUYING GREEN GIFTS The green movement has spawned all sorts of new products advertised as being healthier or better for the environment. Websites tout everything from organic cotton bathrobes to eco-friendly handbags. In fact, environmentalism (the old term for being green) is a long-standing tradition (just ask your hippie parents). Being green is neither new nor does it require the purchasing of *any* consumer goods. In fact, one of the best ways to go green is to *forgo* purchasing goods, especially the ones you don't need.

In fact, the better way to make a difference to our planet is by reducing your consumption of natural resources, not by buying a gift bearing the label "green." This means using your bike or public transportation instead of hopping in your car. It means lowering your house's thermostat by a few degrees in the winter and putting on a sweater. It means eating more vegetables and less meat (because the raising of beef consumes a lot of energy and produces a lot of greenhouse gases). None of these practices have much to do with holiday giving, but they make a much bigger impact on our planet.

One way in which to choose "greener" or eco-friendly gifts is to buy ones that were made locally. This cuts down on the environmental cost of shipping products from factories overseas. A locally made product is less likely to contain toxic chemicals (although of course it is no guarantee). You are also supporting your local businesses and craftspeople.

Another green gift idea is to give consumable items, such as food. For example, organic fruits, vegetables, and meats are better for the planet and our health, but many people find that these foods are expensive. (See Chapter 2 for ways to save when eating organic.) This year, why not give gift cards for food markets that sell organic produce. Or, if you know the recipient loves beef, give a cut of meat from a grass-fed animal.

Valentine's Day

The holiday of lovers is also a big holiday for the little ones in our lives. Each year, children and their adults trade more than one billion paper valentine cards. Candy and flowers round out the holiday traditions. Let's look at some eco-friendly choices for both your children's classmates and grown-ups alike.

CLASSROOM CARD EXCHANGES   One of the annual traditions in elementary schools is to trade Valentine's Day cards. Many of us grew up with the tradition of exchanging preprinted cards, on which we simply scrawled our names 30 times and then handed them out to our classmates. These preprinted, impersonal cards are convenient but somehow empty of feeling.

Perhaps to combat this emptiness, in recent years some parents have upped the ante and now send small bags of candy. If your child's school has a similar tradition, remember that you don't need to do something (especially if it is bad for the environment and children's health) just because everyone else is doing it.

If you do want to add something special to your child's valentine, there are lots of ways that you can do so without promoting tooth decay or creating piles of candy wrappers. You could send school supplies that you know children can use, such as holiday-themed pencils or boxes of crayons. Don't give plastic miniature toys, however, which will quickly become junk and end up in the garbage. Mention to the teacher or school principal your concerns about too much candy in schools.

As for the impersonal preprinted cards festooned with cartoon characters, why not skip them this year and have your child make his own cards for his friends? Give him some colored paper scraps from a previous project, a few markers, and some stickers, and you'll be surprised how creative and fun making Valentine's Day cards can be.

GROWN-UP GIFTS   For the grown-ups in our lives, it is customary to give flowers or chocolate on Valentine's Day. Yet most flowers available in North America in February were grown in South America and shipped on planes or trucks at the expense of pollution-generating fossil-fuel consumption. These flowers are usually grown with pesticides and sprayed with preservatives. Much of the chocolate on the market was grown on farms where impoverished children do much of the labor for minimal wages. (See the Mother's Day section for more on flowers, and the Easter section for more on chocolate.)

Here are some tips on reducing your impact this Valentine's Day:

- ✓ Buy recycled-paper cards or make your own from recycled paper.
- ✓ Send your Valentine's Day cards by e-mail.
- ✓ Buy organically grown or fair-trade flowers. (See Mother's Day.)
- ✓ Choose fair-trade or USDA-organic chocolate. (See Easter.)
- ✓ Think outside the chocolate box: Is there something that your sweetie might enjoy more than a box of chocolates? Find another way to show your love this year.

Spring Holidays

After months of short, dark wintry days, we welcome the pastel colors and images of baby bunnies and chicks that fill store advertisements each spring. The season offers the opportunity to celebrate the annual reawakening of Earth. Let's honor Mother Nature with customs that emphasize conservation and renewal.

EASTER Easter is a Christian holiday, yet today it is celebrated by many Americans with a decidedly secular emphasis on worldly goods, such as candy-filled baskets and chocolate bunnies. Many schools, stores, and institutions now use the term, "spring holiday," but we are still accustomed to referring to the holiday with the terms Easter baskets, Easter eggs, and Easter dresses.

Whatever terms you use, children love the traditions of dyeing or painting eggs and hunting for eggs and gift-filled baskets. We parents face the challenge of coming up with inventive and playful experiences that don't overload our little ones on sugar or require buying cheap plastic items that are poisoning our planet and that our children quickly lose interest in. Here are some suggestions:

Dye eggs the natural way: Choose all natural food dyes rather than chemical ones. Combine 4 cups of water with 2 tablespoons of white vinegar and one of the colorful natural dyes listed below. Bring to a boil and simmer for 30 minutes. Cool the mixture and place your boiled eggs (organic, certified humane, vegetarian-fed, or cage-free that came in nonpolystyrene packaging) in the dye for another 30 minutes.

Create colors the natural way:

PINK fresh or dried beets, pomegranate juice, red onion skins, rhubarb stalks (chopped), frozen raspberries

BLUE/PURPLE boiled red cabbage, frozen blueberries, frozen blackberries

GREEN spinach

BROWN coffee, tea

ORANGE paprika, chili powder

YELLOW turmeric, cumin, orange rind, lemon rind

Instead of plastic grass, try compostable wheatgrass or recyclable raffia. Or have your children plant wheatgrass seeds about two weeks before Easter in a basket-size pot. Place on a sunny windowsill and by Easter your child will have a nice soft bed of grass on which to put the eggs. Your child can decorate the pot by painting it and adorning it with ribbon.

Plastic Easter eggs should be saved and reused from year to year. Or try wrapping your goodies in colorful paper. It may be possible to find cardboard eggs at some craft shops.

Stuff your child's Easter basket with art supplies, playing cards, or toys you know he or she will use. Add candy and chocolate in accordance with your views on how much candy your child should be eating. When selecting candy and chocolate, look for Fair-trade Certified chocolate and candy that is free of artificial dyes and preservatives.

THE FACTS

People spend nearly as much money on Easter candy as on Halloween candy, according to the National Retail Federation's 2008 numbers.

SWEET DECEPTION: CHOCOLATE Chocolate is a favorite of children and adults alike. It comes from the cocoa plant (*Theobroma cacao*) and grows well in shady areas in the fertile soils under the forest canopy trees. This environment provides a home to numerous plants and insects, including pollinators and natural predators of the insects that eat cocoa leaves. Growing cocoa can be done without overly disturbing forests and wildlife corridors.

Unfortunately, many growers, under pressure to produce more cocoa, are turning to clear-cutting forests to grow hybrid varieties that thrive in full sun. This more intensive agriculture demands more chemicals and farming practices that contribute to soil erosion and loss of soil fertility.

In the cocoa-growing region of Côte d'Ivoire (Ivory Coast), it is common for children to work on the family plantation instead of going to school. According to the U.N.'s International Labour Organization, about a third of school-age children living in cocoa-producing households have never attended school. Several organizations are working to provide fair prices that encourage farmers to continue to plant shade-grown cocoa. By receiving fair wages, growers can continue to grow their crop in the shade and conserve the larger forest ecosystem, while earning wages that allow them to reduce their dependency on child labor.

See Eco-Tip: Deciphering Chocolate Labels, below, for suggestions on buying planet- and people-friendly chocolate.

ECO-TIP: DECIPHERING CHOCOLATE LABELS

Organic chocolate is becoming a popular option in the U.S. Sales of organic chocolate were up 49 percent in 2006 over the previous year. Although more than $70 million worth of organic chocolate was purchased in the U.S., it is a small fraction of the $6 billion global chocolate market. Fair-trade chocolate makes up about one percent of this global market. Here are the labels you are likely to encounter:

✓ **USDA-Certified Organic,** *www.ams.usda.gov*: The USDA mandates that certified organic chocolate be from cocoa grown without synthetic pesticides and herbicides on land that has been well-managed to control soil erosion and maintain soil health. Look for the USDA-Certified Organic label.

✓ **Fair Trade Certified,** *www.transfairusa.org*: Products with this certification must contain cocoa obtained entirely from plantations where workers were paid a fair price and worked under fair labor conditions. The Fair Trade Certified label is bestowed by a nonprofit organization called TransFair USA, which is a member of Fairtrade Labelling Organizations International (FLO). The certification also requires that growers avoid hazardous agrochemicals such as DDT, methyl parathion, and lindane, as well as conduct environmental impact assessments, properly use and store agrochemicals, conserve soil and water, and avoid genetically modified organisms (GMOs). Fair-trade certification is available in the U.S. for coffee, tea, cocoa and chocolate, fresh fruit, flowers, sugar, rice, wine, and vanilla.

✓ **Rainforest Alliance Certified, *www.rainforest-alliance.org*: This certification indicates that the cocoa was grown using policies that protect the environment and promote worker health, social justice, and community development. Growers may not use pesticides that are banned by the U.S. Environmental Protection Agency (EPA), the European Union, or those listed by the nonprofit environmental group Pesticide Action Network on its Dirty Dozen list. Certified farms must pay wages that are at least as much as the local minimum wage and take steps to reduce the involvement of children in the growing and harvesting, unless it is a tradition to have children help with the harvest and it does not interfere with education. A product can bear the Rainforest Alliance Certified seal if at minimum 30 percent of the product is from certified sources, but the percentage must be indicated below the seal.**

EASTER EGG HUNT A time-honored tradition is the Easter egg hunt. Today this involves hunting for brightly colored plastic eggs, each one containing small pieces of candy. If you are trying to cut down on candy, why not put small amounts of change—quarters, dimes, nickels, or pennies—in each egg. Your children can collect the money, and, depending on their age, have a lot of fun adding it up. You can have them put some of the money in the bank, give some to charity, and the rest they can save for a toy or book they've been wanting.

Another idea is to put clues in the Easter eggs. Each clue should lead to the next egg. This is more challenging and more fun than just hunting around the yard for eggs. Eventually the clues lead to an Easter basket containing a quality gift such as a book, gardening tools, a homemade puppet, or art supplies. (Try to find a gift your child will treasure.) Or give a "coupon" for some much needed parent-child time.

When you find eco-friendly alternatives to commercialized holiday traditions, you are creating family traditions that can be passed down through generations. For example, why not start the tradition of making an annual holiday craft? Make your own chocolate eggs instead of buying them. Make Easter sock puppets and decorate them as chicks, bunnies, or ducks. Then have the children host a puppet show for the adults. Older children may enjoy hiding eggs for the adults to find. Or, do a charitable act as a family, like planting trees, clearing trails, or helping out in a soup kitchen.

GREEN ON A SHOESTRING

If you have a daughter, you've no doubt been tempted by the becoming frocks that hit the stores each spring. Before you buy, think carefully about the need for such a dress. Is your daughter going to be attending several spring parties where dressing up is required? Or will that dress just end up getting stained with wet grass and mud at the town's annual Easter egg hunt? Shop according to your child's needs. You may be able to find gently used clothes at thrift and consignment shops or hold a kids' clothing swap with your neighbors.

AN "ECO-KOSHER" PASSOVER Kosher meats have always had a reputation for being of high quality. A growing number of families are now extending the traditional Jewish value of protecting the planet to foods they serve at their table. Families are choosing locally grown, organic foods and providing meals that are both nutritionally and spiritually healthy.

The tradition of mindful eating reflects values such as acting as Earth's caretaker and being aware of where food comes from. Some families have chosen to grow foods at their homes or in community gardens. Others have joined cooperative farms or are purchasing foods from farmers markets.

Judaism is not the only religion that has embraced sustainable food provenance. In recent years the Presbyterian Church (USA) and the Unitarian Church have run programs or trainings that bring together faith and food.

EARTH DAY Earth Day is a great time to reflect on all that has been given to us by our planet. See Chapter 5 for eco-friendly activities for children of all ages. Or check out these suggestions:

- ✓ Share nature with children: If you volunteer with a scout troop, incorporate Earth Day into your activities.
- ✓ Go on a family hike: Bring along a guide book that will help you identify birds, blossoming trees, or spring flowers.

✓ Plant trees: Many communities have tree-planting programs in April to celebrate Arbor Day. The exact date of Arbor Day varies according to the best time to plant trees in each state. Check *ArborDay.org* for your state's date. You can also request seedlings at *ArborDay.org* for planting in your yard.

✓ Prepare a garden: Break ground on a new garden, or revive last year's plot.

✓ Join a community Earth Day activity such as picking up trash at a local park. To find events in your area, check www.*EarthDay.net*, www.*EPA.gov/ EarthDay*, or the Nature Conservancy's website, *www.nature.org*.

✓ Take a walk in your neighborhood. Pick up any trash you find.

✓ Try to avoid using your car all day. Walk or bike instead.

✓ Make crafts from items that would have been trashed, such as a flowerpot from an old yogurt container.

✓ Spring clean. Clear out the basement. Donate your old household appliances to a local thrift store. Or have a garage sale and donate the proceeds to a nature-oriented charity.

✓ Plan an Earth Day potluck dinner on your block. Block parties build community spirit and help neighbors get to know each other. Exchange tips on composting, chemical-free lawn care, or recycling. Help spread the word about making greener choices.

✓ Make it Earth Day everyday by reducing your consumption of natural resources, reusing items instead of buying new ones, and recycling the things you no longer need.

Mother's Day and Father's Day

Anyone who has raised kids knows that children have no idea how much parents do for them, from infancy when we spend endless nights rocking them to sleep, to adolescence when we spend sleepless nights wondering what time they'll get home and whether the car will be in one piece. Teach your children to honor Mother's Day and Father's Day, and of course don't forget the grandparents.

MOTHER'S DAY Mother's Day has become a big commercial holiday, with page after page of store ads arriving at the door to tell you about big savings on jewelry, bath products, clothes, and handbags. Yet most moms simply want to be recognized for their hard work and told they are loved. They may enjoy a day off from mom-type duties, or a special excursion with Dad and the kids.

Homemade gifts are great for moms, who love to display and treasure their children's artwork. Encourage the kids to use recycled materials. They could make a vase from a tomato sauce jar. Cards for Mom can be made from scrap paper or computer paper used on only one side.

A sure Mom-pleaser is the gift of doing some of her household chores. Older children could clean the house, top to bottom. Provide the kids with natural plant-based soap and vinegar instead of strong cleaning products. See Chapter 1 for suggestions on eco-friendly cleaning supplies. When kids clean up without having to be reminded, that is a real treat for Mom.

Breakfast in bed for Mom is a tradition in many households. If Mom is a coffee-drinker, make a cup of shade-grown coffee to warm up her morning. Stock the kitchen with whole wheat toaster waffles for the younger kids. Older children could make pancakes from scratch. Choose real maple syrup instead of the high-fructose corn syrup variety. Yes, it costs more, so try to use as little as possible. Or spread jam and pour honey over your waffles or pancakes.

If your children simply must splurge and buy Mom a gift, help them access the growing number of online stores offering green gift ideas such as organic cotton clothing, less toxic beauty supplies, aromatherapy, and more. If you are helping your child pick out a gift, look for durable materials and lasting quality. Make sure the store accepts returns, too, so that Mom can take the item back if it is something she doesn't like or cannot use.

Flowers are a popular choice for moms on their special day. Don't rush to the florist, however, without first considering where the flowers came from and what chemicals they were grown with.

Many flowers available in U.S. markets in May were grown in South America and flown north at great costs in terms of fossil fuels consumed and greenhouse gases emitted. These flowering beauties would be virtually impossible without chemical interventions. Herbicides keep the massive flower plantations clear of weeds. Insecticides prevent pests from chewing unsightly holes in leaves and petals. Preservatives keep flowers looking fresh during transit.

Many of the people who are getting the highest exposure to these pesticides on flower plantations are children and young women of childbearing age, according to the International Labor Rights Forum (ILRF). Pesticides can cause skin rashes, respiratory problems, eye problems, and neurological problems. When workers become too sick to work, they are often sent home rather than given medical treatment. Children who work in the flower fields are usually poor and are often malnourished, which can make them more susceptible to pesticide toxicity. The miscarriage rate is higher in women working in flower fields than it is in the general population, according to the ILRF.

The United States has banned many of the toxic chemicals used in the flower fields of South America, but these countries sometimes have trouble enforcing bans and laws that require workers wear protective clothing, gloves, and eyewear. Pesticide residues can persist on petals, stems, and leaves, right through to the day when your child picks out the flowers at the florist shop.

If flowers are a must for you, it is now possible to buy organically grown florist-quality flowers online and have them shipped anywhere in the nation. Several certification programs have cropped up that ensure consumers the flowers were grown according to eco-friendly standards. These include:

- ✓ Veriflora, *www.veriflora.com*: Flowers and potted plants are certified to have been grown using farming practices that build soil, use fewer chemicals, generate fewer greenhouse gas emissions, and promote an equitable and healthy workplace for farm workers.

- ✓ Fair Trade Certified, *www.transfairusa.org*: Ensures that flower workers make a living wage, are able to send children to school, use sustainable farming methods, and receive benefits such as 12 weeks paid maternity leave and child care.

- ✓ USDA-Certified Organic, *www.ams.usda.gov*: Flowers were grown according to USDA National Organic Program standards, which prohibit the use of synthetic pesticides and herbicides.

- ✓ Florverde, *www.florverde.org:* Requires the safe use of fertilizers, integrated pest management, and water conservation. Child labor is prohibited and safe working conditions must be in place.

GREEN ON A SHOESTRING

Buying organic flowers via the Internet is not likely to fit the budget-conscious green consumer. If you must give fresh flowers, consider the options:

✓ Check your phone directory for local nurseries that grow flowers in greenhouses.

✓ Buy a potted plant that has been grown in a greenhouse, preferably from a local farmer.

✓ Find an organic flower grower near you by visiting the website Local Harvest at *www.localharvest.org.*

✓ Help your child plant bulbs in the fall that will be blooming around Mother's Day.

FATHER'S DAY Fathers are notoriously hard to buy gifts for. Instead, why not make Dad breakfast in bed on his special day. When breakfast is over, engage Dad in a walk, bike ride, fishing trip, or outing to a nature preserve or the beach. The best gift is the gift of spending time together. Create a family tradition such as taking a day trip to a national park, the seashore, or the grandparents' house.

If you must buy a gift, skip the usual items unless Dad really does need a new belt or tie. Appeal to his frugal side and get him some solar patio lights. Is he a coffee drinker? Try certified fair-trade or organic coffee. Is he into gadgets? Get him a solar-powered flashlight or hand-cranked radio. Or, better yet, have the kids make homemade gifts such as a barbecue apron or T-shirt that says "World's Best Dad."

Service gifts are just right for dads, too. Your teen may want to give the gift of mowing the lawn (if he or she doesn't already do it). Dad may appreciate help with a project he has been working on around the house. Don't forget to give him some quiet time to read the paper and drink coffee.

Summer Holidays

Summer holidays are family favorites. Many families choose one of these holidays as the day for their annual family reunion. Favorite activities include parades, music festivals, campouts, and of course, fireworks on the Fourth of July.

OUTDOOR COOKING What summer holiday would be complete without outdoor cooking? Three out of four households own an outdoor grill or smoker, according to the Hearth, Patio, and Barbecue Association. Yet not all outdoor grills are created equal when it comes to their environmental impact. Here is a rundown of the three main options: gas grills, electric grills, and charcoal grills.

GAS GRILL A grill that runs on liquefied petroleum gas (LPG) is your most environmentally friendly option. These grills produce the least amount of the greenhouse gas carbon dioxide, and they produce less soot and other respirable particles than do charcoal grills.

ELECTRIC GRILL Outdoor electric grills release the fewest pollutants at the time of grilling, so your backyard air will stay the cleanest. However the manufacture and transport of electricity release carbon dioxide and other emissions into the air. Given that 50 percent of the nation's electricity is generated from coal, electric grills are big polluters.

CHARCOAL GRILL These grills produce the highest amounts of pollutants directly into the air of your backyard barbecue party. Charcoal and wood smoke contains particles of soot that can worsen asthma attacks and cause respiratory irritation. These grills also release volatile organic compounds (VOCs), some of which are linked to cancer. Most charcoal-users douse charcoal in lighter fluid, which generates additional polluting chemicals.

If you must use charcoal, look for natural charcoal briquettes or wood lump made from well-managed forest sources. If you choose wood lump charcoal, make sure it is made from whole wood pieces rather than processed wood that may contain formaldehyde. Avoid conventional charcoal made with additives such as sodium nitrate and petroleum products, and easy-to-light brands that have been soaked in lighter fluid, since some experts suggest that burning these kinds of charcoal may release toxic by-products into your food. To get charcoal started without lighter fluid, use natural wood lighters or lighter cubes.

THE FACTS

On the Fourth of July, Americans who grill will burn the equivalent of 2,300 acres of forest and consume enough energy to power a town the size of Flagstaff, Arizona, according to the ORNL analysis.

When it comes to greenhouse gas pollution, the gas grill is the clear winner. Operating a gas grill for an hour emits 5.6 pounds of carbon dioxide while a charcoal grill sends up about 11 pounds. An electric grill creates about 15 pounds of carbon dioxide due to the environmental cost of producing electricity, according to a 2003 study by scientists at the U.S. Department of Energy's Oak Ridge National Laboratory (ORNL).[2] A 2009 study found that charcoal created a carbon footprint that was nearly three times greater than that of liquid propane gas when the environmental costs of creating charcoal are included.[3]

If you are looking for zero-emission cooking, and you live in a sunny part of the country, consider trying a solar cooker or solar grill. These cookers typically feature a reflective surface that directs the sun's energy toward your meat and vegetables while making no noxious greenhouse gases. You can buy solar cookers or make one yourself. Since beef, poultry, and fish can harbor dangerous bacteria, and other pathogens, make sure the food is fully cooked before eating.

FRIENDLIER FIREWORKS What would the Fourth of July be without fireworks? Better for the environment, for one thing. Fireworks delight many children (and scare the pants off others), but today's fireworks are not very eco-friendly.

So what is so bad about fireworks? Aerial fireworks, that is, the ones used in overhead displays, contain perchlorate, a chemical that speeds up burning and is commonly used in rocket fuel. Several studies have linked perchlorate to reduced production of thyroid hormone, which in turn can affect growth and development in children.

When the fireworks explode, perchlorate is released and falls back toward the ground. If the fireworks displays are held over lakes or other bodies of water, the perchlorate falls into the water. A study of water samples collected from one lake after a fireworks show found that the perchlorate level was a thousand times higher than normal.[4]

Another problem with fireworks is that they derive their colors from heavy metals such as copper and barium, which have been linked to adverse health effects. And they produce smoke and other toxic combustion products and particulate matter that float down to Earth where we humans can inhale them.

Eco-friendlier fireworks do exist, but most cities and organizations across the nation don't use them because they cost more than perchlorate-containing fireworks, which are usually made overseas using inexpensive labor under inadequate safety provisions. See The Science Behind It for more on Earth-friendly fireworks.

Many people object to fireworks displays because they disturb wildlife. A display in a California coastal town disrupted the nesting of several species of seabirds.

Home fireworks are a popular tradition in many areas, but five states have banned them due to the potential for injuries and deaths. In 2008, roughly 7,000 people were injured when using personal fireworks, according to the U.S. Consumer Product Safety Commission (CPSC). The injuries were mainly clustered in the 15- to 19-year-old range. Young children should not be allowed to handle fireworks. As with municipal fireworks, home fireworks generate toxic pollutants. The best eco-friendly and child-safe choice is to forgo home fireworks.

GREEN DICTIONARY

PERCHLORATE

A component of rocket fuel and fireworks that has been detected in drinking water and groundwater in 35 states, according to the EPA. It has also been detected in cow's milk and infant formula. It interferes with iodide uptake into the thyroid gland, potentially causing harm to fetuses, newborns, and children.

Although not Earth-friendly, fireworks shows are an American institution and are not going away any time soon. If you are concerned about the environmental or health impact of fireworks, here are some suggestions:

- Make your concerns known to your municipality. You may not be the only person concerned about the environmental impact of fireworks. Tell them that more eco-friendly alternatives exist (See The Science Behind It).
- Reduce your exposure to firework pollutants by watching them from a far distance.
- If you find pieces of firework packaging after the show, alert your municipality (or the party responsible for the display). Do not let children handle them because they contain traces of toxic chemicals.

Buy Nothing Day

No book on eco-friendly living would be complete without a section on Buy Nothing Day. Many Americans have this day off, but you won't find it marked on any calendar. Buy Nothing Day is held the day after Thanksgiving. Retailers call it Black Friday, the day when deep discounts lure shoppers from their postprandial slumbers and out to the malls and big box stores in the early morning.

To celebrate this holiday, all you have to do is avoid malls and stores on one of the country's biggest shopping days of the year, and, literally, buy nothing. Not a hard task if you don't like crowds, but it could be tough if you really wanted to scoop up the deep discounts that retailers have begun offering.

The goal of the holiday, say its advocates, is to encourage family togetherness and stewardship of our planet while discouraging rampant consumerism. It is a great time to reflect on how reducing what we buy is good for the planet. It is also a great time to reconnect with relatives who you haven't talked to in a while.

Buy Nothing Day was started nearly two decades ago and has caught on in 65 countries around the world. Some people celebrate it by holding demonstrations at malls where they cut up credit cards.

Tips for celebrating Buy Nothing Day:

✓ Play football with relatives at the park.
✓ Rake fall leaves with the kids.

✓ Take a family walk or hike at a park, nature preserve, or around the neighborhood.

✓ Play board games like chess or checkers.

✓ Sort through old family photos together.

Take Action

▸ Keep birthday parties simple, especially when children are young and are unlikely to notice how many guests were invited or what food was served.

▸ Choose eco-friendly themes and follow through with reusable tableware, napkins, and decorations.

▸ Send invitations and thank-you notes by e-mail instead of sending paper versions.

▸ Help lessen the number of unwanted gifts your child gets by suggesting that guests donate money or needed items to a charity of your child's choice.

▸ Tie charitable giving to the theme of the party, such as a rain forest–themed party teamed with donations to an animal-preservation fund.

▸ When wrapping presents, use reusable birthday-themed bags that you buy or make at home with help from your child. Or make wrapping paper out of old magazines, maps, or scrap cloth.

▸ Make a healthier cake at home using natural ingredients and icing made with food-based dyes instead of artificial ones.

▸ Choose to give party favors that children will use and enjoy such as books or art materials rather than cheap plastic toys.

▸ Get creative and help your child make his or her own Halloween costume out of items you have around the house.

▸ Consider giving out healthier treats or noncandy gifts this Halloween.

▸ Have your child trade his or her trick-or-treating candy for a more worthwhile item, such as a new book.

▸ Serve a healthier turkey this year by choosing one that is USDA-certified organic. Look for a fresh (not frozen) bird. Pile plates high with nutritious fall vegetables.

▸ Go light on holiday lights or skip them altogether. If buying new ones, chose LED lights or consider solar-powered lights.

▸ Forgo the artificial Christmas tree for a live one or a containerized one that you can plant outside after the holiday.

▸ Choose locally grown flowers over ones grown in South America, or give a potted plant that will blossom in the spring.

▸ Consider making your own gifts this year or giving the gift of service or time.

▸ Use food-based dyes to color eggs without chemicals.

▸ Make Earth Day meaningful by planting trees, clearing trails, or picking up beach trash.

▸ Choose a cleaner-burning grill for your summer cookouts.

THE SCIENCE BEHIND IT

The Science of Fireworks

Our nation's fascination with fireworks goes back to before the time of the Revolutionary War. Today's fireworks are more sophisticated but still work on the same principles of the rockets of yore.

The brilliant lights we see each July are created using pyrotechnic rockets. Each rocket contains propellant, chemical binders, fuel, oxygen producers (oxidizers), and colorants. The propellant sends the rocket into the air, the chemical binders keep everything together, the fuel and oxidizer create the explosive burst, and the resulting heat causes the colorants to vaporize and produce brilliant colors in the sky.

Today the oxidizer of choice is perchlorate because it is more chemically stable than previous materials and performs better in terms of safety, reproducibility, and cost. Today's colorants are primarily made from metals, some of which are toxic. Copper creates blues and greens, sodium creates yellow, barium makes green, and strontium is used for red.

Perchlorate has been linked to thyroid hormone problems, and some of the metals are toxic, so the race is on to find more environmentally friendly alternatives.

One such alternative is already available at DMD Systems in New Mexico. These pyrotechnics were invented by rocket scientists formerly of the U.S. Department of Energy's Lawrence Livermore National Laboratory. The fireworks are based on nitrocellulose, a material that burns cleaner and creates a lot less smoke than traditional fireworks make. Many of the fireworks that DMD Systems produces require little or no perchlorate and less of the metal colorants.

So far the nitrocellulose pyrotechnics have been used primarily for indoor shows where smoke and toxic chemicals could endanger or annoy the crowds. The higher price tag of these low-smoke and low-perchlorate materials, however, has prohibited towns and cities across the nation from adopting them for their annual shows. Instead, the towns continue to buy perchlorate-containing pyrotechnics made overseas. With increasing interest in green technologies, assisted by stronger environmental regulations and consumer demand, we may just see cleaner-burning fireworks at our local Fourth of July celebrations in the near future.

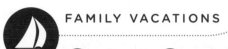

FAMILY VACATIONS

Going Green When Getting Away From It All

THE FAMILY VACATION IS AN AMERICAN TRADITION. PARENTS NEED a respite from workplace pressures, and kids benefit from the opportunity to explore new places and face new challenges. For some kids, those challenges may include saying "hello" in a foreign language, while for others it may be simply eating in a restaurant other than the familiar chains.

Whether your idea of a family vacation is packing the kids in the car for a multistate trip to the national parks, or jetting to a Caribbean island to escape the winter blues, you will be consuming fossil fuels and other resources. Even the increasingly popular "staycation" requires some energy use.

Being green doesn't mean huddling at home, however. You *can* satisfy your travel lust and still tread lightly on the planet. You may have to give extra thought to where to go, how to get there, where to stay, and what to do. Choosing more responsible ways to travel can be intensely rewarding, providing experiences that you wouldn't have had by staying in gated resorts that cater to every whim. (Of course, there are eco-friendly gated resorts, too.)

Traveling with kids presents special challenges. You will want to make sure that the destination has child-friendly activities and adequate health care facilities. You may be looking for services such as babysitting so that you and your spouse can finally get in that much needed date-night. Travel time will likely be a major consideration, since long plane flights and car trips can be tedious for youngsters.

Today many companies offer eco-friendly tour packages, and it is easier than ever before to select a company that can arrange your green travel plans.

Or you can plan a trip yourself, saving dollars along with saving the planet's resources. Whatever your family's tastes and budget, you can find ideas to cut your global eco-footprint in this chapter.

Trains, Planes, and Automobiles

Americans love to travel, whether by car, plane, or train. Vacation travel consumes considerable amounts of fuel and generates significant amounts of the greenhouse gas carbon dioxide. So what is the best way to get to your vacation destination? Let's look at the options.

THE GREAT AMERICAN ROAD TRIP The car trip is the quintessential American vacation. Even if you never took a car trip as a child, you probably can envision the endless landscape rolling by, the occasional bouts of car sickness, the chorus of "Are we there yet?" and the fights with siblings over window seats, radio stations, and just about anything else that can be fought over.

Despite all the inconveniences of the car trip, no one form of transportation offers as much freedom as the automobile. Want to take a day excursion to a little-known historical monument? Easily done. Fancy a stop at that quirky roadside attraction? No problem. Americans are addicted to the freedom of going where we choose, when we choose.

For many families the choice to drive is an economical one. Driving is often cheaper than flying, depending on the distance and proximity to airports. It may even be faster once you factor in driving to the airport and waiting in long security lines.

Driving may be the only choice in regions of the country poorly served by airports, train stations, and bus lines. If you have young children, bringing your own car provides a convenient place to stow portable cribs and other gear that babies need.

Yet few American standbys take their toll on the environment the way the automobile does. Transportation is the second leading source of greenhouse gas emissions in the United States, second only to electricity generation. Cars, SUVs, minivans, and light-duty trucks make up almost two-thirds of these emissions, while freight trucks, aircraft, trains, and watercraft make up the rest, according to the U.S. Environmental Protection Agency (EPA).

ECO-TIP: CHOOSING A GREENER CAR

If your car is a gas-guzzler, what should you do? The best way to cut emissions is to stop using your car and jump on public transportation or your bicycle for most of your needs. That isn't a practical solution for most Americans.

Experts don't recommend replacing your car solely to improve your carbon footprint. The manufacture of cars plus the infrastructure associated with them contributes roughly a third of the greenhouse gases generated over your car's lifetime according to a 2009 study by researchers at the University of California, Berkeley.[1] Buying a brand-new car may save on emissions from operating the car but not from manufacture and infrastructure. Buying a new car is only right if you were planning on replacing your old vehicle anyway.

Once you've decided to buy a new or used car, you'll want to put a lot of thought into which model to purchase. Consult safety records and reliability ratings from consumer groups. Keep your eye out for tax incentives that might reduce the cost of buying a fuel-efficient vehicle. Gas mileage is the biggest determinant of how much carbon dioxide your car will emit. It is also the main factor in how much it will cost you to fuel up. Here are some websites for evaluating new car purchases:

- *www.epa.gov/greenvehicles:* This site helps you find the cleanest and most fuel-efficient vehicles.

- *www.fueleconomy.gov:* Contains many helpful pieces of information, including a place to look up the fuel economy of your current vehicle. The site will also tell you how many tons of carbon dioxide per year your car generates.

- *www.hybridcars.com:* Covers information on hybrid gas-electric vehicles as well as other alternative fuel vehicles. The site has a page where you can compare your current vehicle to a hybrid one.

- *www.greenercars.org:* Ranks cars by their entire life cycle impact, from manufacture through gas usage.

When you are replacing a gas-guzzler, it is more important than you think to consider even seemingly small improvements in gas mileage. That is because our standard measure of fuel economy, miles per gallon, is a little misleading when it comes to telling how much gas our cars use (and therefore how much greenhouse gases they generate and how much money you'll spend on gas) per mile driven.

In fact, it is better for the environment to upgrade from an SUV that gets 10 mpg to one that gets 20 mpg, than it is to upgrade from a sedan that gets 25 mpg to a hybrid vehicle that gets 50 mpg. To find out why, see The Science Behind It at the end of this chapter.

IMPROVE YOUR GAS MILEAGE THROUGH BETTER DRIVING

Your choice of vehicle is not the only factor that determines how your driving affects the environment. Your fuel consumption will suffer when you carry heavy loads, take short trips in cold weather, stop and go on city streets, use the air conditioner, and drive up hills. Your driving habits also affect fuel consumption. Here are some tips for improving your gas mileage from the U.S. Environmental Protection Agency (EPA):

- ✓ Drive sensibly. Aggressive driving wastes gas. Rapid acceleration, speeding, and braking use far more gas than moderate acceleration and braking. According to the EPA, aggressive driving can lower your gas mileage by 33 percent at highway speeds and by 5 percent around town. This is like paying an extra 12 to 81 cents per gallon for gas.
- ✓ Observe the speed limit. For most cars and light trucks, gas mileage is highest at speeds between 35 mph and 60 mph. According to the EPA, each 5 mph you drive over 60 mph is like paying an additional 24 cents per gallon for gas.
- ✓ Avoid idling. An idling car gets 0 mpg, yet still generates carbon dioxide and other pollutants.
- ✓ Use cruise control for driving on flat roads. Cruise control keeps your speed constant, which helps save gas, but it is not as effective in hilly terrain.
- ✓ Don't use the four-wheel drive unless you need it. Engaging all four wheels makes the engine work harder.
- ✓ Remove cargo racks from the top of the car. These can create drag, which makes the engine work harder to maintain the speed.
- ✓ Use a bike or walk for short errands. Using your car for short trips means

GREEN ON A SHOESTRING

Many families buy SUVs or minivans because they occasionally go on trips or haul heavy stuff, then regret it when gas prices spike. Instead, consider buying an eco-friendly car for everyday use (or no car at all if you live near public transportation) and renting a gas-guzzler for the occasional off-road camping trip or other adventure.

that the engine never gets up to proper operating temperature, so fuel mileage is suboptimal.

Keeping your car properly maintained also optimizes gas mileage:
- ✓ Keep tires inflated to the levels recommended in the owner's manual of your vehicle. Maintaining the proper pressure can improve gas mileage by around 3.3 percent.
- ✓ Keep engine properly tuned.
- ✓ Use the recommended grade of motor oil.

CAR SEAT SAFETY If you are taking a multistate car trip, check the car seat regulations of each state you'll be visiting. Car seat requirements vary from state to state. Many states require children to be in a booster seat until they reach age eight or weigh 80 pounds. Two states, Wyoming and Tennessee, require that children be in a booster seat until their ninth birthday, although in Tennessee that requirement is waved if the child is taller than four feet nine inches in height. Car seat laws change often so your best bet is to visit the state's website for current information. The Insurance Institute for Highway Safety maintains an easy-to-use map of car seat laws at *www.iihs.org/laws/childrestraint.aspx*.

The American Academy of Pediatrics recommends that children use a booster seat until the adult seat belts fit correctly (usually when the child reaches about four feet nine inches in height and is between 8 and 12 years of age). Oregon is currently the only state that uses only the height rather than an age/weight standard. Whatever your home state's requirements, consider using the more stringent policy.

> **THE FACTS**
>
> Letting your car idle during short stops to drop kids at school does *not* help fuel economy. It actually uses fuel and generates more pollution, according to the EPA.

BACKSEAT BLUES: KEEPING KIDS BUSY On long car trips, parents are tempted to resort to videos. While videos can be good ways to pass the time, too much screen time robs kids of opportunities to be creative. Here are some fun car games for those long rides:
- ✓ Name that tune: Hum the first line of a song and have the children guess the song.
- ✓ 20 questions: One player thinks of an object and the others take turns asking yes/no questions.
- ✓ Rhyming games: Start a poem with a single line such as "I have a friend named Ray" and have your child provide the next line, such as "and he came over to play," and go back and forth.
- ✓ Cliffhanger: One person starts a suspenseful story with a title such as "The Scariest Night Ever." When she gets to a suspenseful part she says, "and then..." and the next player has to continue the story.

✓ Alphabet search: Find the letters of the alphabet on road signs and license plates.

✓ Play "I spy with my little eye..." using objects you can see from the car.

✓ Sing turn-taking songs like "Who Stole the Cookie from the Cookie Jar?"

✓ Bring along activity books that include mazes and fill-in-the-blank sections.

✓ Play audiobooks such as the childhood classic *Charlotte's Web* by E. B. White (Listening Library, 2002).

✓ Break up the trip with frequent stops. Look for parks that have playgrounds.

Several good books are available that are packed with car games. Check online retailers or your local library.

FLY THE NOT-SO-ECO-FRIENDLY SKIES The skies may be friendly on some airlines, but many people are surprised to find out how unfriendly air travel is to the environment. Not only are commercial jet liners fuel hogs, on par with automobiles in terms of fuel consumption per passenger mile, but they also emit pollutants at high altitudes where they have a greater impact than do similar emissions on the ground.

A typical commercial jet has a 25- to 30-year life span, so while today's engineers are working on making jets more fuel efficient, plenty of older planes will crowd the skies for some time to come.

The primary environmental concern is that aircraft generate a large amount of carbon dioxide (CO_2), a global warming gas. Aircraft also emit long streams of water vapor in the form of jet contrails, as well as sulfur dioxide (SO_2) and particles of soot. These also contribute to climate change. Other pollutants include nitrogen oxides (NOx), which contribute to smog and are lung irritants.

Aircraft emissions make up about 12 percent of the carbon dioxide released by the United States each year (and 10 percent of the U.S. total greenhouse gas emissions), according to EPA sources.[2] Globally, that figure is about 2 to 4 percent of global greenhouse gas emissions, according to the International Civil Aviation Organization (ICAO). However, Climate Action Network Europe says that figure could be as much as 9 percent if all types of climate-changing emissions are accounted for. The amount of emissions from aviation is expected to grow around 3 to 4 percent per year, according to ICAO.

On the ground, the concentration of planes taking off and landing make airports some of the worst land-based air pollution sources around. According to one study, New York City's two major airports are two of the city's biggest emitters of volatile organic compounds (VOCs) such as the cancer-causing

GREEN DICTIONARY

GREENHOUSE GAS

A gas capable of warming the Earth's temperature by trapping the sun's energy in the Earth's lower atmosphere. Carbon dioxide is only one greenhouse gas. Others include methane, nitrous oxide (N_2O), hydro-fluorocarbons, perfluorocarbons, and others.

chemical benzene. The constant stream of cars and buses entering and exiting the airports contributes to this pollution: According to the EPA, automobiles and buses produce 56 percent of VOCs at airports, while aircraft give off roughly 33 percent.

ECO-TIP: MAJOR SOURCES OF GREENHOUSE GASES

Transportation is the second largest contributor to greenhouse gases in the United States. The following shows the percentage by sector in 2007.

Sector	Percent of total greenhouse gases
Electricity generation	34%
Transportation	28%
Industry	20%
Agriculture	7%
Commercial	6%
Residential	5%

Source: 2009 U.S. Greenhouse Gas Inventory Report http://www.epa.gov/climatechange/emissions/usinventoryreport.html

DRIVE OR FLY? The energy efficiency of a transportation mode depends on not how many passengers it theoretically can carry but how many it actually does carry. A full plane, while uncomfortable, is better for the environment than one that is 70 percent full. A car loaded with a family of four on a vacation is more environmentally friendly than one carrying a single commuter to work.

Comparing driving to flying depends on many factors, including the plane's make and model, size, wind and other weather conditions, and how many passengers and how much baggage it carries.

A car's greenhouse gas emission depends not only on the car design—its weight, aerodynamic design, and horsepower—but also on the number of people and suitcases it carries, whether air-conditioning is on, and whether it is being driven in stop and go traffic or on a bucolic highway. Long-distance car travel usually requires sleeping in hotels and eating in restaurants, activities which have their own environmental consequences.

These many factors make it difficult to compare planes to cars, but studies have found that flying creates two to ten times more climate-warming effects per person per mile than driving in a car does, once all the emissions from aircraft are included.[3]

TRAINS AND BUSES Ah, the romance of the rails. The rhythmic sway of the cars. The rattle of the wheels. The savings of greenhouse gases.

Trains are a relatively eco-positive way of transport. A train uses about roughly half the energy and generates less than a third of the greenhouse gas emissions as a large commercial aircraft, according to the 2009 U.C. Berkeley study.

Unfortunately few domestic vacationers find train travel to suit their needs. The lack of high-speed rail lines in the United States makes rail travel a slow and leisurely endeavor. Yet traveling by train gives families the opportunity to see parts of the landscape that few people see, and many of the routes offer unparalleled views of the ocean or mountains.

THE FACTS

Buses are an environmentally friendly option—as long as they have enough passengers. A bus with five or fewer people is less energy-efficient than an SUV, according to a 2009 study by scientists at the University of California, Berkeley.

TRAINS FOR TOTS Train aficionados—many of whom are children—will love riding the train, but high-spirited kids may resort to racing down the aisles to get out their excess energy. Here are some tips for traveling on trains with children:

- ✓ Bring lots of board games, toys, and distractions. Try some of the games listed on page 337.
- ✓ Take lots of walks up and down the train. Visit the observation car and the snack car. Talk with the conductor.
- ✓ Eat in the dining car if there is one.

Buses are a much overlooked form of transportation for family vacations. When full, they are a very eco-conscious method of travel, consuming far less fuel and generating less pollution than driving a personal automobile or flying. When choosing to go by bus, you'll have to consider factors such as trip duration, your child's ability to sit still for long periods of time, and how you'll get around when you get to your destination.

Greener Lodgings

Choosing a hotel is often about location, but that doesn't mean you have to ignore environmental impacts. A number of hotel chains have implemented eco-friendly practices and energy-saving programs. Your choices of where to stay are looking better and better.

KITCHEN TABLE TALK

Should You Pay for Carbon Offsets?

You want to take that dream vacation to Europe, but the idea of generating 3,000 pounds of carbon dioxide per family member is holding you back. One option that has sprung up in the last few years is to offset your carbon dioxide production by donating money to a climate-friendly project that is working to reduce the amount of greenhouse gases emitted into the environment.

These "carbon-offsets" can be "purchased" at numerous Internet sites. (Your purchase is actually a donation to support a greenhouse gas reduction project.) At these carbon-offset sites, you enter your travel itinerary, and the site calculates how much carbon dioxide your flight will generate and charges you accordingly. The longer the flight, the more carbon dioxide produced and the higher the cost of the carbon-offset.

The amount you pay depends on how far you plan to travel, but it will also depend on which carbon-offset company or site you use. Your flight to Europe might cost $17.85 at one carbon-offset calculator whereas another site charges five dollars more for the exact same flight itinerary. These differences reflect uncertainties in the models that the organizations use to calculate the amount of aircraft greenhouse gases as well as differences in the price per ton of CO_2.

Of course you'll want to go with a site that is certified as using the most accurate assumptions about how to calculate the offset for your European flight. One of the best certifications available is fittingly called "The Gold Standard," so look for carbon-offset companies that use this standard.

Whichever site you choose, before you click, you'll want to know that your hard-earned cash really is going to climate-change positive activities. The best activities to invest in, according to climate researchers at Tufts University, are ones that help us transition away from using fossil fuels. These include projects that foster the development of renewable energy, such as wind farms or solar power, or increase the energy efficiency of the transportation sector.

The Tufts researchers recommend against purchasing carbon-offsets for carbon sequestration projects such as preserving forests. Although protecting forests is a worthy goal, these projects are not proven to reduce the amount of carbon dioxide in the atmosphere.

When evaluating websites that offer carbon-offsets, ask:

1. Does the company invest in projects that truly reduce emissions and at the same time benefit local populations and ecosystems?

2. Are your emissions calculated correctly?

3. How is your money used?

4. Does the company work transparently?

5. Does the company use third-party verification to ensure that they are doing what they claim?

For more information on choosing a carbon-offset program, see the consumer handout *Flying Green: How to Protect the Climate and Travel Responsibly* published by the Tufts University Climate Initiative and available at *www.tufts.edu/tie/carbonoffsets/TCI-offset-handout.htm.*

ECO-LODGING Whether you crave the intimacy of an inn or the expansiveness of a large resort, you'll find many hotels and lodges that have set green goals. How well these establishments achieve these goals will depend on their commitment, ownership, management, and philosophy.

To really reduce your ecological footprint, your best option may be to choose a small, energy efficient inn or lodge that is dedicated to treading lightly on the planet. You may find a small eco-friendly hotel that serves locally grown organic food, or perhaps a family-owned (and family-friendly) bed-and-breakfast.

When considering where to stay, don't overlook the transportation options. You may be able to find a centrally located resort where you can park your car and not drive for the entire week, going everywhere on foot, by bike, or on public transportation. Some hotels provide bikes or rent them for a small fee.

If you prefer to stay in a large hotel, look for ones that have in place a substantial green program. Hotels are our home away from home, but their multiguest nature makes them big resource-guzzlers. Compared to your home, a typical hotel uses far more water, electricity, and goods per person.

We guests are often complicit in this wastage. While we may conserve resources at home, we feel entitled to be pampered at hotels, so we take longer showers, leave lights on, and utilize single-use plastic bottles of shampoo (or stow them in our luggage). In addition to paying for wasteful guest behaviors, hotels must expend energy on heating, cooling, and lighting public spaces even when they are not in use.

Many hotels are now advertising that they are making positive improvements to their environmental impacts. Some hotels have a dedicated commitment to preserving the environment, while others are exploiting "green public relations" opportunities while enjoying the cost savings. Most hotel chains are making positive changes that result in true improvements in resource utilization and waste disposal.

Eighteen states have some sort of ecological or energy-saving lodging program. The EPA has an ENERGY STAR certification for the hospitality industry. Green Seal *(www.greenseal.org)* has a hotel certification program that certifies smaller nonchain hotels and lodges. The Rainforest Alliance certifies sustainable tourism operators *(www.rainforest-alliance.org/tourism.)* Several websites maintain lists of environmentally friendly hotels and inns.

Another option is to look into house-swapping or apartment-swapping with a family who wants to stay at your place while you go to theirs. If you want to go to Paris, for example, you could connect with someone who wants to take a vacation the same week in your hometown of San Francisco. Two services that help vacationers plan home exchanges for a fee are the International Home Exchange at *www.intervac.com* and *HomeExchange.com.*

SOME OF THE CHANGES HOTELS MAKE WHEN THEY GO GREEN:
- ✓ Offer the option of not changing the sheets and towels every day.
- ✓ Replace conventional bulbs with low-energy usage lighting options such as compact fluorescent lights (CFLs) and light-emitting diodes (LEDs).
- ✓ Install solar panels to generate electricity.
- ✓ Heat pools with passive solar water systems.
- ✓ Conserve water by installing low-flow showerheads and toilets.
- ✓ Cut back on the amount of bleach they use to keep towels white.
- ✓ Recycle beverage containers, cardboard, and paper.
- ✓ Use natural pest control.
- ✓ Landscape grounds in native vegetation that can thrive with existing rainfall amounts.

If the hotels you stay in are not taking these steps, let the management know about your concerns. The more they hear from customers, the more hotels will start making positive changes.

Camping

Camping is a low eco-impact vacation that can help your child come to love nature, but it is not without its challenges. These include how to keep your toddler from eating dirt, how to keep your little darlings from becoming blood meals for mosquitoes and ticks, and how to make sure your baby gets a good night's sleep so that you can too. Let's take a look at how to make your camping vacation a success.

STARTING OUT SMALL Camping with children can be rough at first, but it is a skill that improves with practice. Your first excursion might be to pitch the tent in the backyard for a night. If all goes well, you'll likely feel empowered to pack up the family, baby and all, and head for a state or national park.

If that backyard foray doesn't go well, however, you might be permanently discouraged from trying it again, at least until your "baby" is studying for the SAT. You risk missing out on years of camping fun. Don't let one bad night convince you to give up on camping permanently. Try it again in a few years when your child is out of diapers and begging you to let her help set up the tent.

Once you've conquered the backyard, the next step is to take a camping trip at a park that is not too far from home. Book two nights, since sometimes it takes children more than one night to become accustomed to sleeping in a tent. If the first night goes reasonably well, you can usually count on a more relaxed and enjoyable second night. If the first night is a disaster, you can drive home in just a few hours.

Most children relish the idea of sleeping in a tent under the stars, but they also crave security. When parents are anxious, kids pick up on it. Pick a campsite that is within your comfort zone. If that is in the backyard, so be it. Start small and build your child's camping muscles along with yours. If your child's introduction to camping is too strenuous or scary, he or she is unlikely to want to repeat it any time soon.

If you are an avid camper or backpacker, you may be tempted for your child's first camping experience to be in the wilderness rather than a campground. But be forewarned: You are likely to have better results if you introduce car camping first. Children will be reassured by the presence of a community of campers. They will be thrilled just to be sleeping outdoors. Delay wilderness expeditions with children until they are old enough to learn survival skills such as basic first aid, making an impromptu shelter, and coping with emergencies, should their adult companion (yes, you!) become hurt.

Perhaps one of the most important things to pack in your camping gear is a good attitude, one that allows you to roll with whatever punches the trip packs. Rainy weather, thunderstorms, mosquitoes, biting gnats, and winds so strong they nearly blow over the tent are just some of the emergencies you might encounter—and conquer.

TIPS FOR HAPPY CAMPING WITH CHILDREN:
- ✓ Involve your children in the selection of the national park or other camping location.
- ✓ Build anticipation by renting videos, reading books, and looking at maps of the area you'll be visiting.
- ✓ Choose a campground with family-friendly amenities like a playground or swimming area.
- ✓ Have your children help plan meals and pack the gear before the trip.
- ✓ Assign your children responsibilities such as setting up the sleeping bags in the tent, fetching water, and washing up after meals.
- ✓ Attend ranger-led hikes and campground presentations. Learn about the natural history of the area, from how the landscape was formed to what sorts of grasses, flowers, and trees grow there.
- ✓ Let your children stay up past their usual bedtimes. Show them the constellations and explain the phases of the moon.

GEARING UP FOR THE TRIP The old saying goes that there is no such thing as bad weather, just bad clothing. The same goes for camping gear. Most common emergencies can be dealt with if you come prepared. Establish contingency plans for common emergencies. If a thunderstorm rolls in, will you ride it out in the tent or car? Or head for a hotel, or home? If someone gets hurt, how will you get emergency services? Do cell phones work at the campground or will you need to drive or walk to a ranger station?

When camping with children, you may not know what preparations you need to make until after the emergency has happened. Let's face it, babies and toddlers need so many items from diapers to pacifiers to feel comfortable, and it may be virtually impossible to pack everything you need.

Since you may not pack everything you need, you may want to camp in easy distance from a store, a *big* store. Campground stores usually sell camping gear and food—not baby items. When planning your trip, check the driving distance to the nearest town and its supermarket.

Once your children emerge out of the toddler years, camping gets much easier. You won't need to pack as much gear, for one thing. Your children will most likely be sounder sleepers who don't need multiple trips to the bathroom at night. They will be at the perfect age to absorb lessons about making as little impact as possible on the surroundings.

Any camping book can provide a list of the basic items you'll need to pack, but you may need additional gear depending on your location and the time of year. For example, if you'll be pitching your tent in the sandy dunes of North Carolina's Outer Banks, you'll need extra long tent poles to keep your tent rooted to the ground in case of high winds. If you are camping in the Sierra Nevada mountain range, you'll need to camp in a campground that provides bear-proof food lockers, or have brought along some rope to hang your food bag high in a tree. Consult campground and park brochures and follow the advice. Don't just assume that the proverbial *it*—whether bears or bad weather—won't happen to you.

WHAT NOT TO FORGET Camping books can provide you with a complete list of items to bring, but here are a few that can make your life easier with children:

✓ Stuffed animal or other sleeping companion.

✓ Pillows to make the tent a cozy retreat.

✓ Extra clothes in case children get wet.

✓ A clothesline on which to dry clothes that got wet.

✓ Insect repellent or insect-proof clothing.

✓ Flashlights for night hikes and shadow play inside the tent. One flashlight per child will help children feel secure and prevent fights over the lights.

✓ Games and toys for playing inside the tent in case of bad weather or when kids are tired after a long hike.

✓ Sporting equipment such as a soccer ball or baseball and gloves can keep kids occupied between hikes.

✓ Air mattresses—especially for parents who have lost the childlike ability to sleep anywhere.

✓ Warm clothing: Check nighttime temperatures before leaving on the trip. It may get colder than you think.

ECO-TIP: PROTECT NATURAL AREAS WHILE HIKING

- **Stay on trails. If the trail is narrow, walk in a single file rather than widening the trail.**

- **Don't take shortcuts when climbing or descending on a switchback trail. Cutting switchbacks contributes to erosion.**

- **Pack it in, pack it out: Pack out all garbage, including used toilet paper.**

- **Pick up after picnics: Get the kids to comb your picnic site so that you leave it cleaner than when you found it.**

SAFETY FIRST Having small children is no reason not to try camping. But when small children are underfoot, you will have to pay more attention to safety issues.

SAFETY ISSUES

✓ A first-aid kit is a must when camping with children. Bring it along on hikes.

✓ Hats, sunscreen, and sun-protective clothing are essential. See Chapter 6 for recommendations on sun protection.

✓ When you arrive at the campsite, spend several minutes discussing with your children the safety rules of the camp, including fire safety, storing food promptly to discourage animals, and always staying within sight of an adult.

✓ Teach children to keep a safe distance from fire rings. Keep lighter fluid, matches, and sharp kitchen utensils out of reach of children.

✓ Carry more snacks than you think you'll need. Children get very hungry when hiking. You can package healthy high-calorie snacks such as nuts and dried fruit at home in small bags or containers.

✓ Teach your children to recognize hazardous plants such as poison oak and poison ivy.

✓ Warn your children about the dangers of wading into swiftly moving rivers and other water bodies. Tell them never to swim without an adult present.

TIPS FOR HIKING WITH CHILDREN:

✓ Hold young children's hands when hiking on trails with steep drop-offs.

✓ If you are planning to do a lot of hiking, condition your children in advance of the trip by taking them on long walks in the neighborhood.

✓ When hiking with children, make sure they are drinking enough water and are not getting overheated. In hot climates, hikes are best done early in the morning before the sun is at full strength.

✓ Have a plan for what to do if you get separated from your children. Tell your child that if he or she gets lost, the best person to ask for help is a uniformed ranger and if none are present, ask a mom with her own children.

✗ Avoid overloading children with heavy things to carry. You risk ruining their enjoyment of the activity and making them overtired. On your return trip, you may be carrying not only the gear but your child, too.

TEACH SURVIVAL SKILLS AS YOUR CHILDREN GET OLDER Older children should be taught survival skills, especially if you plan to hike in wilderness areas. These include:

✓ What to do if he or she gets lost.

✓ How to recognize edible plants and berries.

✓ How to start a fire.

✓ Catching and cleaning fish.

ECO-FRIENDLY MOSQUITO AND TICK REPELLENTS

Mosquito bites can make little campers (and their adults) miserable. These pesky insects can inflict itchy bites and carry diseases such as West Nile virus. Ticks can transmit Lyme disease and other debilitating diseases such as Rocky Mountain spotted fever.

Most major brands of mosquito and tick repellent contain a chemical called DEET (N,N-diethyl-meta-toluamide), which the EPA considers to be safe if used as directed. However, the chemical has been shown to harm brain cells in laboratory animals and has been reported to cause seizures in children. It is also mildly toxic to aquatic wildlife, according to the EPA.

Picaridin is another chemical found in some repellents, but it is not as effective as DEET. Another chemical product you may see for sale, specifically targeting ticks, contains the pesticide permethrin, which may irritate the skin and is toxic to cats and fish. Permethrin should never be applied to the skin but rather sprayed on clothes, according to the EPA.

One of the best defenses is to wear long, lightweight pants and long-sleeve shirts, especially at dawn and dusk when mosquitoes are most active. But mosquitoes can bite through lightweight clothing, and in hot weather, layering your clothes is not an option, and you may have to resort to repellents. (See more on protecting against ticks in Chapter 4.)

Before grabbing a bottle of conventional mosquito repellent off the store shelf, consider trying a natural repellent. Two that are registered by the EPA for use in mosquito repellent are oil of lemon eucalyptus and oil of citronella. Natural brands also may include soybean oil, coconut oil, geranium oil, and other ingredients. Note that natural oils *do not* protect against ticks.

If you are looking for a DEET-free brand, make sure it also does not contain other harmful ingredients such as phthalate-based fragrances. See the Environmental Working Group's Skin Deep Cosmetics Safety Database, *www.cosmeticsdatabase.com*, to investigate individual brands.

IF YOU MUST USE A DEET-BASED BRAND, HERE ARE SOME TIPS:

✓ Follow all directions on the product label.

✓ Try a brand that contains the lowest percentage of DEET available.

✗ Do not use a brand that contains more than 30 percent DEET on children.

✗ Avoid spraying DEET near the eyes, nose, and mouth. Don't spray DEET where children may accidentally inhale it.

✓ Put the repellent on your children rather than letting them apply it themselves.

✗ Avoid getting repellent on children's hands because they frequently put their fingers in their mouths.

✗ Do not use DEET-based repellents near wounds or cuts.

✗ Never use DEET-based brands on pets or on children younger than two months of age.

Source: American Academy of Pediatrics

Cruising

Cruise ships were once the domain of the retiree, but oceangoing excursions have found popularity among families in recent years. Several cruise lines specialize in keeping children entertained with plenty of activities, giving parents the well-earned opportunity to read a novel or just take a nap poolside—

activities some couples haven't engaged in since their first child was born. But cruising gets a bad rap from environmentalists, and with good reason. Let's take a look at the issues so that you can decide if cruising is right for your family.

FLOATING CITIES Cruise ships are like small floating cities, and as such they consume vast amounts of diesel fuel, resources, and fresh water, and in return churn out sewage, food waste, toxic chemicals, and greenhouse gases. According to the ocean protection advocacy group Oceana, the average cruise ship carrying 3,000 passengers and crew generates an amount of greenhouse gases and other air pollution roughly equal to the emissions made by 12,000 automobiles *each day.*

In addition to air pollution, the 3,000-person cruise ship generates 25,000 gallons of sewage from toilets and 143,000 gallons of wastewater from sinks, showers, and kitchens (collectively known as gray water) each day. It is perfectly legal for cruise ships to dump raw sewage directly into the ocean as long as the ship is 3 or more miles offshore. The dumping of raw sewage contributes to coral reef destruction, the killing of marine mammals, harmful algal blooms, and oxygen-depleted dead zones.

Each cruise ship generates about 7 tons of garbage and solid waste each day. Although ships are supposed to incinerate the trash and dump the ashes, some operators have incurred fines for dumping garbage into the ocean. The garbage may contain plastics that marine wildlife mistake as food or become entangled in, leading to the deaths of turtles, seals, seabirds, and other wildlife.

The typical cruise ship also periodically dumps several thousand gallons of bilge water, which collects at the bottom of the ship's hull and contains oil, grease, and contaminants. These toxic substances can kill or sicken marine mammals, fish, and birds. Cruise ships also take up and dump millions of gallons of ballast water, which they use to control how high or low the ship sits in the water. Several invasive marine species have spread to new parts of the world by traveling in ballast water.

The laws that govern how cruise ships dispose of sewage waste vary according to the vessel's distance from shore. For example, U.S. federal law states that vessels must chemically treat sewage before dumping it when the ship is within 3 miles of shore. Outside 3 miles, ships are free to dispose of untreated human sewage except in the Alexander Archipelago in Alaska. Ships can dispose of untreated gray water (from laundries, kitchens, and showers) in any waters except the state waters of California and Alaska, which have enacted laws banning the practice.

Oceana is lobbying for uniform regulations that cover the air and water pollution generated by cruise ships. In addition to trying to pass more uniform environmental protection laws, Oceana is working with cruise lines to voluntarily clean up their emissions—and their images.

If you are still thinking about taking a cruise after learning about their many environmental failings, you'll be relieved to know that cruise lines are improving in response to revised fuel-efficiency standards, pressure from environmental groups, and consumer demand. Here are some of the changes taking place:

✓ **ENERGY SAVINGS** Cruise lines are updating ship engines with more energy-efficient models, reducing the amount of diesel fuel they use and the carbon dioxide they emit, and installing recapture systems to reduce other pollutants. Other steps include coating the exterior of the ship with silicone paint to reduce drag, using shore-based power when in port to minimize running the ship's electrical generators, and covering windows with a tinted film to keep rooms cooler and reduce the load on air conditioners. Still other energy-saving steps include installing LED and CFL lights. Some ships sport solar panels that generate electricity or use solar heating systems to keep pools warm.

✓ **REDUCING WASTE** Many ships collect and recycle glass, aluminum, and some kinds of plastic. They also recycle scrap metal, wood pallets, cardboard, and many other items that the customer never sees. Some ships even collect used cooking oil and donate it to farmers for use in generating biodiesel to power heavy machinery. At least one cruise line has eliminated all disposable tableware and plastic water bottles in favor of biodegradable and reusable versions. Several cruise lines have begun replacing chemical disinfection of sewage with more advanced wastewater treatment technology.

✓ **MINIMIZING IMPACT** Some cruise ships feature onboard desalinization plants that turn seawater into drinking water. Others are reusing gray water to wash decks and water plants. Most ships have some sort of system for separating oil from bilge water before it is dumped. Some ships have filtration systems to make sure that ballast water does not contain foreign marine species that may establish themselves in a new port. Some ships use only locally sourced food and fish that is sustainably harvested from the sea. Many ships now offer environmental education classes to guests who want to learn about how the ship is reducing its impact on the environment. Some lines use environment-friendly cleaning supplies and stock guest bathrooms with biodegradable soaps and shampoos.

CRUISING'S OTHER IMPACTS Water and air pollution are not the only legacies of cruise ships. These massive ocean liners need piers to efficiently load and off-load passengers. Many of the existing piers in tropical cruise destinations are not suitable for cruise ships, and countries that crave cruising dollars are often eager to build new piers in pristine areas. Building piers can destroy natural ecosystems containing coral reefs and mangrove swamps that provide home to numerous species of fish and other marine animals and plants.

Building a pier is not the only environmental impact, however. Cruise ship passengers are another. Large cruise ships carry about 3,000 people, many of whom disembark in port to visit historical sites or take part in water sports such as snorkeling, scuba diving, or sailing. The result is a massive and intense burst of human activity in shops, restaurants, sensitive historical sites such as ruins, and delicate coral reefs. While the shops and restaurants can gear up for the feast-or-famine routine of cruise tourism, the fragile ruins and reef ecosystems have a much harder time recovering from hordes of people, many of whom may have missed the instructions about not touching reefs, plants, and animals.

If you are considering a cruise because you want to see cultural, historical, and ecologically fragile sites, consider taking a land-based trip instead of a cruise. Most port stops last only long enough to skim the surface of what an island or country has to offer. If you care about protecting coral reefs and seeing them in their full beauty, as well as having enough time to explore and enjoy them, you may want to avoid the cruise experience.

If you are committed to going on a cruise, here are some tips for enjoying your cruise while reducing your impact:

- Look for an environmentally friendly cruise line by checking the company's website. Review the cruise ship company's environmental policies. For a quick overview see the cruising page at *www.greenyour.com*.
- Don't let your eyes be bigger than your stomach. Avoid overloading your plate at buffets with food that ends up going to waste.
- Choose shore excursions that involve walking, biking, or nonmotorized boating.
- Turn out lights in your stateroom, take shorter showers, take stairs instead of elevators, and keep other eco-friendly habits in place while on vacation.
- Toxic chemicals generated on ships are usually from activities such

as dry cleaning and photo developing. Avoid these activities while on board.

✓ If you love the water, consider a sailing vacation, which is likely to use less fuel and generate less waste. Look for an eco-friendly sailing outfitter online.

✓ Learn more about Oceana's efforts to clean up the cruising industry at *www.oceana.org* and visit EPA's Cruise Ship Discharges site at *www.epa .gov/owow/oceans/cruise_ships*.

Beaches and Lakes

A visit to the beach offers endless hours of fun for children. If you don't live near a coast, your favorite summer cool-off spot may be a nearby lake. Your family may enjoy renting a cabin along a lakeshore, occupying a large beach house with extended family, or pitching a tent in a lakeshore campsite or at a beach.

BEACH ETIQUETTE Although the ocean seems vast, we now know that the trash and toxic substances we dump can and do come back to haunt us. Pollution causes injury and illness to seabirds, fish, seals, and other marine mammals. Algal blooms can choke out sea and lake life.

Enjoying a beach or lakeside vacation should always start with lessons about how to protect the quality of the water we are visiting. We can start by explaining to our children how the trash we accidentally leave at the beach gets pulled into the water and disintegrates into small pieces that fish view as food. We can talk about the importance of using the bathroom before we go into the water to make sure we don't accidentally leave anything behind (an especially relevant issue when you have small children).

The most common beach pollutants are bacteria and viruses from untreated sewage that runs into waterways during and after heavy rains. Stormwater runoff also contains pet droppings, farm animal manure, pesticides, fertilizers, and other chemicals that run off from lawns, driveways, streets, roofs, and construction sites. Other sources are dysfunctional septic systems, waste generated by boaters and beachgoers, and waterfowl waste. However, in many cases, public health officials cannot point to a single breach or contamination episode when they detect high bacteria levels. These "nonpoint" sources of pollution cannot be isolated so they are difficult to fix.

THE FACTS

Between 1980 and 2003, the coastal population of the U.S. grew by 33 million, and by 2015 it is projected to increase by another 19 million, according to the National Oceanic and Atmospheric Administration (NOAA).

SOME COMMON WATER CONTAMINANTS ARE:

× Sewage—Untreated sewage from sewer system overflows causes bacterial growth that can sicken swimmers.

× Toxics—Chemicals dumped by factories can be very persistent. Polychlorinated biphenyls (PCBs), for example, still contaminate many waterways.

× Fertilizers—Natural and synthetic fertilizers are food for algae. The abundance of food causes harmful algal blooms and dead zones.

× Pesticides—Although designed to kill insects, some of these chemicals attack the same biological systems found in fish and amphibians.

× Oil—Whether it leaks from a tanker or runs off city streets into storm drains, oil is harmful to seabirds and other marine life.

× Trash—From polystyrene takeout containers to plastic grocery bags, just about every sort of trash has ended up in the ocean.

WHAT YOU CAN DO TO REDUCE WATER CONTAMINATION:

✓ When boating, use toilets instead of going in the water. Dispose of waste by chemical treatment or pumping the waste out into a disposal system.

✓ At home, maintain your septic system to prevent overloads.

✓ Forgo using synthetic chemical fertilizers and pesticides on your lawn and garden.

✓ Never dump chemicals or motor oil into storm drains. Teach your children not to throw trash on the streets. It washes into storm drains and eventually onto beaches.

✓ Lobby your civic leaders to upgrade aging storm-water and sewer systems.

WHEN AT THE BEACH, LIMIT YOUR IMPACT WITH THESE TIPS:

✓ At the beach, make sure the little ones wear snug-fitting swim diapers to avoid accidents.

✓ Use bridges and walkovers to cross the dunes rather than walking on sensitive vegetation.

✓ Dispose of all trash. Pick up any additional trash you see.

✓ Clean up after your pet at the beach.

✓ Use the beach's restroom instead of the ocean.

✓ Cut the rings of plastic six-pack holders so that seabirds, fish, turtles, and seals don't get tangled in them.

✓ Refrain from touching or disturbing beach plants, marine wildlife, and birds.

BEACH CLOSINGS A closed beach can spoil a vacation. By far the largest contributor to beach closings is high bacteria levels. In aging sewer systems, a big storm can flush untreated or partially treated sewage into overflow pipes that lead to water bodies.

When raw sewage gets in the water, along with the sewage comes human viruses and bacteria that can make you or your children ill. These illnesses include diarrheal diseases, skin rashes, eye infections such as pinkeye, respiratory infections, and even meningitis and hepatitis. Usually the main symptom is diarrhea. But diarrhea can be quite serious in young children and the elderly, sometimes requiring hospitalization.

The incidence of swimming-acquired infections has been increasing steadily over the years, according to the Centers for Disease Control and Prevention (CDC). Of the 62 waterborne disease outbreaks detected in 2004, about one-third were caused by bacteria, one-quarter were caused by parasites, viruses accounted for about a tenth, and chemicals or toxins about one-twentieth of all diseases reported. (The causes for the remainder are unknown.)

Unfortunately there is no single government agency that collects data and rapidly publishes beach advisories. You will have to become familiar with the jurisdiction that oversees the beach you plan to visit. One place to try is the area health department. Or try the Natural Resources Defense Council's Testing the Waters website, which publishes an annual map of beach closures at *www.nrdc.org*. The EPA's Beach Advisory and Closing On-line Notification (BEACON) site may help but the information is not always current. See *www.epa.gov/beaches*.

COMMON SENSE RULES TO AVOID CONTAMINATED BEACHES:

✓ Look for posted signs at the beach that ban swimming or advise caution.

✓ Swim at beaches that have monitoring systems in place and have strict closure and advisory procedures.

✓ Choose a beach that is away from urban areas and in open waters rather than in enclosed bays with little water exchange.

✗ Avoid swimming near pipes that carry water from storm drains to the ocean or lake.

✓ Wait 24 hours after a heavy rain before swimming. Rainwater can push contaminants through the storm drains and into beach water.

✓ If the beach smells or you see trash floating in the water, don't swim there.

✗ Don't go underwater, swallow water, or open your eyes underwater.

✓ Contact local health officials to report contamination if you suspect it.

THE FACTS

Swimmers are at least partially responsible for beach contamination. Levels of bacteria climb after increased beach use during the weekends.

RED TIDE Harmful algal blooms, sometimes known as red tides, occur naturally but they can be made worse by an influx of nutrients from fertilizer runoff,

GREEN DICTIONARY

WATERSHED
An area of land that drains into a single lake, river, ocean, or other body of water.

inadequately treated sewage, and manure from farms. The development of shoreline into condominium complexes, golf courses, and marinas has contributed to the rise in contaminated storm water and nutrient-rich fertilizer runoff from landscaping.

This nutrient overload can spur the growth of toxic algal species that turn the water red for days, weeks, or even months. The algae produce toxins that can cause human diseases characterized by rashes, diarrhea, fever, cramping, aches, chills, dizziness, tingling and numbness around the mouth, and cardiovascular and respiratory effects. For example, the algae *Pfiesteria piscicida*, discovered in North Carolina in 1991, is associated with skin and neurological damage as well as memory loss.

Red tides are occurring more often, found researchers at the University of Miami. The culprit is often the marine alga *Karenia brevis*. This species appears to be spreading northward from its usual habitat in the waters off Florida, the Carolinas, and the southern coastal states on the Gulf of Mexico. Dolphins and manatees are two mammals that have been killed by red tide blooms and the toxins they produce.

WHAT YOU CAN DO ABOUT RED TIDES:
✓ Forgo using synthetic fertilizers on your own property.
✓ Maintain your septic system.
✓ Buy organic produce, which is grown without synthetic fertilizers.
✓ Limit your consumption of meat produced on industrial farms that do not control animal waste.
✓ Do your part to support the preservation of coastal areas.

Ecotourism

Traveling should not involve ruining the environment that we come to see.

Yet so often it seems that the infrastructure that makes tourism possible—

from hotels to highways—involves the tearing up of sensitive wetlands, the

paving over of animal habitats, and sometimes even the relocation of human

populations. That is where ecotourism comes in.

ECOTOURISM DEFINED Ecotourists try to preserve local resources while restricting their impact on the environment and its inhabitants. In addition, ecotourism involves contributing to conservation efforts, making sure that tourism dollars stay in communities, and assisting (or at least not detracting from) the livelihood of indigenous peoples.

Ecotourism hotels and lodges protect and sustain the environment in a number of ways. They may run on solar power, serve locally provided foods, be built with consideration of local land ownership rights and animal migration patterns, hire local labor, and buy locally produced goods. Additionally they may have systems in place to control pollution, use less water, refrain from running bright lights at night, and avoid using landscaping pesticides and herbicides.

The International Ecotourism Society (TIES) defines tourism as travel that:
- ✓ Minimizes the impact of the traveler on her/his environment.
- ✓ Builds positive cultural and environmental awareness and respect.
- ✓ Directly benefits conservation efforts.
- ✓ Financially benefits local people and economies.
- ✓ Raises awareness of a country or region's political, environmental, and social climate.

In practice, that could mean choosing to stay at a comfortable solar-powered lodge instead of a multistory hotel with a mazelike network of swimming pools. Although you may not be able to swim up to the bar, your lodge may have other benefits, like being quiet enough to hear the sounds of wildlife at night. Many ecotourism lodges are able to provide all the luxuries of a five-star hotel, including high-quality bedding and gourmet meals.

TIPS FOR FINDING ECOTOURISM RESORTS AND PROVIDERS:
- ✓ Get personal recommendations from friends or on Internet travel sites.
- ✓ Consult guidebooks, especially ones aimed at ecotourists or low-budget travelers.
- ✓ Look for certification from an ecotourism agency.

FAMILY-FRIENDLY ECOTOURISM Ecotourism has a reputation for being only for young backpacking adults who are looking to explore the world after graduating from high school or college. In fact, ecotourism can be quite family-friendly.

TIPS FOR ENJOYING ECOTOURISM WITH THE WHOLE FAMILY:
- ✓ Involve the kids in choosing the destination. That way, they'll be excited about the amenities the resort or lodge provides.

GREEN ON A SHOESTRING

You don't have to go to a certified ecotourism lodge to have an ecotourism vacation. Reducing your impact can also be done by staying in a locally owned, traditional hotel instead of a newly built resort. Or you might decide to camp instead of staying in a hotel.

✓ Choose a destination with adequate access to medical care.

✓ Look for resorts or lodges that advertise that they are family-friendly.

✓ Call or e-mail the lodge to find out whether they have specific amenities that you may need. Are there any playgrounds nearby, or other places for active toddlers to run out their energy?

✓ Encourage your child to keep a journal in drawings or words to document his experience.

✓ On your trip, show your children examples of how your resort or lodge is conserving energy, minimizing pollution, reducing the use of water, and contributing to the betterment of the local economy.

ECO-SKEPTICISM Ecotourism has its critics, however. Some people decry the term as a mere marketing gimmick to assuage the guilt of rich travelers. You'll have to do some homework to find out how well a specific hotel or resort manages to combine the preservation of the environment and enhancement of local communities with the need to satisfy the discerning traveler. Many ecotourism operators start out with the best of intentions and later find they cannot live up to some of their promises. Other resorts are indeed guilty of blatant greenwashing.

TIPS ON AVOIDING GREENWASHING When evaluating an operator, here are some tough questions to ask:

• What policies are in place to reduce waste and water consumption?

• Where do you get most of the food served in dining rooms from? Is it from local sources? Is it organically grown?

• Do you use pesticides or herbicides on your landscaping?

• If it is a new or large resort, what was on the site before it was built?

• Does the building use energy-conservation methods or renewable energy such as solar or wind power?

• Do you provide education programs to help visitors understand the eco-system and culture of the area?

HOME AND AWAY Ecotravel can be foreign or domestic. The United States has many sensitive ecosystems that need protecting, including the Florida Everglades. It is possible to find numerous ecotourism opportunities within the U.S. as well as overseas. In each case, look for tour providers that are mitigating the impacts of tourism on natural environments and cultural sites.

Another way to broaden your childrens' horizons is through geotourism, a term coined by National Geographic's Center for Sustainable Destinations (*www*

SLOW TRAVEL

The slow travel movement emphasizes quality relaxation time over rushing from one attraction to the next. Slow travel might involve biking or walking rather than driving when exploring a new town or national park. You might stay with family or friends instead of in a hotel, or stay in a family-owned inn. You could seek out local cuisine instead of eating at chain restaurants.

.nationalgeographic.com/travel/sustainable). Geotourism encourages respect of the natural environment but adds the dimension of respect for and interaction with the region's history, culture, and heritage. The idea is that tourism can be a beneficial force in a region by bringing not only an influx of tourist dollars but also a cultural exchange.

Geotourism involves actively engaging with area residents and contributing to their well-being through the purchase of goods and services. The cultural exchange between tourists and the communities they visit can benefit the community and help tourists grow personally as they see and experience the living customs of other peoples. When they return home, geotourists share the stories of their experiences, thereby enlightening friends and family members about the way people live in other parts of the world.

This type of cultural ambassadorship provides a formative experience for children. The opportunity to exchange experiences with children of other cultures and income levels can become an unforgettable life experience that teaches tolerance, understanding, and a desire to help others.

The Center for Sustainable Destinations has developed a statement of principles that governments and tourism agencies can implement to help achieve the goal of protecting the environment, culture, and character of a region. Through this program, many countries have committed to promoting environmentally and culturally sensitive tourism. The center posts "destination scorecards" in partnership with *National Geographic Traveler* magazine to highlight places that are following these principles.

TIPS ON ECO-TRAVEL TO OTHER COUNTRIES:

✓ Learn greetings in the local language.

✓ Use the travel as an opportunity to learn about the history and culture of the region.

✓ Treat local inhabitants with respect.

✓ Dress appropriately when visiting religious and cultural sites.

✓ Get permission before photographing people, homes, and religious and cultural sites.

✓ Choose restaurants and services owned by local business people.

✓ Select souvenirs made by local craftspeople.

✓ Refrain from distributing candy or money to children. Instead make a donation to a local school or other appropriate organization.

✓ Use eco-travel as an opportunity to educate your children about the need to preserve natural resources and promote equality among peoples.

✓ Read up on the history and culture of the region before you visit.

Volunteer Vacations

Volunteer vacations are overseas or domestic trips to places where you can devote your experience and elbow grease to helping other people or improving the environment. You might lend a hand at a nature preserve or teach a skill you possess. Sometimes called voluntourism, these programs have become increasingly popular over the last several years.

CHILDREN WELCOME Perhaps you've dreamed of taking such a trip, but figured you'd have to wait for the children to grow up, go to college, and get good jobs before you'd have the time. The good news is that many of these programs not only allow children to accompany parents, they also find volunteer jobs and activities for the kids.

These missions can range in duration from one to several weeks. Many of these organizations offer overseas experiences, while others offer the opportunity to help improve environmental conditions within the U.S. Often no special skills are required.

One of the first questions to ask when planning a volunteer vacation is: domestic or international?

Domestic trips allow children and their parents to help others without filling out passport applications and usually without getting additional vaccinations. There are numerous opportunities for helping improve the environment at wildlife preserves, parks, and wilderness areas.

International trips offer the opportunity to engage in cross-cultural exchange. Families may live in the community they are helping, eat local foods, and learn a few words of a new language. Children can learn values such as tolerance, compassion, flexibility, and patience. These unique opportunities can give children a sense that they can make a difference in the world through the work they do.

IS INTERNATIONAL VOLUNTOURISM RIGHT FOR YOUR FAMILY? Here are some questions to ask yourself:

- How do you and your children handle emergencies? Are you the type of person who falls apart if you get a flat tire, or do you stay calm in the face of mishaps?

GREEN DICTIONARY

VOLUNTOURISM
A vacation that involves contributing skills and labor to an important cause such as preserving the environment or helping improve people's lives.

- Can you and your children be flexible about what you eat, what you wear, and where you sleep? When living with a host family you'll probably have to be flexible about food and accommodations.
- Does your family work well as a team? Will power struggles between parents and teens derail your ability to get a job done, or can you put minor squabbles aside and work together?
- Do you have the ability to put aside personal discomfort to get a job done? If it rains and your clothes get soaked, can you keep working with a smile on your face?
- How well do you and your children interact with people from other backgrounds? Do you have an open mind and open heart about becoming friends with people who have had very different life experiences?

FINDING A VOLUNTOURISM PROVIDER

- Check faith-based options: Your religious organization may offer overseas or domestic volunteer opportunities.
- Search the Web: You can find many organizations using common search engines.
- Consult the International Volunteer Programs Association (IVPA), which maintains a list of organizations that arrange for overseas volunteers. Visit their website at *www.volunteerinternational.org*.
- Search the Internet or browse your local bookstore for books that offer lists of organizations. One is *The 100 Best Volunteer Vacations to Enrich Your Life* by Pam Grout (National Geographic, 2009).

ASSESSING A VOLUNTOURISM PROVIDER Numerous charitable and for-profit organizations send volunteers overseas. Finding the right one for you will take some homework. When checking out organizations, ask:

- Is the organization nonprofit or for-profit? What are the administrative costs versus the amount spent on programs? You can look up nonprofit charities at *www.charitynavigator.org*.
- What is the project's purpose? What is the history of the project, and has it been successful?
- What medical care will be available in case my child or I get sick?
- What are the policies in case of trip cancellations?

One last note: Helping the environment does not require leaving the country or even your own community. Volunteer work is a popular option for families whose vacations involve staying right at home. Read on.

Staycations

With the ebbs and flows of the economy, a lot of families are adjusting their travel plans. The "staycation," where you spend your leisure time visiting local sites and enjoying your own backyard, is an increasingly popular option. Maybe you are adjusting to a new economic situation, or you've always been the type that likes to putter around the yard and visit local attractions. Staycations can serve as positive educational experiences for children, exposing them to historical attractions, museums, and natural environments.

Staycations are generally a positive experience for the environment, too. You won't be flying anywhere, so you won't generate a lot of greenhouse gases. You won't be staying at resorts that were carved out of Everglade wetlands or pristine forests. You'll be consuming the same amount of resources you always do, and perhaps even less so if you are not commuting to work during your vacation.

STAYCATION IN STYLE Here are some options for fun-filled staycations:

STAY LOCAL, REALLY LOCAL Explore the wonders that exist right outside your door, within walking or biking distance. Have you ever toured your neighborhood on foot? You'll probably notice a lot of things you haven't seen before. There may be a vacant lot at the end of your block, or a patch of woods you've never entered. You may be able to walk or bike to shops or the ice cream store. Start with small trips and build up your children's endurance for walking and biking around your town.

HISTORICAL SITES Civil war battlefields, settler homesteads, and Spanish missions are just some of the historical sites that our nation affords. Have you explored the historical sites in your area? Your children may have only seen these on the occasional field trip from school. Why not make a point of visiting the historical sites in your area this summer?

BACKYARD CAMPING If you have a patch of dirt in the backyard, you can go backyard camping (see the camping section in this chapter for ideas).

If you live in an apartment, you could set up the tent in the living room. Don't have a tent? Let the children build a fort out of sofa cushions or an old cardboard box and allow them to spend the night there.

THE SHORE If you live in a coastal state, why not make a day trip to the shore? If possible, choose a beach that is part of a state park that has an interpretive center, so your children can learn about tide pool creatures, shorebirds, and how to conserve and protect these natural areas.

MUSEUMS Child-centered museums are wonderful places for learning about nature and science. Many feature interactive exhibits that can help children understand concepts such as biodiversity and conservation.

AQUARIUMS AND ZOOS Aquariums provide a cool and inviting place to take refuge on a hot summer day. Zoos offer the opportunity to learn about animals, and what we can do to protect their habitats. Go early in the day when animals are more active.

VOLUNTEER STAYCATIONS Consider devoting part or all of your vacation to helping those in need. Look for volunteer opportunities in your area. One resource is VolunteerMatch *(www.volunteermatch.org),* an organization that provides a search engine that matches volunteers with local agencies in need of volunteers. Another is *serve.gov,* a comprehensive clearinghouse of U.S. volunteer opportunities.

Summer Camps

Schools are out, and your energetic youngster is climbing the walls. Wouldn't it be great if he or she could climb a boulder at summer camp instead? Summer programs are an increasingly popular option for all families, and are pretty much a necessity in single-parent households and two-parent dual-income households. Let's take a look at the options.

When shopping for a summer program, look for one that keeps kids busy *and* teaches them to respect and protect their environment. You may be able to find summer day programs offered by local nature preserves, zoos, parks and recreation departments, your child's school, community organizations such as the YMCA, and science museums. If you are sending your child to spend a week or more at an overnight camp, look for one that teaches environmental conservation.

DAY CAMPS AND PROGRAMS Whether you live in the city, suburbs, or countryside, you will likely find several programs that have nature, science, or the environment as their emphasis. Some of the topics may be:

PROTECTING WILDLIFE Why are species endangered, and what can we do to protect them?

ANIMAL HABITATS What sorts of animals live in the surrounding area, what are their habitats, and what foods do they eat?

FOREST ECOLOGY What types of trees grow nearby, and what can we do to conserve and protect forests?

STREAM ECOLOGY What tiny creatures live in your region's streams? What do they eat? How do our choices (using pesticides and fertilizers, for example) affect stream health?

BIRDING How can we identify birds by their appearance and songs?

WILDFLOWERS AND VEGETATION How does the climate affect what grows in your area, and how are human activities contributing to climate change?

SOLAR ENERGY How can the sun power our vehicles, warm our water, and cook our food? Projects include making solar-powered cars, robots, or ovens.

CONSERVATION How can our everyday choices improve the health of the planet? Kids may visit organic farms and recycling centers.

ECO-TIP: HEALTHY CAMPERS ARE HAPPY CAMPERS
When at camp, you'll want your child to eat well, get plenty of exercise, and continue the good habits of recycling and caring for

the planet. Before signing your child up, some good questions to ask are:

- **What outside activities will be offered?**

- **Are healthy foods and snacks provided, or will lunch be sent from home?**

- **Does the facility recycle and if not, why not?**

- **Are videos shown, and if so, are they nature programs or commercial movies?**

AWAY FROM HOME Overnight camps immerse your child in the wilderness, but do they offer a wilderness experience? Just because a camp is located down a dirt road doesn't mean that it is an eco-conscious establishment. Do your homework and choose a camp that provides wilderness education and operates using sound ecological practices.

When selecting an overnight camp, some questions to ask are:

- What sort of environmental education does the camp provide? Is the camp focused on outdoor sports such as canoeing and horseback riding, or do the children learn about nature, science, resource conservation, and the importance of preserving animal habitats?

- What is the camp doing to lessen its environmental impact? Does the camp use disposable plastic water bottles and picnic ware? Does the camp recycle? Does it use pesticides and chemical fertilizers to maintain its grounds? What steps are they taking to conserve energy?

- What food is served and where is it from? Does the camp use locally sourced vegetables and fruits, or is the food from a large food service company? Is the menu made up only of traditional kid fare—French fries, chicken nuggets, and pizza—or does it offer a variety of entrees? Are snacks prepackaged potato chips or something that is healthier and doesn't create garbage?

- Does the camp have a policy on electronic handheld gadgets like cell phones and games? Many camps prohibit these devices because they detract from the nature experience and distract other children. Some camps limit the hours they can be used. Others offer computer time for e-mail and games. Check on the policy and make sure it matches your views on the use of electronics at camp.

GREEN ON A SHOESTRING

You may be able to get a discount on your child's camp tuition by volunteering to teach a skill at the camp. For example, you might give lessons on how to plant a garden, save energy at home, recognize flowers and trees, or identify birds.

Take Action

▸ When choosing a vacation destination, consider trips that allow your children to learn about the natural world in ways that don't involve using a lot of natural resources.

▸ When driving, adjust your driving habits to maximize your fuel efficiency.

▸ If it is time to replace your car, consider buying a fuel-efficient hybrid for everyday driving. You can rent a larger vehicle for occasional weekend trips.

▸ Take into consideration the amount of greenhouse gases your trip will generate.

▸ Incorporate walking, biking, and hiking into your vacation rather than driving to each attraction.

▸ Why not take the train this year instead of flying? Your kids may love it.

▸ When selecting a hotel, ask about the hotel's commitment to reducing its environmental impact.

▸ Choose an older hotel rather than a big resort built on an environmentally sensitive area.

▸ Check into ecotourism and try to select a dedicated organization rather than one engaged in greenwashing.

▸ Teach your children to be good hotel guests and turn off lights, take short showers, and turn off the air conditioner if it is not needed.

▸ Consider taking a volunteer vacation aimed at helping wildlife or restoring natural environments in another part of the country or the world.

▸ Opt for a "staycation" this year. You'll reduce your environmental impact while learning more than you ever dreamed about your local environment.

▸ Look into all the ways you can help the environment in your own part of the country during your staycation.

▸ Before booking a cruise, consider the ecological impact of cruise ships on ocean water quality, marine organisms, and fragile shore environments.

▸ When evaluating summer camps and programs, ask not only what ecology lessons are taught, but also whether the camp follows eco-sound practices such as recycling and conserving water.

THE SCIENCE BEHIND IT

The Miles per Gallon Illusion

Which do you think will save more fuel: upgrading from a 10 mpg car to a 20 mpg car? Or upgrading from a 25 mpg car to a 50 mpg car?

If you said the second option, you'd be wrong. If you said both options would save the same amount of fuel, you'd also be wrong. That's because "miles per gallon" does not tell us as much about fuel use and savings as we think it does.

Researchers call this the mpg illusion. Miles per gallon tells you how many miles you travel on a single gallon of gas. But it doesn't directly tell you how much gas you use for your typical amount of driving. That is what you really want to know, so that you can compare two cars and find out how much gas, money, and emissions you'll save by upgrading to a more fuel-efficient car for your driving needs.

To make that comparison, you need to know how much gas each car uses per mile, or gallons per mile (gpm). It is easy to convert mpg into gpm. Let's say you own a pickup truck that gets 10 mpg, meaning that it travels 10 miles on one gallon. In gpm, your pickup consumes 1 gallon every 10 miles.

Your pickup that consumes 1 gallon every 10 miles logically consumes 5 gallons every 50 miles. In contrast, a Toyota Prius that gets 50 mpg consumes 1 gallon every 50 miles. You can easily see that your vehicle uses 4 more gallons than the Prius does to go the same distance.

But how does this help us compare two cars for your driving needs? Let's find out.

Let's say that you want to replace your 10 mpg pickup with a hybrid SUV that gets 20 mpg. Your pickup uses 1 gallon to go 10 miles so it consumes 10 gallons to travel 100 miles. The new SUV slurps up 1 gallon every 20 miles so it will consume 5 gallons every 100 miles. For your 100-mile journey, your pickup guzzles 10 gallons of gas while the new SUV sucks down only 5 gallons. Your upgrade from a 10 mpg clunker to a 20 mpg SUV saves you 5 gallons of gas for every 100 miles you drive.

Now let's say that your other car is a compact that gets 25 mpg (one gallon takes you 25 miles, so four gallons takes you 100 miles) and you are thinking of upgrading to a hybrid that gets 50 mpg (one gallon takes you 50 miles, so two gallons takes you 100 miles). To go 100 miles, your compact car requires 4 gallons while the new hybrid would require only 2 gallons. Your upgrade from a 25 mpg to a 50 mpg car saves you 2 gallons per every 100 miles you drive.

So, switching from a 10 mpg to a 20 mpg vehicle saves 3 gallons more gas (per 100 miles) than switching from a 25 mpg to a 50 mpg vehicle. Improvements at the low end of the mpg range make bigger impacts on gasoline usage than the improvements at the high end.

These improvements can make a big impact on your wallet and on the planet, too. For every 100 gallons of gas burned, about one ton of carbon dioxide is released into the atmosphere. Upgrading from a car that gets 20 mpg to one that gets 25 mpg will keep one ton of carbon dioxide out of the atmosphere each year (based on an average driving total of 10,000 miles per year).

Of course, the best improvements could be had if people would switch from heavy SUVs to super-efficient Priuses: Switching from a 10 mpg car to a 50 mpg car would save a whopping 8 gallons for every 100 miles of driving.

Unfortunately it is unrealistic to expect all SUV drivers to switch to compact or midsize sedans. Many people buy a car based on family size and other considerations. A Prius won't work for every family. But this example shows that tremendous fuel savings (and carbon dioxide reductions) are possible by upgrading to a hybrid SUV or replacing a low-mileage SUV with a higher performing minivan.

If all this math seems confusing to you, check out the gpm calculator at *www.gpmcalculator.com*. You can enter your car's mpg and the site will conduct gpm comparisons against the vehicles of your choice.

For more details see *www.mpgillusion.com* and learn more about this revelatory research by Duke University economists Richard Larrick and Jack Soll.

CHAPTER 1: THE HOME FRONT

1 Landrigan, Philip J., et al. 2004. "Children's Health and the Environment: Public Health Issues and Challenges for Risk Assessment." *Environmental Health Perspectives* 112:257–265.

2 Jusko, Todd A., et al. 2008. "Blood Lead Concentrations <10 µg/dL and Child Intelligence at 6 Years of Age." *Environmental Health Perspectives* 116:243–248.

3 Bellinger, D. C., et al. 2008. "Very low lead exposures and children's neurodevelopment." *Current Opinion in Pediatrics* 20:172–177.

4 Hansel, Nadia N., et al. 2008. "A Longitudinal Study of Indoor Nitrogen Dioxide Levels and Respiratory Symptoms in Inner City Children with Asthma." *Environmental Health Perspectives* 116:1428–1432.

5 Braun, Joe M., et al. 2006. "Exposures to Environmental Toxicants and Attention Deficit Hyperactivity Disorder in U.S. Children." *Environmental Health Perspectives* 114:1904–1909.

6 Winickoff, Jonathan P., et al. 2008. "Beliefs About the Health Effects of 'Thirdhand' Smoke and Home Smoking Bans." *Pediatrics* 123:e74–e79.

7 Karr, Catherine J., et al. 2007. "Health Effects of Common Home, Lawn, and Garden Pesticides." *Pediatric Clinics of North America* 54:63–80.

8 Barr, D. B., et al. 2005. "Concentrations of Selective Metabolites of Organophosphorus Pesticides in the United States Population." *Environmental Research* 99:314–326.

9 Nalyanya, Godfrey, et al. 2009. "German Cockroach Allergen Levels in North Carolina Schools: Comparison of Integrated Pest Management and Conventional Cockroach Control." *Journal of Medical Entomology* 46:420–427.

10 Bornehag, Carl-Gustaf, et al. 2004. "The Association Between Asthma and Allergic Symptoms in Children and Phthalates in House Dust: A Nested Case-Control Study." *Environmental Health Perspectives* 112:1393–1397.

11 Manori, J., et al. 2004. "Urinary Levels of Seven Phthalate Metabolites in the U.S. Population from the National Health and Nutrition Examination Survey (NHANES), 1999–2000." *Environmental Health Perspectives* 112:331–338.

12 Sjödin, A., et al. 2008. "Serum Concentrations of Polybrominated Diphenyl Ethers (PBDEs) and Polybrominated Biphenyl (PBB) in the United States Population: 2003–2004." *Environmental Science and Technology* 42:1377–1384.

13 Lunder, Sonya, and Renee Sharp. 2003. "Toxic Fire Retardants (PBDEs) in Human Breast Milk." Environmental Working Group.

14 Toms, Leisa-Maree L., et al. 2008. "Higher Accumulation of Polybrominated Diphenyl Ethers in Infants Than in Adults." *Environmental Science & Technology* 42:7510–7515.

15 National Public Radio (NPR). July 10, 2009. "Central Valley Disconnect: Rich Land, Poor Nutrition." *Morning Edition.*

16 USDA Natural Resources Conservation Service. July 2003. "National Resources Inventory 2001: Urbanization and Development of Rural Land."

CHAPTER 2: GREEN AND LEAN

1 American Heart Association, et al. 2006. "Dietary Recommendations for Children and Adolescents: A Guide for Practitioners." *Pediatrics* 117:544–559.

2 Sacks, Frank M., et al. 2009. "Comparison of Weight-Loss Diets with Different Compositions of Fat, Protein, and Carbohydrates." *New England Journal of Medicine* 26:859–873.

3 von Hippel, P. T., et al. 2007. "The Effect of School on Overweight in Childhood: Gain in Body Mass Index During the School Year and During Summer Vacation." *American Journal of Public Health* 97:696–702.

4 Johnson, F. M. 2002. "How Many Food Additives Are Rodent Carcinogens?" *Environmental and Molecular Mutagenesis* 39:69–80.

5 Schab, David W., and Nhi-Ha T. Trinh. 2004. "Do Artificial Food Colors Promote Hyperactivity in Children With Hyperactive Syndromes? A Meta-Analysis of Double-Blind Placebo-Controlled Trials." *Journal of Developmental and Behavioral Pediatrics* 25:423–434.

6 McCann, D., et al. 2007. "Food Additives and Hyperactive Behaviour in 3-Year-Old and 8/9-Year-Old Children in the Community: A Randomised, Double-Blinded, Placebo-Controlled Trial." *Lancet* 370:1560–1567.

7 Schonwald, Alison. February 2008. "ADHD and Food Additives Revisited." *American Academy of Pediatrics Grand Rounds* 19:17.

8 Karstadt, M. L. 2006. "Testing Needed for Acesulfame Potassium, an Artificial Sweetener." *Environmental Health Perspectives* 114:A516.

9 Soffritti, M., et al. 2007. "Life-Span Exposure to Low Doses of Aspartame Beginning During Prenatal Life Increases Cancer Effects in Rats. *Environmental Health Perspectives* 115:1293–1297.

10 Lim, U. 2006. "Consumption of Aspartame-Containing Beverages and Incidence of Hematopoietic and Brain Malignancies." *Cancer Epidemiology, Biomarkers & Prevention* 15:1654–1659.

11 Abou-Donia, Mohamed B., et al. 2008. "Splenda Alters Gut Microflora and Increases Intestinal P-Glycoprotein and Cytochrome P-450 in Male Rats." *Journal of Toxicology and Environmental Health* A 71:1415–1429.

12 Apelberg, B. J., et al. 2007. "Determinants of Fetal Exposure to Polyfluoroalkyl Compounds in Baltimore, Maryland." *Environmental Science and Technology* 41:3891–3897.

13 Fei, Chunyuan, et al. 2009. "Maternal Levels of Perfluorinated Chemicals and Subfecundity." *Human Reproduction* 24:1200–1205.

14 Lund, K. H., and J. H. Petersen. 2006. "Migration of Formaldehyde and Melamine Monomers from Kitchen- and Tableware Made of Melamine Plastic." *Food Additives and Contaminants* 23:948–55. and Bradley, E. L., et al. 2005. "Survey of the Migration of Melamine and Formaldehyde from Melamine Food Contact Articles Available on the U.K. Market." *Food Additives and Contaminants* 22:597–606.

15 Begley, T. H., et al. 2005. "Perfluorochemicals: Potential Sources of and Migration from Food Packaging." *Food Additives and Contaminants A* 22:1023–1031.

CHAPTER 3: GREEN FOODS

1 The Pew Commission on Industrial Farm Animal Production. 2008. *Putting Meat on The Table: Industrial Farm Animal Production in America.*

2 Starmer, Elanor, and Timothy A. Wise. 2007. "Feeding at the Trough: Industrial Livestock Firms Saved $35 Billion from Low Feed Prices" (Policy Brief No. 07–03). Global Development and Environment Institute.

3 Institute of Medicine. 1999. *The Use of Drugs in Food Animals: Benefits and Risks.* National Academy Press, Washington, D.C.

4 U.S. Department of Health and Human Services Agency for Toxic Substances and Disease Registry (ATSDR). 2000. "Public Health Statement for Polychlorinated Biphenyls (PCBs)."

5 ATSDR. 1998. "Public Health Statement for Chlorinated Dibenzo-p-dioxins (CDDs)."

6 ATSDR. 1999. "Public Health Statement for Mercury."

7 See Table 2 in Winter, Carl K., and Sarah F. Davis. 2006. "Organic Foods." *Journal of Food Science* 719:R117–R124.

8 Lu, Chensheng, et al. 2008. "Dietary Intake and Its Contribution to Longitudinal Organophosphorus Pesticide Exposure in Urban/Suburban Children." *Environmental Health Perspectives* 116:537–542.

9 Karr, Catherine J., et al. 2007. "Health Effects of Common Home, Lawn, and Garden Pesticides." *Pediatric Clinics of North America* 54: 63–80.

10 Hayes, T., et al. 2003. "Atrazine-Induced Hermaphroditism at 0.1 Ppb in American Leopard Frogs (Rana Pipiens): Laboratory and Field Evidence." *Environmental Health Perspectives* 111:568–575.

11 Villanueva, C., et al. 2005. "Atrazine in Municipal Drinking Water and Risk of Low Birth Weight, Preterm Delivery, and Small-For-Gestational-Age Status." *Occupational & Environmental Medicine* 62:400–405.

12 Beaulieu, J. J., et al. 2009. "The Effects of Season and Agriculture on Nitrous Oxide Production in Headwater Streams." *Journal of Environmental Quality* 38:637–646.

13 See page 23 in U.S. Department of Agriculture. 2007. "Pesticide Data Program Annual Summary."

14 Pollak, M. 2008. "Insulin and Insulin-Like Growth Factor Signaling in Neoplasia." *Nature Reviews Cancer* 8:915–928.

CHAPTER 4: LIVING WELL

1 Harris, Gardiner. October 31, 2008. "The Safety Gap." *New York Times Magazine. and* Government Accountability Office. September 2008. "Better Data Management and More Inspections Are Needed to Strengthen FDA's Foreign Drug Inspection Program" (GAO-08-970).

2 Aiello, A. E., et al. 2007. "Consumer Antibacterial Soaps: Effective or Just Risky?" *Clinical Infectious Diseases* 45:S137–S147.

3 Donn, Jeff, et al. March 10, 2008. "AP: Drugs found in drinking water." Associated Press.

4 Bjørling-Poulsen, M., et al. 2008 "Potential Developmental Neurotoxicity of Pesticides Used in Europe." *Environmental Health* 7:50.

5 Government Accountability Office. January 2009. "Dietary Supplements: FDA Should Take Further Actions to Improve Oversight and Consumer Understanding" (GAO-09-250).

6 Levin, Myron. February 8, 2005. "1991 Memo Warned of Mercury in Shots." *Los Angeles Times.*

7 Jefferson, Tom, et al. 2004. "Adverse Events after Immunisation with Aluminium-Containing DTP Vaccines: Systematic Review of the Evidence." *Lancet Infectious Diseases* 4:84–90.

8 Madsen, Kreesten M. 2002. "A Population-Based Study Of Measles, Mumps, and Rubella Vaccination and Autism." *New England Journal of Medicine* 347:1477–1482.

9 Gilbert, Steven G., et al. February 20 (revised July 1), 2008. "Consensus Statement on Environmental Agents Associated with Neurodevelopmental Disorders." Collaborative on Health and the Environment's Learning and Developmental Disabilities Initiative.

10 Hertz-Picciotto, I., and L. Delwiche. 2009. "The Rise in Autism and the Role of Age at Diagnosis." *Epidemiology* 20:84–90. *and* Brown, Phyllis. January 7, 2009. "U.C. Davis M.I.N.D. Institute Study Shows California's Autism Increase Not Due to Better Counting." U.C. Davis M.I.N.D. Institute press release.

11 Korrick, S.A., et al. 2008. "Polychlorinated Biphenyls, Organochlorine Pesticides and Neurodevelopment." *Current Opinion in Pediatrics* 20:198–204.

12 Braun, Joe M. 2006. "Exposures to Environmental Toxicants and Attention Deficit Hyperactivity Disorder in U.S. Children." *Environmental Health Perspectives* 114:1904–1909. *and* Froehlich, Tanya E. November 23, 2009. "Association of

Tobacco and Lead Exposures with Attention Deficit/Hyperactivity Disorder." *Pediatrics* 10:1542.

13 LoGiudice, Kathleen, et al. 2003. "The Ecology of Infectious Disease: Effects of Host Diversity and Community Composition on Lyme Disease Risk." *Proceedings of the National Academy of Sciences* 100:567–571.

14 Naseri, Iman, et al. 2009. "Nationwide Trends in Pediatric *Staphylococcus aureus* Head and Neck Infections." *Archives Otolaryngology: Head & Neck Surgery* 135:14–16.

15 Aiello, A. E., et al. 2008. "Effect of Hand Hygiene on Infectious Disease Risk in the Community Setting: A Meta-Analysis." *American Journal of Public Health* 98:1372–1381.

16 Zock, Jan-Paul, et al. 2007. "The Use of Household Cleaning Sprays and Adult Asthma: An International Longitudinal Study." *American Journal of Respiratory and Critical Care Medicine* 176:735–741.

17 Litonjua, A. A., and S. T. Weiss. 2007. "Is Vitamin D Deficiency to Blame for the Asthma Epidemic?" *Journal of Allergy Clinical Immunology* 120:1031–1035.

18 Beggs, Paul John, and Hilary Jane Bambrick. 2005. "Is the Global Rise of Asthma an Early Impact of Anthropogenic Climate Change?" *Environmental Health Perspectives* 113:915–919.

19 Infante-Rivard, C., and J. E. Deadman. 2003. "Maternal Occupational Exposure to Extremely Low Frequency Magnetic Fields During Pregnancy and Childhood Leukemia." *Epidemiology* 14:437–441.

20 Sadetzki, S., et al. 2008. "Cellular Phone Use and Risk of Benign and Malignant Parotid Gland Tumors: A Nationwide Case-Control Study." *American Journal of Epidemiology* 167:457–467.

21 Hardell, L., et al. 2009. "Epidemiological Evidence for an Association Between Use of Wireless Phones and Tumor Diseases." *Pathophysiology* 16:113–122.

22 Zahm, S. H., and M. H. Ward. 1998. "Pesticides and Childhood Cancer." *Environmental Health Perspectives* 106:893–908.

23 Carozza, Susan E., et al. 2008. "Risk of Childhood Cancers Associated with Residence in Agriculturally Intense Areas in the United States." *Environmental Health Perspectives* 116:559–565.

24 Rudant, Jérémie, et al. 2007. "Household Exposure to Pesticides and Risk of Childhood Hematopoietic Malignancies: The ESCALE Study (SFCE)." *Environmental Health Perspectives* 115:1787–1793.

25 Shim, Youn K., et al. 2009. "Parental Exposure to Pesticides and Childhood Brain Cancer: U.S. Atlantic Coast Childhood Brain Cancer Study." *Environmental Health Perspectives* 117:1002–1006.

26 National Research Council Committee on Fluoride in Drinking Water. 2006. *Fluoride in Drinking Water: A Scientific Review of EPA's Standards*. National Academies Press, Washington, D.C.

27 Bassin, E. B., et al. 2006. "Age-Specific Fluoride Exposure in Drinking Water and Osteosarcoma (United States)." *Cancer Causes and Control* 17:421–428. and Douglass, C. W., and K. Joshipura. 2006. "Caution Needed in Fluoride and Osteosarcoma Study." *Cancer Causes and Control* 17:481–482.

28 The American Dental Association. 2006. "Professionally Applied Topical Fluoride: Executive Summary of Clinical-Based Professional Recommendations."

29 U.S. Department of Health and Human Services National Toxicology Program. 2008. "The NTP-CERHR Monograph on Bisphenol A."

30 U.S. Centers for Disease Control and Prevention. 2005. "Third National Report on Human Exposure to Environmental Chemicals: Spotlight on Mercury."

31 DeRouen, Timothy A., et al. 2006. "Neurobehavioral Effects of Dental Amalgam in Children: A Randomized Clinical Trial." *Journal of the American Medical Association* 295:1784–1792.

32 Needleman, Herbert L. 2006. "Mercury in Dental Amalgam: A Neurotoxic Risk?" *Journal of the American Medical Association* 295:1835–1836.

33 Luby, S. P., et al. 2005. "Effect of Handwashing on Child Health: A Randomised Controlled Trial." *Lancet* 366:225–233.

CHAPTER 6: BABY STEPS

1 Kosemund, Kirstin, et al. 2009. "Safety Evaluation of Superabsorbent Baby Diapers." *Regulatory Toxicology and Pharmacology* 53:81–89.

2 Alberta, Lauren, et al. 2005. "Diaper Dye Dermatitis." *Pediatrics* 116:e450–e452.

3 U.K. Environment Agency. 2008. "Science Report: An Updated Lifecycle Assessment Study For Disposable And Reusable Nappies."

4 ATSDR. 2007. "Public Health Statement for Polybrominated Diphenyl Ethers (PBDEs)."

5 World Health Organization International Program on Chemical Safety. 2000. "Tetrakis (Hydroxymethyl) Phosphonium Salts." *Environmental Health Criteria* 218:61–108.

6 American Academy of Pediatrics Policy Statement. 2005. "Breastfeeding and the Use of Human Milk." *Pediatrics* 115:496–506.

7 Greer, Frank R., et al. 2008. "Effects of Early Nutritional Interventions on the Development of Atopic Disease in Infants and Children: The Role of Maternal Dietary Restriction, Breastfeeding, Timing of Introduction of Complementary Foods, and Hydrolyzed Formulas." *Pediatrics* 121:183–191.

8 Grummer-Strawn, Laurence M., and Zuguo Mei. 2004. "Does Breastfeeding Protect Against Pediatric Overweight?" *Pediatrics* 113:e81–e86.

9 Lucas, A., et al. 1992. "Randomized Trial of Early Diet in Preterm Babies and Later Intelligence Quotient." *Lancet* 339:261–264.

10 Schwarz, E. B. 2009. "Duration of Lactation and Risk Factors for Maternal Cardio-vascular Disease." *Obstetrics & Gynecology* 113:974–982.

11 LaKind, Judy S., et al. 2008. "The Heart of the Matter on Breastmilk and Environ-mental Chemicals: Essential Points for Healthcare Providers and New Parents." *Breastfeeding Medicine* 3:251–259.

12 Forste, Renata. 2008. "Are U.S. Mothers Meeting the Healthy People 2010 Breastfeeding Targets for Initiation, Duration, and Exclusivity? The 2003 and 2004 National Immunization Surveys." *Journal of Human Lactation* 24:278–288.

13 Rozman, Karl K., et al. 2006. "NTP-CERHR Expert Panel Report on the Repro-ductive and Developmental Toxicity of Soy Formula." *Birth Defects Research B: Developmental and Reproductive Toxicology* 77:280–397.

14 Badger, Thomas M., et al. 2009. "The Health Implications of Soy Infant Formula." *American Journal of Clinical Nutrition* 89:1668S–1672S. *and* Core, Jim. January 2004. "Study Examines Long-Term Health Effects of Soy Infant Formula." *Agri-cultural Research Magazine.*

15 Osborn, David A., and John K. H. Sinn. 2006. "Soy Formula for Prevention of Allergy and Food Intolerance in Infants." *Cochrane Database of Systematic Reviews* 4:CD003741.

16 Osborn, David A., and John K. H. Sinn. 2006. "Formulas Containing Hydrolysed Protein for Prevention of Allergy and Food Intolerance in Infants." *Cochrane Database of Systematic Reviews* 4:CD003664.

17 Environmental Working Group. November 26, 2008. "EWG: Infant Formula Companies Should Come Clean on Melamine, BPA" (news release). *and* Environ-mental Working Group. December 2007. "EWG Guide to Formula."

18 Martin, Andrew. November 26, 2008. "Melamine Traces Found in U.S. Infant For-mula." *New York Times.*

19 Schiera, Joshua G., et al. 2009. "Perchlorate Exposure from Infant Formula and Comparisons with the Perchlorate Reference Dose." *Journal of Exposure Science and Environmental Epidemiology* 10:1038.

20 Lu, Chensheng, et al. 2008. "Dietary Intake and Its Contribution to Longitudinal Organophosphorus Pesticide Exposure in Urban/Suburban Children." *Environ-mental Health Perspectives* 116:537–542.

21 Whitaker, Robert C. 2004. "Predicting Preschooler Obesity at Birth: The Role of Maternal Obesity in Early Pregnancy." *Pediatrics* 114:e29–e36.

22 Stothard, Katherine J., et al. 2009. "Maternal Overweight and Obesity and the Risk of Congenital Anomalies: A Systematic Review and Meta-analysis." *Journal of the American Medical Association* 301:636–650.

23 Burros, Marian. January 23, 2008. "High Mercury Levels Are Found in Tuna Sushi." *New York Times*.

24 Swan, S. H., et al. 2007. "Semen Quality of Fertile U.S. Males in Relation to Their Mothers' Beef Consumption During Pregnancy." *Human Reproduction* 22:1497–1502.

25 Environmental Working Group. March 5, 2007. "Bisphenol A: Toxic Plastics Chemical in Canned Food."

26 Calafat, A. M., et al. 2008. "Exposure of the U.S. Population to Bisphenol A and 4-Tertiary-Octylphenol: 2003–2004." *Environmental Health Perspectives* 116:39–44.

27 National Intitutes of Health National Toxicology Program. September 2008. "NTP-CERHR Monograph on the Potential Human Reproductive and Developmental Effects of Bisphenol A" (NIH Publication No. 08 – 5994).

CHAPTER 7: PLAY TIME

1 Cox-Foster, Diana, and Dennis vanEngelsdorp. April 2009. "Solving the Mystery of the Vanishing Bees." *Scientific American Magazine*.

2 Linebarger, Deborah L., and Dale Walker. 2005. "Infants' and Toddlers' Television Viewing and Language Outcomes." *American Behavioral Scientist* 48:624–645.

3 Primack, Brian P., et al. 2009. "Association Between Media Use in Adolescence and Depression in Young Adulthood." *The Archives of General Psychiatry* 66:181–188.

4 Hamer, M., et al. 2009. "Psychological Distress, Television Viewing, and Physical Activity in Children Aged 4 to 12 Years." *Pediatrics* 123:1263–1268.

5 Christakis, Dimitri A., et al. 2009. "Audible Television and Decreased Adult Words, Infant Vocalizations, and Conversational Turns: A Population-Based Study." *Archives of Pediatrics and Adolescent Medicine* 163:554–558.

6 California Environmental Protection Agency. January 2007. "Evaluation of Health Effects of Recycled Waste Tires in Playground and Track Products produced for the Integrated Waste Management Board by the Office of Environmental Health Hazard Assessment."

CHAPTER 8: SCHOOL DAYS

1 Joshi, Anupama, Marion Kalb, and Moira Beery. 2006. "Going Local: Paths to Success For Farm to School Programs." National Farm to School Program Center for Food and Justice, Occidental College, and Community Food Security Coalition.

2 Klemmer, C. D., et al. 2005. "Growing Minds: The Effect of a School Gardening Program on the Science Achievement of Elementary Students." *HortTechnology* 15:448–452.

3 Barros, Romina M., et al. 2009. "School Recess and Group Classroom Behavior." *Pediatrics* 123:431–436.

4 Reynolds, D., and R. I. Nicolson. 2007. "Follow-Up of an Exercise-Based Treatment for Children with Reading Difficulties." *Dyslexia* 13:78–96.

5 Solomon, Gina, et al. January 2001. "No Breathing in the Aisles: Diesel Exhaust Inside School Buses." Natural Resources Defense Council and the Coalition for Clean Air.

CHAPTER 9: EARTH-FRIENDLY FESTIVITIES

1 Luangtongkum, T., et al. 2006. "Effect of Conventional and Organic Production Practices on the Prevalence and Antimicrobial Resistance of *Campylobacter spp.* in Poultry." *Applied and Environmental Microbiology.* 72:3600–3607.

2 Walli, Ron. July 3, 2003. "Fourth of July No Picnic for the Nation's Environment" (news release). Oak Ridge National Laboratory.

3 Johnson, Eric. May 8, 2009. "Charcoal Versus LPG Grilling: A Carbon-Footprint Comparison." *Environmental Impact Assessment Review* 29:370–378.

4 Wilkin, R. T., D. D. Fine, and N. G. Burnett. 2007. "Perchlorate Behavior in a Municipal Lake Following Fireworks Displays." *Environmental Science & Technology* 41:3966–3971.

CHAPTER 10: FAMILY VACATIONS

1 Chester, Mikhail V., and Arpad Horvath. 2009. "Environmental Assessment of Passenger Transportation Should Include Infrastructure and Supply Chains." *Environment Research Letters* 4:024008.

2 See Table 11.6 of U.S. Department of Energy. 2009. *Transportation Energy Data Book,* 28th edition.

3 European Federation for Transport and Environment and Climate Action Network Europe. 2006. "Clearing the Air: The Myth and Reality of Aviation and Climate Change."

FURTHER READING

HOME

Berthold-Bond, Annie. *Home Enlightenment: Practical, Earth-Friendly Advice for Creating a Nurturing, Healthy, and Toxin-Free Home and Lifestyle*. Rodale Press, 2008.

Frumkin, H., L. Frank, and R. Jackson. *Urban Sprawl and Public Health*. Island Press. 2004. Establishes the link between sprawling communities and poor health. Discusses how to design, plan, and build healthy communities.

Sandbeck, Ellen. *Green Housekeeping*. Scribner, 2006. A comprehensive resource for safer, less toxic cleaning solutions that you can make at home.

CHILDREN AND TOXIC CHEMICALS

Gavigan, Christopher. *Healthy Child, Healthy World*. Penguin, 2007. Presents detailed ways in which parents can create a healthy and environmentally sound home.

Landrigan, P., H. Needleman, and M. Landrigan. *Raising Healthy Children in a Toxic World*. Rodale Press, 2001. A detailed look at the toxins in our every day lives and how we can protect our children.

HEALTHY AND SUSTAINABLE EATING

Earle, Sylvia. *Sea Change: A Message of the Oceans*. Ballantine Books, 1996. Earle chronicles the depletion of fisheries against the backdrop of the resiliency of the oceans.

Institute of Medicine. *Food Marketing to Children and Youth: Threat or Opportunity?* National Academies Press, 2006. An in-depth look at how food marketing affects children's health.

Nestle, Marion. *What to Eat*. North Point Press, 2007. A commonsense guide to choosing healthy foods. Informative on food additives, artificial sweeteners, organic versus conventional foods, and how to find fresh, whole-grain bread.

Pollan, Michael. *In Defense of Food*. Penguin, 2008. Nutrition science, with its focus on individual nutrients packaged in processed foods, has not made us healthier. Pollan urges us to return to eating simple, traditional, real foods.

————. *The Omnivore's Dilemma: A Natural History of Four Meals*. Penguin Press, 2006. A fascinating look at how our nation produces food today.

Schlosser, Eric. *Fast Food Nation*. Harper Perennial, 2005. A riveting examination of the beef industry and the practices behind the creation of the typical fast-food meal.

Weasel, Lisa H. *Food Fray: Inside the Controversy over Genetically Modified Food*. AMACOM, 2008. A summary of the issues surrounding genetically modified foods.

HEALTH

Levy, Stuart B. *The Antibiotic Paradox: How the Misuse of Antibiotics Destroys Their Curative Powers.* Da Capo Press, 2002. A comprehensive exploration of how superbugs are spreading due to overuse of antibiotics in medicine.

Mitman, Gregg. *Breathing Space: How Allergies Shape Our Lives and Landscapes.* Yale University Press, 2007. It explains how land-use patterns have enabled the spread of allergen-producing plant species.

Sears, Robert. *The Vaccine Book.* Little, Brown & Co., 2007. A thorough overview of the safety and effectiveness of pediatric vaccines, as well as outlining the major controversies associated with vaccines.

Shu, Jennifer, editor. *Baby & Child Health: The Essential Guide From Birth to 11 Years.* American Academy of Pediatrics, 2004. A commonsense reference for handling common children's health issues.

RAISING AN ECO-MINDED CHILD

Lewis, Barbara. *The Kid's Guide to Service Projects: Over 500 Service Ideas for Young People Who Want to Make a Difference.* Free Spirit Publishing, 2009.

Martin, Laura C. *Recycled Crafts Box.* Storey Publishing, 2004.

McKay, Kim, and Jenny Bonnin. *True Green Kids: 100 Things You Can Do to Save the Planet.* National Geographic Society, 2008.

Pollan, Michael. *The Omnivore's Dilemma for Kids: The Secrets Behind What You Eat.* Dial, 2009.

Savedge, Jenn. *The Green Teen: The Eco-Friendly Teen's Guide to Saving the Planet.* New Society Publishers, 2009.

BABY

Greene, Alan. *Raising Baby Green: The Earth-Friendly Guide to Pregnancy, Childbirth, and Baby Care.* Jossey-Bass, 2007.

Imus, Deirdre. *Growing Up Green: Baby and Child Care.* Simon & Schuster, 2008.

Planck, Nina. *Real Food for Mother and Baby: The Fertility Diet, Eating for Two, and Baby's First Foods.* Bloomsbury USA, 2009.

TOYS

Brown, Stuart, and Christopher Vaughan. *Play: How It Shapes the Brain, Opens the Imagination and Invigorates the Soul.* Avery, 2009.

Guernsey, Lisa. *Into the Minds of Babes: How Screen Time Affects Children From Birth to Age 5.* Basic Books, 2007.

Louv, Richard. *Last Child in the Woods*. Algonquin, 2007.

McDonald, Libby. *The Toxic Sandbox: The Truth About Environmental Toxins and Our Children's Health*. Perigee, 2007.

SCHOOLS

Frumkin, Howard, Robert J. Geller, I. Leslie Rubin, and Janice Nodvin, editors. *Safe and Healthy School Environments*. Oxford University Press, 2006.

Linn, Susan. *Consuming Kids: The Hostile Takeover of Childhood*. The New Press, 2004.

McClendon, Marie, and Christy Shauck. *The Healthy Lunchbox*. American Diabetes Association, 2005.

GREENER CELEBRATIONS

Colwell-Lipson, Corey, and Lynn Colwell. *Celebrate Green! Creating Eco-Savvy Holidays, Celebrations and Traditions for the Whole Family*. The Green Year, 2008.

Sander, Jennifer Basye, Peter Sander, and Anne Basye. *Green Christmas: How to Have a Joyous, Eco-Friendly Holiday Season*. Adams Media, 2008.

Weisman, Carol. *Raising Charitable Children*. F. E. Robbins & Sons Press, 2006.

GREEN TRAVEL

Gendler Silverman, Goldie. *Camping With Kids*. Wilderness Press, 2005.

Grout, Pam. *The 100 Best Volunteer Vacations to Enrich Your Life*. National Geographic, 2009.

Rasheed de Francisco, Fawzia. *The Rough Guide to Travel with Babies and Young Children*. Rough Guides, 2008.

U.S. GOVERNMENT AGENCIES

**Centers for Disease
Control and Prevention**
1600 Clifton Road
Atlanta, GA 30333
(800) 311-3435
www.cdc.gov

Environmental Protection Agency
Ariel Rios Building
1200 Pennsylvania Avenue N.W.
Washington, DC 20460
(202) 272-0167
www.epa.gov

Food and Drug Administration
5600 Fishers Lane
Rockville, MD 20857-0001
(888) 463-6332
www.fda.gov

National Cancer Institute
U.S. Department of Health
and Human Services
6116 Executive Boulevard, Room 3036A
Bethesda, MD 20892-8322
www.cancer.gov

**National Institute of Environmental
Health Sciences**
U.S. Department of Health
and Human Services
P.O. Box 12233, MD NH-10
Research Triangle Park, NC 27709
(919) 541-3345
www.niehs.nih.gov

U.S. Department of Agriculture
1400 Independence Avenue S.W.
Washington, DC 20250
(202) 720-2791
www.usda.gov

ENVIRONMENTAL ORGANIZATIONS

Conservation International
2011 Crystal Drive, Suite 500
Arlington, VA 22202
(800) 429-5660; (703) 341-2400
www.conservation.org

Environmental Defense Fund
257 Park Avenue South
New York, NY 10010
(800) 684-3322; (212) 505-2100
www.edf.org

Environmental Working Group
1436 U Street N.W., Suite 100
Washington, DC 20009
(202) 667-6982
www.ewg.org

Greenpeace
702 H Street N.W.
Washington, DC 20001
(800) 326-0959
www.greenpeace.org

Natural Resources Defense Council
40 W. 20th Street
New York, NY 10011
(212) 727-2700
www.nrdc.org

Rainforest Alliance
665 Broadway, Suite 500
New York, NY 10012
(212) 677-1900
www.rainforest-alliance.org

Sierra Club
85 Second Street, 2nd Floor
San Francisco, CA 94105
(415) 977-5500
www.sierraclub.org

Washington Toxics Coalition
4649 Sunnyside Avenue North
Suite 540
Seattle, WA 98103
(206) 632-1545
www.watoxics.org

Worldwatch Institute
1776 Massachusetts Avenue N.W.
Washington, DC 20036-1904
(202) 452-1999
www.worldwatch.org

CHILDREN'S HEALTH ORGANIZATIONS

Children's Environmental Health Network
110 Maryland Avenue N.E., Suite 505
Washington, DC 20002
Telephone: (202) 543-4033
www.cehn.org

Collaborative on Health and the Environment
Institute for Children's
Environmental Health
c/o Commonweal
PO Box 316
Bolinas, CA 94924
www.healthandenvironment.org

Columbia Center for Children's Environmental Health
100 Haven Avenue
Tower III, Suite 25F
New York, NY 10032
(212) 304-7280
www.mailman.hs.columbia.edu/ccceh

Healthy Child Healthy World
12300 Wilshire Boulevard, Suite 320
Los Angeles, California 90025
(310) 820-2030
www.healthychild.org

ONLINE DATABASES OF CHEMICAL TOXICITIES

Agency for Toxic Substances and Disease Registry
Centers for Disease Control
and Prevention
4770 Buford Highway N.E.
Atlanta, GA 30341
(800) 232-4636
http://www.atsdr.cdc.gov/phs

Center for the Evaluation of Risks to Human Reproduction
National Institutes of Health
U.S. Department of Health
and Human Services
P.O. Box 12233, MD NH-10
Research Triangle Park, NC 27709
(919) 541-5021
http://cerhr.niehs.nih.gov/chemicals/

Environmental Protection Agency
Integrated Risk Information Center
c/o EPA Docket Center
Mail Code 28221T
EPA-West Building
1301 Constitution Avenue N.W.
Washington, DC 20005
(202) 566-1676
www.epa.gov/iris

International Programme on Chemical Safety
World Health Organization
United Nations Environment Programme
International Labour Organisation
135 Hunter Street East
Hamilton ON L8N 1M5
Canada
(905) 572-2981
www.inchem.org

National Pesticide Information Center
Oregon State University
333 Weniger Hall
Corvallis, OR 97331-6502

(800) 858-7378
www.npic.orst.edu

TOXNET Toxicology Data Network
National Library of Medicine
U.S. Department of Health
and Human Services
Two Democracy Plaza
Suite 510
6707 Democracy Boulevard
MSC 5467
Bethesda, MD 20892-5467
(301) 496-1131
toxnet.nlm.nih.gov

HOME DESIGN AND ENERGY USE

Active Living by Design
Gillings School of Global Public Health
University of North Carolina
400 Market Street
Suite 205
Chapel Hill, NC 27516
(919) 843-2523
www.activelivingbydesign.net

**American Council for an
Energy-Efficient Economy**
529 14th Street N.W.
Suite 600
Washington, D.C. 20045-1000
Phone: (202) 507-4000
www.aceee.org

**Energy Efficiency and
Renewable Energy**
U.S. Department of Energy
1000 Independence Avenue S.W.
Washington, DC 20585
(877) 337-3463
www.eere.energy.gov

Energy Information Administration
1000 Independence Avenue S.W.
Washington, DC 20585

(202) 586-8800
www.eia.doe.gov

Energy Star Program
1200 Pennsylvania Avenue N.W.
Washington, DC 20460
(888) 782-7937
www.energystar.gov

Forest Stewardship Council
11100 Wildlife Center Drive, Suite 100
Reston, VA 20190
(703) 438-6401
www.fscus.org

Healthy House Institute
13998 West Hartford Drive
Boise, ID 83713
(208) 938-3137
www.healthyhouseinstitute.com

Healthy Places
Centers for Disease Control
and Prevention
600 Clifton Road
Atlanta, GA 30333
(800) 311-3435
www.cdc.gov/healthyplaces

**National Association
of Home Builders**
1201 15th Street N.W.
Washington, DC 20005
(800) 368-5242
www.nahb.org

Sustainable Forestry Initiative
1600 Wilson Boulevard, Suite 810
Arlington, VA 22209
(703) 875-9500
www.sfiprogram.org

U.S. Green Building Council
1800 Massachusetts Ave. N.W., Suite 300
Washington, DC 20036
(800) 795-1747
www.usgbc.org

RECYCLING

Earth 911
Global Alerts, LLC
14646 N. Kierland Boulevard
Scottsdale, AZ 85254
(480) 889-2650
www.earth911.org

**Rechargeable Battery
Recycling Corporation**
1000 Parkwood Circle, Suite 450
Atlanta, GA 30339
(678) 419-9990
www.call2recycle.org

TerraCycle Inc.
121 New York Avenue
Trenton, NJ 08618
(609) 393-4252
www.terracycle.net

FOOD & AGRICULTURE

**Center for Science
in the Public Interest**
1875 Connecticut Ave. N.W., Suite 300
Washington, DC 20009
(202) 332-9110
www.cspinet.org

Food Alliance
1829 N.E. Alberta, #5
Portland, OR 97211
(503) 493-1066
www.foodalliance.org

Humane Farm Animal Care
P.O. Box 727
Herndon, VA 20172
(703) 435-3883
www.certifiedhumane.com

**Humane Society of
the United States**
2100 L Street N.W.
Washington, DC 20037

(202) 452-1100
www.hsus.org

Local Harvest
220 21st Avenue
Santa Cruz, CA 95062
(831) 475-8150
www.localharvest.org

Marine Stewardship Council
2110 N. Pacific Street
Suite 102
Seattle, WA 98103
(206) 691-0188
www.msc.org

**Monterey Bay Aquarium
Seafood Watch**
886 Cannery Row
Monterey, CA 93940
(831) 648-4800
www.seafoodwatch.org

National Organic Program
Room 4008-South Building
1400 Independence Avenue S.W.
Washington, DC 20250 0020
(202) 720-3252
www.ams.usda.gov/NOP

Organic Consumers Association
6771 South Silver Hill Drive
Finland, MN 55603
(218) 226-4164
www.organicconsumers.org

Organic Trade Association
P.O. Box 547
Greenfield, MA 01302
(413) 774-7511
www.ota.com

**Pesticide Action Network
North America (PANNA)**
49 Powell Street, Suite 500
San Francisco, CA 94102
(415) 981-1771

www.panna.org
www.pesticideinfo.org

**Pew Commission on Industrial
Farm Animal Production**
901 E Street, NW
Washington, DC 20004
(301) 379-9107
www.ncifap.org

**Food and Agriculture Organization
of the United Nations**
Viale delle Terme di Caracalla
00153 Rome
Italy
(+39) 06 57051
www.fao.org

DRINKING WATER

California Department of Health
Certified Water Treatment Devices
(916) 558-1784
www.cdph.ca.gov

National Sanitation Foundation
789 North Dixboro Road
Ann Arbor, MI 48113-0140
(800) NSF-MARK
www.nsf.com

**Office of Ground Water
and Drinking Water**
Environmental Protection Agency
Ariel Rios Building
1200 Pennsylvania Avenue N.W.
Washington, DC 20460
(202) 272-0167
www.epa.gov/safewater/
consumerinformation

CONSUMER PRODUCTS

Campaign for Safe Cosmetics
(202) 321-6963
www.safecosmetics.org

**Coalition for Consumer
Information on Cosmetics**
P.O. Box 56537
Philadelphia, PA 19111
(888) 546-2242
www.leapingbunny.org

**Consumer Product
Safety Commission**
4330 East West Highway
Bethesda, MD 20814
(301) 504-7923
www.cpsc.gov

**Greener Choices and Consumer
Reports Consumers Union**
101 Truman Avenue
Yonkers, NY 10703
(914) 378-2000
www.greenerchoices.org
www.consumerreports.org

Household Products Database
National Library of Medicine
8600 Rockville Pike
Bethesda, MD 20894
tehip@teh.nlm.nih.gov
hpd.nlm.nih.gov

Skin Cancer Foundation
149 Madison Avenue, Suite 901
New York, NY 10016
www.skincancer.org

HEALTH TOPICS

**Alliance for the Prudent Use
of Antibiotics**
75 Kneeland Street
Boston, MA 02111-1901
(617) 636-0966
www.apua.org

**American Academy of Allergy Asthma
& Immunology**
555 East Wells Street, Suite 1100
Milwaukee, WI 53202-3823

(414) 272-6071
www.aaaai.org

American Academy of Pediatrics
141 Northwest Point Boulevard
Elk Grove Village, IL 60007-1098
(847) 434-4000
www.aap.org

Centers for Disease Control and Prevention
1600 Clifton Road
Atlanta, GA 30333
(404) 498-1515; (800) 311-3435
www.cdc.gov

Institute for Vaccine Safety
Johns Hopkins Bloomberg School of Public Health
615 N. Wolfe Street, Room W5041
Baltimore, MD 21205
www.vaccinesafety.edu

Medical Investigation of Neurodevelopmental Disorders (M.I.N.D) Institute
University of California, Davis
2825 50th Street
Sacramento, CA 95817
(916) 703-0280
www.ucdmc.ucdavis.edu/mindinstitute

National Network for Immunization Information
301 University Boulevard
Galveston, TX 77555-0350
(409) 772-0199
www.immunizationinfo.org

TOYS

Art & Creative Materials Institute
P.O. Box 479
Hanson, MA 02341-0479
(781) 293-4100
www.acminet.org

Guidelines for Safe Use of Art and Craft Materials
California Environmental Protection Agency
Office of Environmental Health Hazard Assessment
1001 I Street
Sacramento, California 95814
(916) 324-2829
www.oehha.org/education/art/getart.html

Green Electronics Council
121 S.W. Salmon Street
Suite 210
Portland, OR 97204
(503) 279-9383
www.greenelectronicscouncil.org
www.epeat.net

My Green Electronics
Consumer Electronics Association
2500 Wilson Boulevard
Arlington, VA 22201-3834
(866) 858-1555
www.mygreenelectronics.org

Recalls.gov
(a "one stop shop" for U.S. government recalls of toys, food, baby gear, etc.)
www.recalls.gov

SCHOOLS

Better School Food
487 E. Main Street
Mount Kisco, NY 10549
(914) 864-1293
www.betterschoolfood.org

Campaign for a Commercial-Free Childhood
53 Parker Hill Avenue
Boston, MA 02120
(617) 278-4172
www.commercialexploitation.org

Clean School Bus USA
Environmental Protection Agency
Ariel Rios Building
1200 Pennsylvania Avenue N.W.
Washington, DC 20460
www.epa.gov/otaq/schoolbus

**Community Action to
Change School Food Policy**
Massachusetts Public Health Authority
434 Jamaicaway
Jamaica Plain, MA 02132
(617) 524-6696 x103
www.mphaweb.org

Farm to School Network
Center for Food & Justice, UEPI
Occidental College
1600 Campus Road, MS-M1
Los Angeles, CA 90041
(323) 341-5095
www.farmtoschool.org

The Healthy School Lunch Campaign
Physicians Committee for
Responsible Medicine
5100 Wisconsin Avenue N.W.
Suite 400
Washington, DC 20016
(202) 686-2210
www.healthyschoollunches.org

Healthy Schools Network, Inc.
110 Maryland Avenue N.E., Suite 505
Washington, DC 20002
(202) 543-7555
www.healthyschools.org

**Shop with a Conscience
Consumer Guide**
SweatFree Communities
30 Blackstone Street
Bangor, ME 04401
(207) 262-7277
www.sweatfree.org

HOLIDAYS AND CELEBRATIONS

Adopt a Species
National Zoo
3001 Connecticut Avenue N.W.
Washington, DC 20008
(202) 633-4800
*nationalzoo.si.edu/Support/
AdoptSpecies*

Birthdays Without Pressure
Family Social Science Department
University of Minnesota
290 McNeal Hall
St. Paul, MN 55108
(612) 625-4752
www.birthdayswithoutpressure.org

Fair Trade Federation
3025 Fourth Street N.E.
Washington, DC 20017-1102
(202) 636-3547
www.fairtradefederation.org

National Wildlife Federation
11100 Wildlife Center Drive
Reston, VA 20190
(800) 822-9919
www.nwf.org

New American Dream
6930 Carroll Avenue
Suite 900
Takoma Park, MD 20912
(877) 683-7326
www.newdream.org

TransFair USA
1500 Broadway, Suite 400
Oakland, CA 94612
(510) 663-5260
www.transfairusa.org

Wildlife Adoption Center
Defenders of Wildlife
1130 17th Street N.W.

Washington, DC 20036
(800) 385-9712
www.wildlifeadoption.org

TRANSPORTATION AND LODGING

Center for Sustainable Destinations
National Geographic Society
1145 17th Street N.W.
Washington, DC 20036-4688
(202) 828-8045
www.nationalgeographic.com/travel/
sustainable

Intergovernmental Panel on Climate Change
c/o World Meteorological Organization
7bis Avenue de la Paix C.P. 2300
CH-1211 Geneva 2
Switzerland
41-22-730-8208
www.ipcc.ch

International Ecotourism Society
1333 H Street N.W., Suite 300E
Washington, DC 20005
(202) 347-9203
www.ecotourism.org

League of American Bicyclists
1612 K Street N.W., Suite 800
Washington, DC 20006-2850
(202) 822-1333
www.bikeleague.org

National Highway Traffic Safety Administration
1200 New Jersey Avenue S.E.
Washington, DC 20590
(888) 327-4236
www.nhtsa.dot.gov

Partnership for Global Sustainable Tourism Criteria
United Nations Foundation

1800 Massachusetts Avenue N.W.
Suite 400
Washington, DC 20036
(202) 887-9040
www.sustainabletourismcriteria.org

Rainforest Alliance Sustainable Tourism
665 Broadway, Suite 500
New York, NY 10012
(888) MY EARTH
www.rainforest-alliance.org/tourism

Sustainable Travel International
835 S.W. William Drive
White Salmon, WA 98672 USA
(800) 276-7764
www.sustainabletravelinternational.org

Travelers' Philanthropy
1333 H Street N.W.
Suite 300 East Tower
Washington, DC 20005
(202) 347-9203
www.travelersphilanthropy.org

GREEN WASHING

Greenwashing Index
EnviroMedia Social Marketing
24 N.W. First Avenue, Suite 275
Portland, OR 97209
(503) 327 8031
www.greenwashingindex.com

TerraChoice Environmental Marketing Inc.
171 Nepean Street, Suite 400
Ottawa, Ontario K2P 0B4
Canada
(800) 478-0399
www.terrachoice.com

National Geographic's *Green Guide* offers simple tips and practical examples on how to make changes that add up to big benefits for your wallet, your family's health, and the planet. Visit the website at *www.thegreenguide.com.*

ABOUT THE AUTHOR

Catherine Zandonella, science editor of the *Green Guide* magazine and website, is a longtime science writer with experience as a researcher and teacher. She holds a B.S. degree in pharmacology from the University of California at Santa Barbara and a master of public health degree from the University of California at Berkeley. She has written for *Nature* and *New Scientist*. She lives in Princeton Junction, New Jersey, and has two children.

ABOUT THE FOREWORD WRITER

Wendy Gordon has been a leader in the green consumer movement, having founded Mothers & Others for a Livable Planet, a pioneering consumer outreach organization, in 1989, and *Green Guide*, the go-to resource for the eco-conscious consumer, acquired in 2007 by National Geographic. Mothers & Others was conceived at the Natural Resources Defense Council, where Gordon was a senior project scientist in the Health Program.

ABOUT THE ADVISORY BOARD

Lynn Goldman, M.D., M.P.H., is principal investigator for the Johns Hopkins University Center for the National Children Study. She conducts research on environmental exposures and adverse health outcomes in newborns. Her work is key in developing regulatory and science policies that address health and environmental risks to children.

Richard Joseph Jackson, M.D., M.P.H., is an international leader in environmental health, focusing on epidemiology, infectious diseases, and toxicology. For 15 years Dr. Jackson worked at the Centers for Disease Control, where he advanced the program in childhood lead poisoning prevention. He is the coauthor of *Urban Sprawl and Public Health*.

Susan Kolodziejczyk is a standards and practices manager for the National Geographic Channel, a member of National Geographic's LEED team, and a steering committee member of National Geographic's GoGreen Initiative.

Emily Main is an online editor at Rodale.com, an environmental health news service. She served previously as senior editor of National Geographic's *Green Guide* magazine and worked at thegreenguide.com for five years.

Paul McRandle is a consulting senior editor for the Natural Resources Defense Council's Simple Steps and Smarter Cities websites, where he covers issues ranging from environmental contaminants to transportation improvements. Previously, he served as the deputy editor of National Geographic's *Green Guide* magazine. He has written on green living issues for *WorldWatch*, *Grist*, and the *Huffington Post*.

Nsedu Obot Witherspoon, M.P.H., is an influential national voice in the area of policy and protection of children's environmental health. She has held significant committee posts in the areas of child care, environmental public health, and housing. She is the author of a chapter on climate change and children's health in *The Way We Will Be 50 Years from Today: 60 of the World's Greatest Minds Share Their Visions of the Next Half Century.*

AUTHOR ACKNOWLEDGMENTS

Heartfelt thanks go to my editor at National Geographic, Garrett Brown, for many hours of dedication to this project. I would also like to thank Susan Tyler Hitchcock for stewarding this book through its earliest stages.

This book is the culmination of many years of dedication to making our planet a greener, healthier place by the writers and editors at *The Green Guide* magazine. I express my deep gratitude to Paul McRandle and Emily Main for their editorial expertise and their commitment to improving the health of the planet and its people through their work at *The Green Guide*. I'd like to thank Wendy Gordon, founder of *The Green Guide,* for her efforts to make the world a healthier place for kids and for her leadership in the green consumer movement. My deep appreciation goes to Mindy Pennybacker for her many years of building *The Green Guide* into a fine publication.

My special thanks go to the reviewers of this book for their instructive comments on early drafts. These include Richard J. Jackson, Emily Main, Lynn Goldman, Susan Kolodziejczyk, Paul McRandle, and Nsedu Obot Witherspoon. I'd also like to thank Gina Solomon of the Natural Resources Defense Council for her review of an early draft and her insightful comments. My thanks go to many others who helped supply material for this book, including Beth Feehan, Richard Larrick, Kyndaron Reinier, Jenn Savedge, Corey Colwell-Lipson, and Darren Naud.

Many people deserve my sincere gratitude for their guidance over the years, including Lana Beckett, Martyn T. Smith, Justin Mullins, John Wilkes, and Robert Irion. I'd also like to thank my father and mother for their unconditional love, my sister for all the long telephone calls, and my brother for being a good friend.

Finally, I would like to dedicate this book to my husband and children. To my husband, I say thank you for years of love and support. Thank you for building a vegetable garden so that our children could have healthy foods, caring for our lawn without synthetic pesticides and fertilizers, and for riding your bike to the train station every day, rain or shine. Oh yes, and thank you for taking out the compost.

To my children, and to all children on our planet, I hope that you will grow up to be part of a generation that views Earth as a place where resources are managed not plundered, where waste is recycled rather than dumped, and where forests are viewed as homes for wildlife rather than areas to be clearcut in the name of progress. Most of all I hope that you will grow to be compassionate beings who think outside the borders of our country to promote healthy and ecologically sound living throughout the world.

GREEN GUIDE
FAMILIES

PUBLISHED BY THE NATIONAL GEOGRAPHIC SOCIETY

John M. Fahey Jr.
President and Chief Executive Officer

Gilbert M. Grosvenor
Chairman of the Board

Tim T. Kelly
President
Global Media Group

John Q. Griffin
Executive Vice President
President Publishing

Nina D. Hoffman
Executive Vice President
President Book Publishing Group

PREPARED BY THE BOOK DIVISION

Barbara Brownell Grogan
Vice President and Editor in Chief

Marianne R. Koszorus
Director of Design

Carl Mehler
Director of Maps

R. Gary Colbert
Production Director

Jennifer A. Thornton
Managing Editor

Meredith C. Wilcox
Administrative Director Illustrations

STAFF FOR THIS BOOK

Garrett Brown
Editor

Susan Tyler Hitchcock
Consulting Editor

Sanaa Akkach
Art Director

Al Morrow
Designer

Karin Kinney
Copy Editor

Jane Sunderland
Proofreader

Mike Horenstein
Production Project Manager

MANUFACTURING AND QUALITY MANAGEMENT

Christopher A. Liedel
Chief Financial Officer

Phillip L. Schlosser
Vice President

Chris Brown
Technical Director

Nicole Elliott
Manager

Rachel Faulise
Manager